PSYCHOLOGY AND

MODERN NURSING SERIES

This Series caters for the needs of a wide range of nursing, medical and ancillary professions. Some of the titles are given below, but a complete list is available from the Publisher.

Revision Notes on Psychiatry
K. T. KOSHY SRN, RMN, BTA, RNT, ARIPHH, MRSH

Theory and Practice of Psychiatric Care
P. T. DARCY RMN, SRN

Textbook of Medicine
R. J. HARRISON ChB, MD

Gerontology and Geriatric Medicine
SIR W. FERGUSON ANDERSON OBE, KstJ, MD, FRCP
F. I. CAIRD MA, DM, FRCP
R. D. KENNEDY MB, ChB, FRCP
DORIS SCHWARTZ

Neurology
EDWIN R. BICKERSTAFF MD, MRCP

Rheumatology
D. R. SWINSON MB, BS, MRCP
W R SWINBURN MB, MRCP

Obstetrics and Gynaecology
JOAN M. E. QUIXLEY SRN, RNT
MICHAEL D. CAMERON MA, MB, BChir, FRCS, FRCOG

MCQ Psychiatry
MARY J WATKINS SRN, RMN

PSYCHOLOGY AND PSYCHIATRY

an integrated approach

Sixth edition

PETER DALLY

MB, FRCP, FRCPsych, DPM

Consultant Psychiatrist, Westminster Hospital, London

MARY WATKINS

SRN, RMN, DipNEd DN (London)

Tutor for In-service Education and Training
School of Nursing, The Bethlem Royal and
Maudsley Special Health Authority, London

HODDER AND STOUGHTON

LONDON SYDNEY AUCKLAND TORONTO

British Library Cataloguing in Publication Data

Dally, Peter
Psychology and psychiatry.——6th ed.——
(Modern nursing series)
1. Psychiatry 2. Psychiatric nursing
I. Title II. Watkins, Mary J. III. Series
616.89'0024613 RC454

ISBN 0 340 37685 6

First printed 1964
Second edition 1967 Reprinted (with corrections) 1969
Third edition 1972 Reprinted 1973, 1974
Fourth edition 1975 Reprinted 1977
Fifth edition 1982 Reprinted 1983
Sixth edition 1986

Photo Typeset by Macmillan India Ltd., Bangalore, 560025

Printed and bound in Great Britain
for Hodder and Stoughton Educational
a division of Hodder and Stoughton Ltd,
Mill Road, Dunton Green, Sevenoaks, Kent,
by Richard Clay (The Chaucer Press) Ltd,
Bungay, Suffolk

Introduction

There has been steady progress and many changes in psychiatry since the first edition of this book appeared 21 years ago. Our understanding of the nature of mental disorders has widened, and particularly the effects of adversity and social and family pressures on people with 'vulnerable' constitutions. Treatment has continued to improve. Psychotropic drugs are still essential at some point at least for most psychotic illnesses, and are useful in many neurotic states. But the importance – and limitations – of other forms of treatment are now recognised, especially behaviour therapy and psychotherapy, both individual and group. Increasingly, nurses are actively participating in these treatments; running groups of all kinds, teaching social skills, and planning and carrying out behavioural programmes.

The role of the psychiatric community nurse is evolving into a dynamic vital one; tracing and supervising those psychiatric patients who are discharged from mental hospitals destined for closure into communities unprepared – and often unwilling – to look after them properly; working hand in hand with local general practitioners and social workers, providing advice, referring patients in need to the psychiatric consultant, intervening to defuse a dangerous crisis situation building up in a family. It is exciting, strenuous and highly responsible work.

This sixth edition has been extensively rewritten. The clinical sections have been brought up-to-date. An entirely new and comprehensive chapter on drug dependence has been written by Dr Ann Dally, a leading expert in this field. And we have added new chapters on pregnancy and puerperal disorders, sexual development and its problems, and bulimia nervosa. The 1983 Mental Health Act is explained in detail. Nursing duties and practices, which have changed so greatly over the last ten years, are described and discussed. All aspects of the nurse/patient relationship are considered here and provide insights and understanding, not only for psychiatric nurses but for others coming into contact with patients; general nurses, social workers, occupational therapists, and teachers.

We have included a new reading list at the end of the book for those wishing to explore a subject in greater depth.

Contents

I

Evolution and Adaptation

All life must adapt to its surroundings. Adaptation to the external environment is necessary for survival. An independent, single living cell, such as an amoeba, must continually search for food, escape from enemies, avoid drying up and remain within certain limits of temperature in order to survive.

Life began with single living cells, in direct contact with their surroundings. Gradually organisms evolved that were composed of many cells, increasingly separated from the exterior. A nervous system developed and allowed communication and co-ordination between different parts of the body. As organisms became more complex, so did the nervous system. It enabled the animal to perceive changes in both the external and the internal environment, and react appropriately to changing events in both. The internal environment of the highly developed organism is much more complicated than the internal environment of a single cell. Not only are there many cells of many different types but there are also body fluids which bathe these cells continuously.

The fact that man has a highly developed internal environment allows him to be free of many of the restrictions of the external environment which limit simpler organisms. Man is able to be mobile. We can live at the North Pole or the Equator and in dry or wet regions. But it is vitally important for our bodies that the internal environment remains steady. The constancy of the internal environment is called *homeostasis*.

Any change is immediately corrected by sensitive mechanisms in the body which act through the nervous system by *reflex action*. Thus, for instance, a fall in blood pressure is corrected by an increased heart rate and a constriction of blood vessels running to the less important structures, such as the skin. This is why a patient suffering from shock is pale. Such changes occur reflexly, and often without our being aware of them.

Although we are now less dependent on the external environment than were our primitive ancestors we still have to obtain food and avoid enemies. In addition a partner has to be found for sexual reproduction. Simple reflex behaviour, although suitable for adjusting the internal environment, is now altogether too crude and unadaptable for dealing with the external environment.

At a certain stage in the evolution of organisms, *instincts* developed, and they reached their peak in the insect world. Instincts are unlearned inherited forms of behaviour, particularly concerned with self-preservation and reproduction. Many insects perform the most complicated pattern of behaviour, which is common to the whole species, and cannot be altered by experience. They seem to be fixed and innate. At this level of evolutionary development, such behaviour is unadaptable. But as the evolutionary ladder is ascended, instinctive behaviour becomes increasingly adaptable and liable to be modified by experience. This tendency reaches its maximum in man, and the human infant is born with few established or fixed patterns of behaviour. A baby can breathe, suck, swallow and perform other actions necessary for life, but in most other respects he is totally dependent on adults for his wants.

It is because of his immature and underdeveloped state at birth and his long dependence on adults that man has become so flexible. At birth his central nervous system is malleable, capable of being moulded in many directions by environmental pressures throughout childhood, and perhaps later to a lesser extent. Family and social influences direct his outlook and influence his behaviour. He still has need for sex, food and other biological necessities, for fundamentally he remains an animal. But the way he satisfies these needs will depend on patterns of behaviour formed in his nervous system during his early years. It is better therefore to speak of human *needs* rather than human *instincts*. However, instinctive behaviour is a phrase commonly used to express the activities aroused by hunger, sexual desire, and other biological needs.

An infant's needs – for example hunger – cause him to become tense and uncomfortable; he then cries and behaves in a characteristically noisy manner. Satisfaction follows feeding and produces the sense of pleasure and relaxation. Feelings of pleasure or 'unpleasure' are known as *emotions* and may be the only emotions a newborn infant has. But as the brain matures, new derived emotions develop. Emotions provide much of the drive behind our behaviour.

Intelligence, which depends on the development of the cerebral cortex, is the main means by which man is able to adapt to his environment. But natural hazards – hunger, warmth and so on – are no longer the most serious problems encountered by most of us. More important we have to adapt to the demands and restrictions of the society in which we live. We need to satisfy our wants and yet take into account the expectations of others.

Emotions and needs

An emotion is a mental feeling associated with often widespread bodily changes. Supposing, for instance, you are anxious, perhaps just before sitting an important examination. Your mouth dries up, your heart rate increases, you feel shivery, faint and sweaty and keep going to the lavatory. Or you feel anger when someone is unnecessarily rude to you, and again your heart beats faster, your face flushes and muscles tense. Fear and anger in these circumstances are appropriate emotions, aroused in most people. Likewise, when someone close to you dies or goes away, you feel sad.

Emotions are sparked off by situations which call for the satisfaction of some need. They provide the motivating force behind the actions taken. In an uncomplicated situation fear results in your running away and escaping; anger causes you to attack your opponent with all your strength. But in our society situations are rarely as simple as this. It may be appropriate to run away from an angry lion or to attack an insect that is annoying you. But it is obviously inadvisable to run away before an examination or to attack your boss when he provokes your anger. Most of us have learnt to inhibit and control our behaviour, although we still feel primitive emotions. However, a few unfortunate people seem unable to control themselves and are easily overwhelmed by their emotional impulses. They run away from the examination room or beat up the boss. Inevitably they find themselves in difficulties and do not easily adjust or conform to society.

Once an emotional need has been satisfied, the feeling of discomfort dies away. However, adult emotions are often complicated and more than one emotion may be involved at any one time. Conflicting needs can result in tension, discontent, sadness and restlessness.

All needs arouse emotional feelings. Often two or more needs are present at the same time and they may conflict with one another. Why, for instance, do most candidates not run from the examination room when their insides 'turn to jelly'? They may be ambitious, and in order to succeed they must pass the examination. They may be conscious of the shame and 'loss of face' that will result from running away. No one likes to be called a coward, to lose the esteem of his companions. For most people the emotion of fear felt before an examination is not strong enough to overcome emotions linked to other needs.

Our sense of identity, the strength of which influences self-confidence and inner security, our values and many of our needs, particularly those concerning relationships with other people, are all acquired in early childhood. How strong these needs are, and the emotional distress that develops when satisfaction is denied them, depends partly on the patterns learnt during childhood.

If an emotion is strong enough it will dominate behaviour until it is satisfied. Take an extreme example, such as the need to breathe, and think what happens when you partially suffocate. You become increasingly frightened, tension builds up and you struggle wildly for breath. If suffocation continues you become panic-stricken and lose all self-control. The bodily accompaniments of fear may last for several minutes after normal breathing has been restored.

The need to breathe is vital for life and cannot be delayed for long. This is why such powerful emotions appear so rapidly and take precedence over any other need at that time. But in a less extreme way emotions are continually determining the way we behave. A heavy smoker who is prevented from smoking for several hours becomes restless, is unable to concentrate on his work, and continually searches for an excuse to go out for a cigarette. Many adolescents are dominated by their need for sexual and aggressive outlets, to free themselves from family restrictions. When these needs are frustrated, as they usually are to some degree, the resulting tensions may lead to antisocial behaviour, promiscuity, or the adolescent becoming a 'dropout'. Some men and women, through promiscuity and other ways, are constantly trying to reassure themselves that they are lovable. When such needs are combined with great ability, their lives may be spent in acquiring vast wealth and property, an end in itself rather than a means to other ends.

Emotions also influence what we perceive. A hungry man notices food which he will overlook at other times. Unsatisfied sexual needs can lead to greater awareness of admiring glances or of an attractive pair of legs. Fear can make you more attentive, but it may also bring about a distortion of perception, such as an illusion. Visualise yourself alone at dusk in a house reputed to be haunted. In your apprehensive state you may easily imagine that a piece of furniture in the shadows is a ghostly figure, or that creaks in the hall are footsteps coming towards you.

At one time emotions were thought to be simply the result of becoming aware of internal bodily changes. According to this theory, if you felt afraid it was because of your dry mouth, rapid pulse and other accompaniments of fear; if you felt sad it was because you wept; if you felt hungry it was because your stomach was contracting. This was the *theory of James and Lange*. Although bodily sensations may certainly modify emotional feelings, it seems unlikely that they are primarily responsible for arousing them. However, some hypochondrial people, acutely conscious of the workings of their bodies, are alarmed and upset by unusual peripheral sensations, for instance extra systoles, and their fear generates further cardiac irregularities and anxiety. There is a good deal of evidence which suggests that emotional feelings arise as a result of activity in the brain itself. Most of the work providing this evidence has been with rats, each with an electrode implanted in a certain area of its brain. Through this a minute stimulating electric current can be given by the rat to itself. Stimulation of certain parts of the brain strongly reinforces behaviour; stimulation of other areas has the opposite effect. Human beings, when particular areas of their temporal lobes are stimulated during open brain surgery, have reported intense feelings of pleasure.

Unsatisfied needs lead to emotional feelings and reactions. It is understandable to feel afraid when charging the enemy, or climbing a difficult rock face, or meeting a dangerous animal in the wild. It is natural to feel grief at the death of a beloved relative, or joy when a much wanted ambition is realised. All these emotions are common to most of us in such circumstances.

Other emotions are less easily understood. For instance, a mouse or a spider can hardly be regarded as a real danger, yet in some people they provoke tremendous fear. But mice and spiders can usually be avoided by city dwellers, so that even when they arouse strong and uncontrollable emotions they are rarely likely to interfere with everyday life.

Sometimes irrational fears of this type may interfere with everyday life. Suppose, for instance, the fear is for open spaces, or for enclosed areas. Both are quite common. A fear of open spaces may simply mean that a person avoids going into the country, which probably no one will notice. However, if it becomes so extreme, that there is fear even of crossing the road, then it is likely to become obvious and seriously interfere with his life. Similarly a fear of enclosed spaces may mean that someone chooses to walk up the stairs instead of using the lift, and this may be regarded as no more than a mild eccentricity; the fear becomes disabling if it leads to an inability to be in a room with the door shut, or even in any small room at all.

Fear of some object or situation, for which there is no reasonable cause, is known as a *phobia*. In some cases this can become widespread and crippling, and develop into a *phobic anxiety state*. Sometimes there is no specific phobia, but merely an all-pervading sense of anxiety which seems irrational and ridiculous, yet cannot be shaken off. Such anxiety often stems from the threatened loss of something important in that person's life. Depression follows the actual loss. Such a threat or loss may be real or 'neurotic', meaning that it stems more from inner fantasies and associations than from real outside circumstances. Depression or unhappiness, of course, is felt by everyone at some time or another, following bereavement say, or a serious disappointment. But sometimes depression may be excessive or unaccountably prolonged. It is abnormalities of the emotions like these that constitute psychiatric disorder.

Thought

Thought refers to any conscious mental activity. It can be controlled and directed purposefully as in *reasoning*, or it may be allowed to take its own course as in *fantasy* thinking. McKellar calls these two types of thinking R-thinking, which is logical and reality adjusted, and A-thinking, which is non-rational and is not subject to checking against external events. A-thinking is most clearly seen in dreams, fantasy and some forms of psychotic thinking. For most of us a comparatively large part of our thinking includes an element of fantasy.

Imagery may be *visual, auditory, kinaesthetic*; in fact, it may involve any of the senses. People vary in the type they most use. One person may be able to recall clearly a picture of what he was doing yesterday. Another may have only a hazy visual image but be able to 'hear' distinctly what was said at tea-time last week. Yet another may picture a game of tennis or football in terms of body movements and sensations. A peculiarly vivid form of visual imagery occurs in children, almost photographic. This is eidetic imagery, which tends to disappear in adult life. Oscar Wilde probably possessed eidetic imagery and as a result was able to mystify people at parties by glancing at a book and then reproducing any part requested.

Much of our thinking occurs in the form of words. For this most of us use auditory rather than visual imagery, but thought can occur without the use of any form of imagery. *Abstract thinking*, for instance, on a philosophical problem connected with beauty or goodness, is particularly likely to occur without imagery. The thinker is then simply *aware* of the train of thought.

In terms of brain structure, the modes of thought of the two halves of the brain differ. The left cerebral hemisphere, in righthanders, controls language and cannot cope, alone, with problems requiring a nonverbal solution. The right hemisphere controls pattern recognition. It is this that allows you to recognise a familiar face or scene. In practice, of course, the two sides work together, and words and patterns interlaced.

Reasoning is mainly concerned with solving problems. It involves not only thought but memory and learning. Thought starts when the problem is recognised and continues until it is abandoned or solved. Reasoning is characterised by controlled purposeful thinking, which excludes irrelevant thoughts and distractions. The need to solve the problem provides the drive motivating the train of thought. When interest flags concentration and persistence diminish. However, it is important to recognise that in practice rational thought and fantasy thinking are rarely clearly separated. The answer to a problem which has hitherto seemed insoluble may suddenly come during a period of relaxation when thoughts are allowed to wander. Most artists and scientists have experienced sudden insight into their work on waking from a night's sleep. Fantasy thinking is intimately bound up with creativity.

Rational thought, concentration and memory are usually disturbed by the presence of strong emotional factors, particularly anxiety. Serious psychiatric disorder also distorts rational thinking.

Fantasy or autistic thought

Fantasy thinking, unlike reasoning, occurs without conscious control or direction. It may well be that fantasy thinking represents some basic activity of the brain, just as during sleep some dreaming always seems to be occurring, whatever the depth of sleep. Most of us indulge in fantasy thinking – for instance, daydreaming – at some time during the day. During such fantasy thinking you are largely cut off from the outside world and from reality. Freud looked upon daydreams and dreaming as 'wish fulfilments', unconsciously directed. Fantasy thoughts certainly provide an outlet for bottled-up aggression and frustrations. Indeed, fantasy is a tremendous safety valve, by means of which we can experience socially forbidden or impossible activities with ease and safety. Fantasy thinking also gives satisfaction to more prosaic needs. On a cold, wet winter day you can dream of the Mediterranean in summer. A hungry man enjoys thinking of food, the thirsty one of sparkling waters, the sexually frustrated of sex. The person who feels a failure in his work dreams of success and acclaim. There is no harm in this unless fantasy takes the place of reality and interferes with adaptation, as it may do in some forms of psychopathy and mental illness.

Fantasy develops in a child along with memory. During the first three or four years fantasy is probably inseparable from the child's play. But from then on, play becomes gradually more 'socialised' and the two slowly begin to diverge. Fantasy thinking reaches its peak in puberty when it is particularly likely to have a sexual colouring, or to be concerned with ambitions. Although fantasy does not generally generate action, adolescent fantasy thinking may provide additional incentives for working and passing exams, and in increasing social activities and confidence.

Sexual fantasies, those connected with masturbation and sexual intercourse, are of particular interest. They often involve sadomasochistic themes, and they inversely reflect outward personality traits. They are particularly important, not only in comprehending sexual deviations, but also in understanding normal sexual relationships and the difficulties that may arise within marriage (see p. 57).

Fantasy thinking and dreaming are closely related, and one may fade into the other on going to sleep or on waking. Fantasy thinking is increased by anxiety or by any condition which interferes with rational thought. Drugs such as marijuana and alcohol, amphetamines and some of the psychotropic drugs (although this will also depend upon the personality of the patient) can all enhance fantasy thinking.

Memory

What is memory? What happens when you try to memorise a poem, or the causes of heart failure, or the ways of bandaging a hand? Why is it so much more difficult to memorise a meaningless jumble of words or numbers than a poem or something which makes sense?

Not only is memory made up of several different mental functions, but there is a difference between a long term, fairly permanent system and a transitory one. Much of what we see or hear needs to be remembered only for a short time, and can then be forgotten. For instance, a telephonist needs to remember a number only for a minute or so; if she tried to memorise numbers for longer, she would soon be in a muddle. Short-term memory is said to involve an 'activity trace', a kind of mirror image of events, which rapidly decays.

When someone is given a list of say 20 *unrelated* words – dog, sea, gut, hat, and so on – he can recall the later words more readily than the earlier ones. But if recall is delayed by asking him to add a column of figures, the later words are as difficult to recall as the earlier ones. In other words, short term memory has been lost or diminished by the delay. Contrast this with learning a meaningful sentence. The individual may not be able to recall the exact words of the sentence, but he can nonetheless give its meaning.

Anything committed to memory must first be learnt. The information is then *stored* or *retained* in the brain, although how this is done is not known. We suppose that some physical change must accompany the imprinting of information on the brain. We call this supposed change a *memory* or *structural* trace. When we wish to remember something, the relevant memory is activated and brought into consciousness. This is known as *recall*. Provided the correct memory trace has been recalled, its appearance in consciousness is accompanied by a sense of recognition. If it is wrong, it is rejected.

Sometimes information may be forgotton, either temporarily or permanently. We have all had the experience of meeting an old friend and being unable to recall his name. Perhaps you have experienced stagefright and forgotten completely the lines you knew by heart so perfectly only a few minutes earlier. The information is still there, since it will certainly be remembered later. In this case anxiety has interfered with recall. Anxious and agitated patients often experience similar difficulties in recalling recently acquired information. Drugs may also interfere with recall, particularly tranquillisers and antidepressant drugs.

The psychologist Thorndike believed that forgetting occurred as a result of *trace decay*, of memories fading through disuse. But this now seems unlikely to be true. Recent evidence, both clinical and experimental, suggests that forgotton memories have become inaccessible rather than decayed. New memories often interfere with old ones. Loss of memory may be due more to '*retroactive inhibition*' than to time itself. Retroactive inhibition is the interference with a memory trace in the brain that occurs as a result of the later learning of similar information. For example, you may remember a shopping list perfectly all day, but after you have learnt the next day's shopping list, you are unable to remember the first.

Retroactive inhibition ceases during sleep. For this reason the best time to learn something that you really want to remember is just before you go to bed, as there is then plenty of time for the information to fix itself firmly in the memory, without interference.

Development of memory

Memory develops slowly and by stages. A baby of a month or two smiles at his mother, but this is a reflex response to a face, and he smiles just as much if shown a paper mask. At this age the child is still unable to *recognise* his mother.

The ability to recognise develops before the ability to *recall*. By the time he is six months old the baby is able to recognise his mother and other people around him, his own hands and feet and his toys in the cot. But he is still unable to recall his mother and familiar beings and objects in their absence. He still lives largely in the present. Recall becomes possible at about the end of a child's first year of life. He can now remember where he put his toys, even though they are not visible. He can also visualise his mother when she is not present. At first the process of recall is unstable, and he can only think back a few minutes. But this interval grows progressively longer, and by the age of four he can recall events that occurred months or as long as a year ago. Past learning can now be recalled for solving new problems and developing conceptual thought.

Memory is not a static process by means of which information is photographed, stored and reproduced unchanged some time later. Memory is an active process, and memories are continually being inhibited, forgotten, modified and distorted. Just as perceptual processes tend to fill in gaps and to reduce unfamiliar perceptions to more familiar and conventional ones, so also memory is biased towards what is familiar. We spoke of the recall of a trace memory, but of course in practice recall is never as simple as this. Trace memories are continually modified by related experiences and emotional attitudes. Recollections are always liable to this type of distortion, and the longer the time between the event and the recall, the greater is the distortion. Unpleasant memories are liable to be *repressed*, particularly those which cause anxiety. The conscious reliving of some repressed incident, by hypnosis or giving the patient intravenous methohexitone sodium or sodium amytal, is sometimes used in the treatment of psychological disorders. Such a method of treatment is known as narcoanalysis; it can result in an outpouring of emotions, known as abreaction.

The physical basis of memory

We still know very little about the physical basis of memory. Hebb's two-stage theory of memory postulates that incoming stimulation sets up reverberatory activity in and between the receptor and effector cells involved. With repeated stimulation and reverberation, structural changes occur, setting up a memory or structural trace. Electric shocks might be expected to interfere with this process, and certainly can be shown to do so in the case of rats. Electro-convulsive therapy (ECT) sometimes has a disruptive effect on recent memory, particularly when given bilaterally (see p. 367).

Visual hallucinations may occur during epileptic disturbances arising from the occipitoparietal area of the cerebral cortex. Vivid memories can also be produced by electrical stimulation of certain parts of the temporal lobe of the brain. From a structural point of view the limbic lobe (see p. 74) seems to be intimately involved with memory. In the *Korsakov Syndrome*, a complication of alcoholism, the patient has difficulty in making new lasting memories. In this condition lesions are found in the *mammillary bodies* and the medial thalamus. The *hippocampus* is linked to the *mammillary bodies* by the *fornix*. Apart from damage to the mammillary bodies, bilateral removal or damage to the hippocampus, or surgical section of the fornix produce similar disturbances of memory. Temporal lobectomy can be followed by profound amnesia going back several years.

Patients with *temporal lobe epilepsy* may experience *déjà vu*, a curious sense of familiarity that they have 'been here before' or lived through the same experience at some earlier stage of existence. This sense of familiarity is never complete and delusions rarely arise. The feeling is experienced by normal people, particularly when fatigued or worried. It can result from the use of certain drugs, particularly marijuana and hallucinogenic drugs, occasionally from excessive use of alcohol. In acute anxiety states it may be associated with depersonalisation. It is a not uncommon symptom in acute psychotic states.

For memory tests, see. p. 101.

Learning

We start to learn as soon as we are born, if not before. How we behave as adults is largely determined by what we learn in our early years. In more ways than one the child is father to the man.

The baby learns that his parents will satisfy his needs. He learns to be clean, and to behave in ways that are acceptable to others. He learns to crawl and walk, to ride a bicycle, to solve arithmetical problems, to recognise danger, to form friendships and cooperate and compete with others, and so on. All learning is concerned with adapting to new situations and problems. Compared with some other animals the human child is born with few instinctive forms of behaviour. His nervous system is like plasticine, waiting to be moulded by environmental influences.

There is still a good deal of disagreement about how learning actually occurs. Much of our information comes from experiments with animals, particularly rats, and it is not always easy to know how much of it applies to humans.

Imprinting

Very rapid learning in animals occurs at certain times during development. The nervous system needs to be developed and to be ready to respond to the stimulus encountered. The learning process is rapid, tenacious and long lasting. This form of learning was studied by Konrad Lorenz in birds, and in its original sense imprinting refers to the attachment which newly hatched birds develop to moving objects, living or inanimate, in their immediate vicinity. Lorenz's early work was with mallard ducklings and grey-lagged goslings. They quickly learn to follow the first moving object they encounter (usually the mother duck or goose) and thereafter only follow the imprinted 'object'. Lorenz showed that the adult sexual behaviour of these birds was also influenced by this early imprinting. There is however controversy as to whether such sexual imprinting arises from the initial imprinting phenomenon or whether it develops separately.

It seems possible that imprinting plays a part in human development and behaviour, both sexual and non-sexual.

Classical conditioning

Relatively simple learning is based on the principle of the conditioned reflex. The Russian physiologist Pavlov was the first to make a detailed study of conditioned reflexes, although it had long been known that two events occurring together in time tend to become linked in the mind. Pavlov studied unconditioned reflexes in dogs, particularly the reflex that causes saliva to drip from the lips when meat is placed in the dog's mouth. He found that when another stimulus, a light or a bell, was given with the meat several times running, the dog would sooner or later produce saliva on this stimulus alone and without the meat. The light or bell had thus become a *conditioned stimulus*, and the salivation that followed when it was given was known as a *conditioned reflex*. The conditioned stimulus had to be reinforced from time to time by combining it with food, otherwise the conditioned reflex tended to fade.

Pavlov put forward a theory of two complementary processes in the nervous system. (1) A process of excitation spreads through the nervous system as conditioned reflexes form. (2) A process of inhibition develops when stimuli are not reinforced, so that eventually no response occurs to them. Pavlov's theory has been elaborated upon by William Sargant in *Battle for the Mind*, which purports to explain certain types of behaviour.

Pavlov's work was taken up and applied in an extreme way to human learning by Watson, an American psychologist. He virtually rejected the idea of anything being inherited through the central nervous system. He declared that an infant is born with a few simple reflexes only, and that these reflex responses become linked to new stimuli by conditioning, and grow steadily more complex. He believed that by proper conditioning any child could successfully be brought up to be anything you chose, whether this be a doctor, soccer star or dustman.

However, classical conditioning gives an acceptable explanation of how certain irrational fears and dislikes can develop through emotional states becoming associated with objects or situations. Watson carried out a famous experiment on a small boy called Albert. He showed him a white rat, and at the same time frightened him by making a loud noise. He repeated this on several occasions, and eventually the boy became afraid of the rat, and cried whenever he saw it. His fear spread to include all white furry animals, and Albert went out of his way to avoid them. White furry animals had become a conditioned stimulus which caused fear. In everyday language he had learnt to fear and to avoid such animals. Many of us have equally absurd fears connected with mice, insects or birds, which we have probably learned like little Albert.

Learning by trial and error

This is more usually known as instrumental or *operant conditioning*. Conditioning is built upon operant behaviour, that is on the normal activities of the animal. Instrumental or operant conditioning consists of rewarding or punishing some acts and not others, thereby directing the animal's behaviour in certain directions. This is based on Thorndike's law of effect. Thorndike, an American psychologist, showed that if you shut a hungry cat in a cage with food placed on the floor outside, the cat stretches and pulls at the bars of the cage until eventually by chance it releases the catch holding the door. Next day the same sort of behaviour may occur, but eventually the cat goes straight to the catch and opens the door. The initial opening of the cage is by chance, but since this action results in satisfying the cat's needs by reducing its hunger, the cat quickly learns to release the catch whenever it is put into the cage. Thorndike's law of effect states that actions which result in satisfaction become stronger, while those which cause no satisfaction are weakened and eventually ignored.

Various methods are available for studying operant conditioning. In the Skinner box the animal learns to obtain food or water by pressing a lever, or by some analogous action. In the T-maze the animal has to find the right turning. Operant learning may be based on a reward system or punishment training.

Both classical and operant conditioning need reinforcement. Whereas in classical conditioning the unconditioned stimulus is the reinforcement, in operant conditioning the reinforcing stimulus is associated with and follows some particular response.

Every mother and school child knows the principle of operant conditioning, rewarding 'good' behaviour, punishing 'bad' behaviour. This is the basis of much of the upbringing, training and education of children, of how they learn to behave and acquire simple skills. The reward need not necessarily be a material one. The approval of someone whom the child loves and respects may be just as good as, if not better than material rewards. B. F. Skinner, of Harvard University, a radical behaviourist, believes that all actions, including mental activity and beliefs, are the result of earlier conditioning, that free will does not exist, and that men are mindless and have no more control over their lives than beetles. Needless to say, many people reject such a materialistic theory.

Learning with insight

The idea that all learning derives from trial and error has been much criticised on the grounds that learning is then entirely automatic. This may well be so in lower animals, but in man and the higher apes *understanding* and *insight* are also involved. Kohler showed that chimpanzees were able to solve problems (such as obtaining an out-of-reach banana) by piling boxes on top of one another or fitting sticks together in an insightful way.

A small child seems to learn at first by trial and error, which is probably a reflection of the child's lack of experience. But before long he adopts a more rational approach to new problems. He no longer acts by trial and error, but picks out recognisable patterns or components of the puzzle or task which he then utilises to gain insight and eventually achieve the solution.

Man can learn more quickly and efficiently than other animals because he has the use of language. By means of words he can construct ways of tackling new problems, selecting only those ways which seem likely to succeed. This, of course, is a sort of mental trial and error, but it is very different from the trial and error behaviour of the cat in the cage.

Exposure learning

Apart from classical and operant conditioning it seems likely that learning also occurs without specific reinforcement, simply from exposure to a particular experience. Thus hungry or thirsty rats rapidly learn to run through a maze when rewarded at the end. A satiated and therefore unmotivated rat does not appear to learn, yet if he is allowed to wander at will through the maze he subsequently learns very quickly. Some people believe in playing classical music as a background to their children's lives, others try to learn a foreign language by playing a tape just before going to sleep, on the same principle.

A number of factors influence learning:

1. *Motivation.* Without motivation there can be no drive to learn. In order to be motivated there must be a need, and therefore an interest in the subject. There may be several conflicting needs, causing ambivalence and indecisiveness over learning. Anxiety sometimes acts as a spur to learning, but if too great its effect is disruptive.

2. *Punishment.* There is still considerable controversy about the value or otherwise of punishment in learning. In general punishment is an effective instrument for avoidance training, both with animals and man. Thus a child learns to wash his hands before meals because otherwise he is not allowed to eat at table. However, if punishment is too severe it provokes such anxiety that learning is inhibited. It only makes matters worse if a frightened child is threatened or punished for wetting his bed. In such a case it is better to reward the child for being dry than punishing him for being wet

(positive reinforcement). But many factors are involved in the efficiency of punishment. Punishment is most effective when it immediately follows the response. And from the point of view of a child, it depends upon how he views the punishment, how consistent, restrictive or permissive his parents and other authority figures are towards him.

3. *Exercise and repetition.* This will increase the rate of learning. *Over*-learning, continuing the learning process for longer than is necessary, fixes what has been learnt more securely in the brain.

Perception

Perception is a process by which we become aware of what is happening around us and in our own bodies. But it is more than just receiving stimuli through our special sense organs: eyes, ears, skin and so on. It is more than just recording stimuli. Perception is an active process of the brain which selects and organises stimuli. The selection and organisation are performed according to inherent properties of the brain and past learning and experience. Percepts are thus also influenced by interest, needs and emotions. In a way you can compare this internal perceptual process with what happens when a lump of clay is modelled. The final result depends upon the structure of the clay and the aims and skill of the modeller, together with his interest and feelings at the time. The lump of clay is transformed as a result of all these factors. In a somewhat similar manner the brain's perceptual processes deal with stimuli that reach it and transform them into recognisable objects and scenes. These are then *projected* out of the brain and back into the environment and perceived there.

Everyone has to learn the *meaning* of *stimuli* or *signs.* A child gradually learns to recognise objects, distance, time and so on by experience. He does this by exploring his environment constantly, by handling and reaching for objects. All the time he is combining and comparing what he sees with what he feels and hears and tastes. He perceives adults and learns that a smile means approval or happiness, and a frown disapproval. He observes closely how people behave in different circumstances and learns to recognise attitudes and intention from expressions and behaviour. As he learns to understand words his development is helped by the use of language.

William James, a famous psychologist of the last century, believed that a new-born child saw the world as 'blooming, buzzing confusion'. This is probably wrong, for it is unlikely that a new-born child is aware of anything except himself, and he is probably incapable of distinguishing himself from things outside himself. For the new-born infant existence probably consists largely of his needs, and whether or not these needs are satisfied. However, the world may well appear to be all confusion to a man, blind from birth, whose vision is suddenly restored by an operation. Imagine you know him well and are by his bedside when the bandages are removed from his eyes for the first time. Will he smile and say, 'You look just as I expected'? On the contrary, although he knows who and where you are from your voice, he will see you only as a blur, without expression, colour or distinguishing features. The receptors in his retina are responding to you, but the impulses travelling from them to his brain are as yet meaningless. Only after a time, with experience and learning, will he come to recognise your features and be able to distinguish you from someone else. Even after learning to recognise you in the hospital ward he may fail to recognise you at first in unfamiliar surroundings. For such a man visual learning is slow compared with that of a child.

It is probable that, as with other functions, there is a *critical period of development* during which perceptual learning is most effective. If, for one reason or another, perception is interfered with during this critical period, subsequent learning is much slower and less effective. We can compare this with what happens in chickens. It is obviously important that chicks should be able to peck efficiently. Experiments suggest that there is a critical period coinciding with the first fourteen days after hatching during which the chick must have pecking experience if he is to develop his powers of pecking adequately. If he is prevented from pecking during the first fourteen days of his life the bird is permanently retarded in pecking compared with his fellow chicks.

But not all perception is due to learning. The internal processes involved in perception depend also on inherent properties of the brain. Much of our knowledge of these inherent properties comes from the work of *Gestalt* (meaning form or pattern) psychologists working in the early half of this century. These workers realised that the perceptual field was organised in such a way that certain unitary parts stood out as wholes; and these segregated themselves from the rest of the field. Thus three dots on a sheet of paper form a triangle.

If more dots are added the triangle is eventually lost. Such a segregated whole is called a *Gestalt*, from which *Gestalt theory* is derived. The distinguishing characteristic of a *Gestalt* is that the segregated whole (in this case the triangle) is more than simply the sum of its parts. As you can see (Fig. 1.1), the shape varies although the parts remain the same.

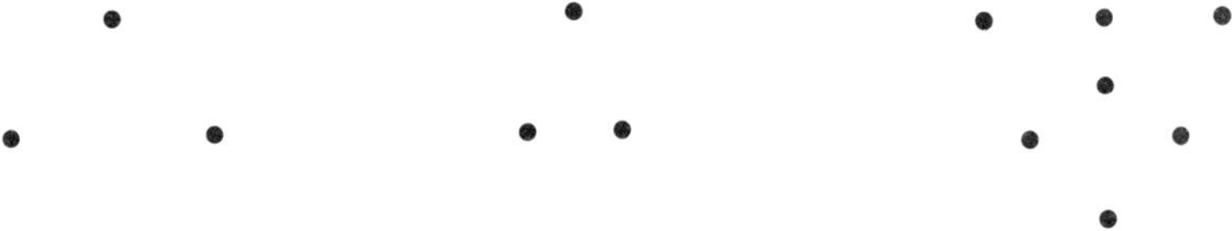

Fig. 1.1 A Gestalt

We have an automatic tendency to transform incomplete percepts into complete ones. The way dots become organised into *Gestalten* is determined by their closeness to one another, by their similarity in shape and size, and by their continuity of direction. No matter what is perceived, the brain tends as far as possible to perceive the most simple and stable geometrical shapes in preference to unstable complicated shapes.

When a child is faced with an unfamiliar jumble of stimuli, he first tends to pick out some bright spot or moving object that stands out from its background. A figure stands out naturally against a shapeless background; for instance, a black triangle drawn on a white piece of paper is sharply outlined. But if the figure is not too different from its background, its contour may be indistinct and it will then be *unstable* and will keep disappearing into the background. This, of course, is the principle upon which camouflage is based, and it also accounts for ghostly appearances at dusk.

Another characteristic of the brain is *perceptual constancy*. The size, shape, brightness and colour of anything remains constant. When you see a man at a distance of a hundred yards the image he makes on your retina must be smaller than the image of a man only ten yards away; yet you perceive them both as similar size (see Fig. 1.2). Because of its past experience your brain automatically adjusts its interpretation of the actual image that is received for the estimated distance.

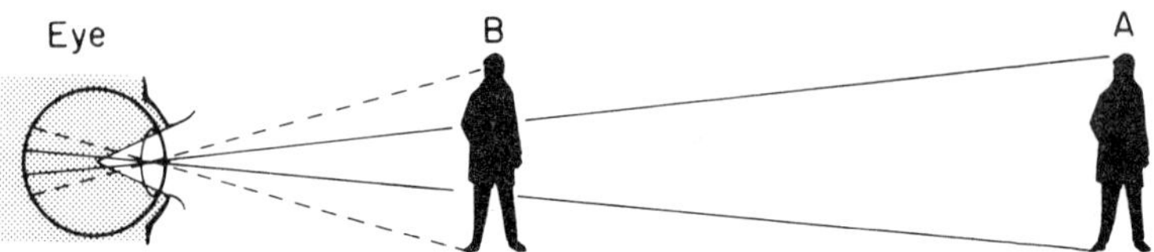

Fig. 1.2 Perceptual constancy

Similarly you perceive a coin as round whether you look at it face or end on. Your experience tells you that it is round and so you perceive it as such. This perceptual constancy produces a basically stable world within which you can appreciate real changes. Without such constancy the external world would be unbearably chaotic.

We mentioned earlier that subjective factors influence perception. For instance, you may easily pick out a familiar figure in a crowd, particularly if you expect to see him; or fail to recognise him when he is unwelcome. There is a tendency on occasion to overlook mistakes in familiar material. You may for instance not see glaring errors in your own writing. People fill in details according to what they expect to find. This often happens in a Court of Law. A witness may, unwittingly and in all honesty, fill in gaps in his account of what happened; the brain may alter the story itself in various ways to make it conform to what is familiar and expected. For this reason two witnesses may, and often do, give honest but differing accounts of an accident.

Emotional attitudes and habits also have considerable influence. If you are afraid or suspicious you are liable to see other people as unfriendly, and to misinterpret innocent remarks and gestures as though they are directed against you. In extreme cases, usually associated with psychiatric illness, a man may misinterpret remarks and gestures so grossly that he may even assault total strangers, believing them to be hostile.

Stereotypes are fixed, over-simplified and generalised conceptions that many individuals have about other people: Jews, women, negroes, the working-class, civil servants, nurses. When these conceptions are unfavourable they are linked with *prejudice*. Many people, not least among the medical and nursing professions, have a stereotyped idea of mental illness. They see the mentally ill as dangerous, unable to control their feelings and behaviour, and morally blameworthy.

Prejudice influences how one person perceives another, and how he behaves towards him. A Nazi, who knew a man to be a Jew, might perceive him as a loathsome villain and exterminate him without mercy. Yet such a man could be kind and considerate to non-Jews. Similar prejudices exist today towards men of different colour and race. Most of us have minor prejudices about the way people speak or eat, certain forms of dress or hair-style, foods and so on, which affect our attitudes and feelings. Many of our prejudices are based not so much on ignorance as upon fear and our own sense of insecurity. For instance, one reason for a person strongly disliking homosexuals may be his own homosexual inclinations, fiercely but precariously kept in check.

Emotions can influence perception in negative as well as in positive ways. Unpleasant incidents are overlooked or conveniently forgotten. If you happen to meet someone you dislike you may fail to recognise him. Or you may misread the date of a dreaded interview and arrive a day late for it.

There is continual rejection and selection of stimuli by the brain. Sometimes perception may be so distorted that an *illusion* is produced. This occurs either because the stimuli are misleading or ambiguous, or because the internal organisation of the brain has broken down. *Illusions* are *errors of perception* which cause stimuli to be wrongly interpreted. We mentioned above how extreme fear or anger, especially when there is lack of perceptual clarity, may do this. Some old people at night, and delirious patients, are particularly liable to suffer from illusions; a piece of fluff on the bed becomes a terrifying animal, a nurse dissolves into a threatening intruder. Illusions and hallucinations are common in the early stages of bereavement; the dead person is heard coming into the house or even speaking, and may perhaps be glimpsed in the hall or the bedroom at twilight. It is important to realise that illusions are not necessarily morbid, and that any of us can experience illusions if conditions are appropriate.

Hallucinations are more abnormal, for these are perceptions that arise without any stimuli at all, and so they can only be perceived by the patient and cannot be shared with others. Often *hallucinations* only occur, or are most troublesome, at night when external stimuli are least. It seems as though the brain has a need for stimulation in order to relate itself adequately to its environment. In *sensory deprivation experiments* volunteers have been cut off, as far as possible, from all sensory stimuli; as a result, they have developed *illusions* and *hallucinations*. Oldish patients operated on for cataract, who have their eyes bandaged for several days postoperatively, not infrequently hallucinate. Rather similar experiences have been described by arctic explorers, long-distance drivers and shipwreck survivors at sea. In these people *hallucinations* and *illusions* sometimes seem to occur as a result of monotony and a lack of fresh stimulation. Hallucinations may involve any of the senses. Many normal people experience hallucinations as they are falling asleep or waking; these are known as *hypnogogic* and *hypnopompic hallucinations* respectively. Auditory hallucinations are more common than visual, and usually take the form of the subject's name being called. Volunteers deprived of sleep may develop a *hypnogogic psychosis*, with auditory and visual hallucinations. Auditory hallucinations, in a setting of clear consciousness, are a characteristic of schizophrenia. Patients with severe psychotic depression sometimes report hearing disjointed words or phrases. Visual hallucinations are common in delirium and states of intoxication, and are not uncommon in hysteria. Temporal lobe lesions can cause visual hallucinations and hallucinations of smell and taste.

Reality. We have explained how perception involves receiving and reorganising stimuli and projecting them back into the environment. We have also mentioned that errors of perception may arise and a man may hear voices and see forms which no one else can hear or see.

How do we know that what we perceive has physical reality? That the external world exists? Most of us take this for granted. What we perceive is familiar and fits into our framework of *reality*. Moreover, as far as we can see, it is accepted and shared by other people. But if we see a devil sitting at the foot of the bed or hear threatening voices coming from the radiator, we are puzzled and frightened. These perceptions are *unreal*, particularly as no one else can see or hear them. But if we go on having these perceptions for some time we may come to accept them as real. When this happens, as in *schizophrenia*, the *sense of reality* is lost and adaptation to the environment becomes disturbed, particularly with other people.

However, it is important to understand that there is no absolute reality. We all have our own personal fantasy world which exists and interacts with what is going on in the outside world. When we are extremely tense, confused, intoxicated or mentally ill, inner fantasies may become for a time more real than what is happening in the outside world.

Development of perception of self and body image

Perception develops along with thinking and memory. At first there is little distinction between self and the external world. Even before birth tactile sensations are constantly travelling from different parts of the body to the brain. After birth, as a child becomes more mobile, he gradually increases his knowledge of his body from tactile sensations. He explores his body with his hands and his self-awareness increases. Vision, hearing, pain, temperature and smell – in fact all the sensory organs – play their part. He develops an awareness of himself.

As he grows and increases his activities, his body image is continually modified. Emotional attitudes and values become attached to this image of his body and its various parts. The expectations and behaviour of his parents, his relationship with them and his early childhood experiences inevitably influence the way he regards himself. Strength and muscular development, beauty, intellectual prowess, or chastity may be praised or devalued according to family values. A man may put tremendous significance on the physical development of his body and spend all his spare time playing games and doing gymnastics. For such a man to be physically disabled by illness or injury, however minor the disability, may be catastrophic and result in severe psychiatric disturbance. Ageing is sometimes not just ignored, but virtually denied, and he continues to exercise at 65 as he did when he was 20. Plastic surgery and hair transplants may make him or her feel better, although to outsiders they may appear ridiculous.

Adults who lose a limb commonly experience the sensation that it is still present. This imaginary limb is known as a *phantom limb*. It is interesting that children born without limbs, or who lose a limb before the age of five, do not develop phantom limbs. Presumably the *body image* is not yet firmly established.

Adolescent girls commonly see themselves fatter than they really are, especially around the hips and thighs. Such body image distortion is pronounced in anorexia nervosa, where fear of fatness is strong; however thin she is, the girl invariably sees herself as too fat and big, and so continues to diet.

Organic factors may form the basis of some symptoms labelled psychiatric. Thus the child may be damaged *in utero* or suffer some minor injury at birth, insufficient to cause cerebral palsy but sufficient to cause sensory deficiencies and interfere with his development and co-ordination. As a result he may be late in learning to read or write, excessively clumsy, unable to ride a bike and so on. The body-image concept normally arises in the second half of the first year and only when this is established can the child respond as a whole appropriately to afferent stimuli. If the development of his body image concept is deficient the child may find it difficult to wash, walk, feed, dress and carry out the most basic functions. A vicious circle may clearly spring up as a result of this and the child be looked upon as psychiatrically disturbed and his disabilities attributed to this, rather than vice versa.

Both constitutional factors and learning are involved in the development of perception. For instance, infants begin to follow the movements of their hands with their eyes from about twelve weeks. This is so even in children blind from birth. But if there is no feedback, the co-ordination of eyes and hands gradually ceases. The child has to compensate through other senses, such as hearing, touch, taste, which may become more developed than normal.

Congenitally deaf children have difficulty with speech. They begin to babble like other children from about three months old, but because they cannot hear themselves or others, learning cannot naturally take over from the babbling stage.

Children have enormous potential for adapting. Thalidomide children, born without limbs, are able to adapt perceptually so well that they are just as competent as normal children on intelligence testing at the age of two. Children with sensory or physical defects need above all to feel secure in order to develop and compensate to the full. Parents of such children may be guilty and ashamed, ignorant of how to help their child. They often need prolonged support. The child must not be overprotected, for he needs new experiences in order to develop. And to learn, he needs the incentive of praise and encouragement from those he loves and respects.

Gender identity

Gender identity refers to an individual's sense of his/her masculinity or femininity. It needs to be distinguished from sexual drive and energy, and sexual preference. For instance, a man can feel himself to be male (male gender), but may consider himself to be a homosexual, bisexual or heterosexual. Most of us are labelled male or female at birth correctly on the strength of our external genitalia, which in turn correspond to an appropriate internal reproductive system. Rarely a mistake is made, and the child whose chromosomes and hormones are male is brought up as a girl, or vice versa. If the mistake is discovered such a child is as likely as not to opt to continue in the sexual role to which he or she has become accustomed. However, the formation of gender is far more complex than this. It is discussed in more detail, along with sexual development on p. 50.

2
Intelligence

Intelligence has different meanings for different people. To an educator it probably means the *ability to learn*; to a biologist it may be the *capacity to adapt*; while psychologists use the word intelligence to mean the *ability to reason* and to think rationally and purposefully. It is the capacity to use experience and knowledge that constitutes intelligent behaviour and enables man to solve problems and to adapt to changing situations. You can, for instance, give a man a perfect set of tools; but unless he has the necessary intelligence, he is unlikely to acquire the skill to use those tools.

Intelligent behaviour is always rational. It differs greatly from instinctive or impulsive behaviour which may seem pointless and harmful. Consider the behaviour of a man who is trying to cross a river. First, he looks for a bridge or a boat; in the absence of these he tries to find a shallow crossing; failing this he starts to build himself a raft, and so on. This behaviour is rational and understandable. But compare this to the behaviour of a wealthy woman who had a quarrel with her husband, went out to a shop, stole a cheap trinket, and was caught and sent to prison. Such impulsive behaviour is purposeless and not understandable at first sight. What is more, it is unadaptable, for it may be repeated time after time, showing that no lesson has been learnt from the experience.

But it is usually impossible entirely to distinguish intelligent from impulsive behaviour. Most human action is, in fact, a mixture of both. Unconscious impulses may provide the drive for apparently intelligent behaviour, and much of our everyday behaviour is based upon habit, prejudices, and emotional likes and dislikes of which we may be hardly aware.

Intelligence often develops unevenly in the growing child and reaches its maximum at about the age of fifteen or sixteen, though perhaps a few years later in some people. It is important to realise that although intelligence is maximum, experience and knowledge are not. Moreover, an adolescent often has limited control over his impulses. Thus, to an adult, adolescent behaviour often seems to be irrational.

As age advances intelligence declines, and this decline is probably slower in people who use their minds. Old people find it harder to learn, and they cannot adapt so readily to change as young people.

In the past 50 years many tests have been developed in an attempt to provide an objective measure of intelligence. Alfred Binet worked with Paris school children and was the originator of these tests. He decided that no single test could measure intelligence and he therefore designed a variety of different tests, using the obvious fact that children become more 'clever' with age. He found that the *average* child at each age could do certain things. For instance, a three-year-old could string at least four beads in two minutes; a six-year-old could count 13 coins, copy a diamond shape, and see what is missing in pictures of incomplete faces; a nine-year-old could describe how wood and coal are alike and how they differ.

Binet tried out his tests on many children and modified them until he eventually knew which could be done by the majority of children in each age-group. The modern *Binet–Simon scale* contains 55 tests. This is made up of five items for each year from three to ten inclusive, 12, 15, and an adult group. The age-group for which the child passes *all* tests is known as the *basal age*; to this is added the number of tests that the child can pass for higher ages. The total gives the *mental age*. For instance, let us consider the performance of a six-year-old child.

4-year tests – 5 *out of* 5 *tests passed* = basal age
5-year test – 3 out of 5 tests passed
6-year test – 2 out of 5 tests passed
7-year test – 0 out of 5 tests passed
Mental Age = basal age (4) $+ (\frac{3}{5} + \frac{2}{5})$ = 5 years

This is then expressed as the *intelligence quotient* (IQ). This is the ratio of

$$\frac{\text{mental age}}{\text{chronological age}} \times 100$$

In this case IQ is $\frac{5}{6} \times 100 = 83$

The *average* child of six has an IQ of $\frac{6}{6} \times 100 = 100$. This child is therefore well below the *average intelligence* of six-year-olds. In practice, the term 'average' includes everyone with an IQ of between 90 and 110.

Numerous tests of intelligence have been designed since Binet's work was published. Tests in common use today are the Stanford–Binet scale for children between 2 and 18, and the Wechsler intelligence scale for children (WISC). For testing of adults the Wechsler Bellevue scale is preferable, the IQ being calculated by comparing the actual score with the expected average score of adults of the same age.

IQ tests are reasonably reliable in that they give a similar result on retesting. However, variations of up to 15–20 points can occur over a five-year period, particularly with a bright child. The IQ is mainly a measure of a child's present status, in relation to children of similar age, and not necessarily a reliable pointer to his future abilities. The growth of intelligence is not a smooth upward curve but consists of spurts and plateaux which may continue into late adolescence. IQ tests measure only what they set out to measure. Nonetheless the IQ correlates positively with actual intellectual activity and scholastic ability, and is a useful practical measure of a person's intelligence.

The Stanford – Binet and the WISC scales are composed of groups of verbal and non-verbal, or performance tests. Verbal tests include general knowledge, comprehension, arithmetical problems, the ability to recognise similarities and dissimilarities, vocabulary range and digit span. Their solution depends to a large degree on a child's education and upbringing. Performance tests, which include assembling jigsaws, completing missing parts of pictures, paper-and-pencil maze tests, are less dependent on educational and cultural factors for their solution. Most people score roughly the same on verbal and performance tests. A marked discrepancy between verbal and performance test scores may result from lack of education, unrecognised deafness or other perceptual deficiencies, psychosis or brain injury. In such cases the child's uneven abilities are liable to create uncertainty and anxiety, both in him and in his parents, which may result later in psychiatric problems.

A number of other factors, apart from cultural, can affect IQ test results. A child may lack motivation to complete the test, and extreme anxiety interferes with his understanding and performance of the test. Practice in IQ tests adds only about five points, but frequent coaching can increase an IQ score by as much as 15–20 points.

Group tests are given to several individuals at once and do not require skilled supervision. For this reason among others, they are less reliable than individual tests. Achievement tests are group tests which measure and compare one child with another in terms of school subjects. The IQ of children under two can be measured by Ruth Griffith's mental development scale. This assesses the child's locomotor development, learning and speech, hand and eye co-ordination and his personal social adjustment. The tester must be specially trained.

Various theories exist as to what exactly is being measured by intelligence tests. Spearman believed that individual differences in tests were due to the presence of one factor common to all tests, which he labelled G or general intelligence, and others specific to the tests involved. This idea has now been modified; specific factors may overlap with one another, to produce group factors. For instance, a brilliant pianist has a high general intelligence (G), high musical ability (the group factor) and a specific factor for the piano.

Distribution of IQ in the population

The distribution of IQ in a population is, for a large sample, a 'normal' one. That is, if the number of people of similar IQ scores is plotted on the scale of intelligence, a symmetrical curve is obtained (slightly skewed to the lower end of intelligence). This suggests that variations in intelligence, like stature and weight, are dependent on many small effects, genetic and/or environmental, opposing or reinforcing one another. Above an IQ of 50 the genetic effects are thought to be due to multifactorial genes scattered throughout the normal population. Below an IQ of about 50, single pathological genes, chromosomal defects, infections of and injury to the brain, are more likely to be responsible.

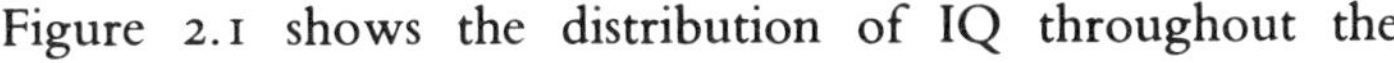

Figure 2.1 shows the distribution of IQ throughout the

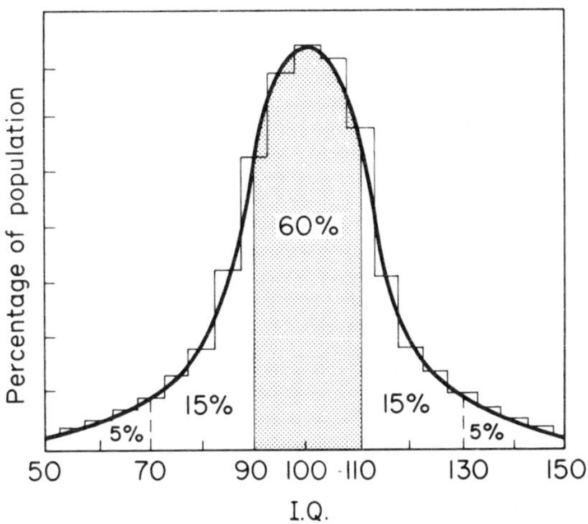

Fig. 2.1 Distribution of IQ throughout the population

population. IQ is sometimes expressed as a percentile. An individual with an IQ of 130 is more intelligent than 96 per cent of the population and therefore falls above the 96th percentile. An IQ of between 90 and 110 is regarded as 'average'; 55 per cent of the population fall within this range. To go into the professional classes you need an IQ of a least 110. Only one per cent have an IQ above 140. To go to University it is advisable to have an IQ of 120 or above.

Education may be a problem for children of very high intelligence. They easily become bored and ordinary education may not give them enough intellectual stimulation. Yet moving them into a class of older children may be difficult, for their *emotional development* may not be sufficiently great to enable them to adjust to older children. Children with average, or with slightly above average IQ, who scrape into Grammar Schools, may be pushed too hard by over-ambitious parents. Educational difficulties may also occur in the child with a low IQ (68–85 per cent) (border line intelligence, see p. 292) who is unable to cope in an ordinary school. He may display behavioural problems until he is transferred to a school which caters specifically for his needs.

The influence of heredity and environment on intelligence

Differences of intelligence between different people are largely due to *genetic* or *hereditary factors*. Intelligent parents tend to have intelligent children. The average IQ for children of professional fathers is 116; for unskilled labourers it is 95. Identical twins have similar IQs. However, *environmental factors* certainly have some influence and identical twins brought up apart show larger differences in IQ than those reared together. Intellectual stimulation from the home is important and may help to explain part of the difference between the children of labourers and professional men. A cultured background stimulates the child and provides maximum opportunity for the child's basic abilities to emerge. Children from better class homes tend to do better than those from families in the lower social groups. Homes of the latter tend to be more crowded, parents are often less interested in their child's efforts, and there is less stimulation generally. Children from small families develop better intellectually than those from large ones. The effect of being one of a one or two child family, compared to a five or more child family, is to show a gain in reading age of 12 months by the age of seven.

Mental handicap

Although people of IQ less than 70 are usually classified as mentally handicapped, it is important to realise that such a classification can never be made simply on the results of a test, but depends on other factors, particularly personality and sociability. After all, in practice a person can only be below normal in relation to his environment. He may be able to adapt normally to one environment but not to another.

There are many varied classifications of degrees of mental handicap. In 1965 the International Classification of Diseases described levels of handicap in grades of retardation:

	IQ
Borderline	68–85
Mild	52–67
Moderate	36–51
Severe	20–35
Profound	below 20

Generally speaking people with an IQ of between 50 and 70 are part of the normal distribution of inherited intelligence. On the whole they come from families of below average IQ. Individuals with IQs below 50 are normally distributed throughout all social classes. This type of mental handicap is often caused by single abnormal genes, by physical agents which damage the unborn child such as rubella or Rhesus incompatibility, or by brain injury or infection (see p. 289).

Assessing intelligence in a patient

A good intelligence is generally associated with a wide vocabulary; conversely people with below average intelligence tend to have a limited vocabulary. It is important for doctors and nurses to realise this association and make due allowance for it when explaining illness or treatment to a patient. Patients may be too frightened to say that they do not understand and, in consequence, may be made more fearful rather than reassured by a well-meant but incomprehensible explanation. It is just as important, however, not to 'talk down' to a patient.

Lastly it should be remembered that (statistically speaking) intelligence is inversely related to neurotic and behavioural disorders; that is, the lower the intelligence, the more frequent these become.

3
Family

The family has come in for much criticism over the centuries, but has not yet been replaced by anything better from the child's point of view. It provides him/her with a more satisfactory environment in which to develop than any tried alternative. At the same time we must recognise that the influences of the family on its members are not always entirely beneficial and may lead to considerable distress and even psychiatric illness.

The way members of families behave and communicate with one another can be seen and described in terms of an active system. This has come to be known as *systems theory*, and it provides a useful means of understanding family reactions. Families can be characterised by lack of boundaries between members so that they become *enmeshed* in each other's problems. Anorexia nervosa not infrequently arises in an enmeshed family, when a daughter (the patient) becomes overinvolved in her mother's marriage difficulties and depression. Other families maintain tight boundaries; emotional expression is restricted and controlled, and family tensions are kept well below the surface, so that to an outsider the family – albeit on the point of explosion – appears to be a contented one. There may be considerable pressures to resist changes within the family, and the illness of one of its members may be utilised to this end. An invalid, demanding parent, fearful of being left alone or with just a spouse, may through her illness prevent children marrying and leaving home, or one of the children may take on a sick role and so keep her parents from quarrelling or even separating.

One parent, mother or father, may overwhelmingly dominate the family, while the other parent clings tenaciously to a submissive, even humiliating role, however much this may outrage her children or close friends, intent on family stability and fearful of change. One child may be the family scapegoat, blamed for whatever goes wrong. Another may be overprotected, a compensation for marital dissatisfaction, or the death of a sibling. Strong ambivalent feelings for a child sometimes result in contradictory or double bind behaviour by a parent. *Double bind* describes an event in which one person gives conflicting signals to another; for instance, a mother holding out her arms to her child demanding a kiss, but in such a way and with such a look, as to repel the child.

It will be apparent that changes in one part of the family system, i.e. sickness, antisocial behaviour, success, failure, pregnancy, will invariably be followed by changes in another part. It is when these changes are of a pathological nature that psychiatric treatment may be required. And for this to be effective the therapist must examine and understand the family system to the maximum.

The battered baby syndrome

At least 3000 infants and children are injured or seriously deprived each year in the UK, and at least 40 of these infants die. The child who is battered, bitten, scalded, burnt and generally abused, is usually between a few weeks and three years old, although he can be much older. Violence tends to be episodic and occurs when one or both parents become tried beyond their endurance by the crying or the negativism of the child. The mortality rate among battered babies is substantial, and a high proportion of the survivors are brain damaged or permanently crippled. Many show emotional difficulties and have problems later in social relationships.

Battering parents come from all social classes. They were commonly abused themselves as children, and perhaps learnt at an early age to react aggressively to difficulties and tension. They tend to be inadequate personalities, unable to tolerate their child's fractious behaviour without resorting to violence. Sometimes a battering parent is psychotic, has postpartum depression, or is mentally impaired (although mental impairment bears no direct relationship to battering). But only about 5 per cent are ill in the strict psychiatric sense. If a parent batters his first-born child, the risk of further children being battered is very high.

Practitioners are often reluctant to diagnose the 'battered baby syndrome', preferring to overlook the possibility. Any suspicion, any delay in bringing the baby for treatment of injuries, twist injuries of the joints, or multiple scattered injuries, should be investigated by a complete skeletal X-ray examination.

A Care and Protection Order may be needed if a child is thought to be at risk. Needless to say, as the American psychiatrist Kempe has reiterated: 'Criminal penalties for battering parents are absolutely useless'.

Social and living conditions

Social conditions contribute to parental reactions, and influence the way children develop. Overcrowding increases after each child, and is particularly likely to affect adversely the one-parent family. Children may encounter hostile neighbours and be frightened to go alone into the streets and the playground. Racial tensions may grow and cause anxiety among coloured children.

Problem families exist in every large urban area, unable to fend for themselves in the manner demanded by society. They may be evicted from their homes for non-payment of rent. If their home is broken up, children are uprooted from their schools, taken from teachers and other trusted people on whom they have come to depend. Or parents may be sent to prison for thieving and their children put into care and protection. It is important to acknowledge that children can have important relationships outside their families which will be shattered if the family is split or moved, sometimes with serious consequences for the child.

It is often difficult for immature and anxious parents to cope with social and cultural pressures, particularly when they move into new and unfamiliar areas, next to people of different social backgrounds. Anxious parents fear their child showing them up, and try to discipline him into behaving 'properly'. The child may react angrily to his parents' sense of shame and inferiority, thus setting up a vicious circle. Parents with fragile psychological defences are liable to break down under such social pressures. And like their children, they then regress in behaviour. Social pressures of this kind on parents are likely to be greater if their children are handicapped, and are singled out for attention by neighbours.

Faced with such a situation a child finds the pressure increasingly hard to tolerate and may gradually become near-psychotic in behaviour. Sooner or later he will have to be removed from this disrupting environment. Social and cultural pressures will have combined to destroy, perhaps permanently, the bond between parents and child.

Depression among working class mothers is common (see p. 204). This is especially so with those who have children under 6 and who do not go out to work. Depression not only limits their emotional involvement with their children, but causes them to be irritable and intolerant to the children's needs and demands. This in turn causes the children to become increasingly disturbed and liable later to become deliquent.

Immigrant children may pose special problems because of the

structures of their families and the way their parents adapt to life here. Pakistani and Indian children are, on the whole, not psychiatrically disturbed and do not seem likely to have serious difficulties later in adult life. When they arrive in this country they usually have relatives waiting to accept and take them into an extended family structure. The child feels reasonably safe and secure from the start.

West Indian children often have a far higher incidence of conduct disorders than white children. This may be related to a number of factors, including lack of early stimulation at home, their large families, unsatisfactory and overcrowded schools, educational retardation, and a high rate of family disruption. Their difficulties are compounded later by scarcity of work and colour prejudices.

4
Maturation and Development

Maturation is development rather than growth. A new-born child has legs but cannot use them for walking. If he is premature he may even be unable to suck. At one year old, though he may be able to take a few steps on his own, he will not be able to talk, and he will still be wet at night. A child of five may 'fall in love', but his feelings and behaviour will be quite unlike those of an adult who has fallen in love, and he will certainly not be capable of adult sexual behaviour.

Maturation occurs progressively. A child who has had a normal full-term delivery can suck, swallow, breathe and carry out functions that are essential for life and growth. This is because his central nervous system, as well as the organs concerned, has matured and developed its organisations sufficiently for these actions to be possible. After birth, the nervous system continues to mature, and there is a corresponding orderly growth of behaviour. Sitting up, standing, walking, sphincter control, language and sexual behaviour can occur only when the nervous system is sufficiently mature to organise them. Until the appropriate stage of maturity has been reached, these things will not be possible, no matter how strong the demand from the environment. Thus, however much a mother wants her child to talk, walk or be dry, and however hard she tries to persuade him in these matters, she will not be successful until his nervous system is sufficiently developed to cope with them. Since there is an enoromous amount of individual variation, one child will learn these things much more quickly than another.

Even when the nervous system is sufficiently mature to learn certain modes of behaviour, these may not in fact occur unless there is suitable stimulation from the environment. No matter how mature his nervous system, a child will not learn Greek unless someone teaches him. For the same reason some people continue to wet their beds throughout their lives simply because they are never taught sphincter control.

There is a rough level of maturity for each age. But it is very rough, because normal individuals can differ so widely from each other.

Infants and young children have characteristic brain-waves, as recorded by *electroencephalogram*. These brain-waves are thought to reflect the still immature organisation of the brain. As the child grows older, the 'immature' waves tend to die out, and they only appear under special conditions. It is interesting to note that in some adults, particularly *psychopaths*, this immature type of record may persist. It is possible that the impulsive, egocentric and childlike behaviour of psychopaths may be related to the lack of maturation of the brain.

There is no convincing evidence showing that a breast-fed infant develops more satisfactorily than a bottle-fed one. Fifty years ago breast-feeding was definitely preferable because less was known about the nutritional needs of infants and also because bottle-feeding was unhygienic. But today, from the point of view of hygiene and nutrition, bottle-feeding is as satisfactory as breast-feeding; with the proviso that artificial feeds contain more starch and may contribute to overweight later. Only about fifty per cent of mothers want to try to breast-feed, and just over one third give up after a week or so. Breast-feeding is not really a reflex action, but has to be learnt by mother and baby, a fact sometimes forgotten by midwives and health visitors. But tactile stimulation does seem to be important, and the amount of handling a child receives is probably much more important than how he is fed. Emotional difficulties and tensions in his mother may be transmitted to the child through the way he is handled.

The infant needs food and comfort. When he is satisfied he feels pleasure. The satisfaction becomes associated with his mother and other people who satisfy his needs. Gradually, by a conditioning process, the mother herself becomes a need; now the infant feels pleasure when she is with him and handling him. He feels unrest when she is absent.

The infant's relaxed contented state is satisfying to the mother, but even more so is the child's smiling. The feedback from the child to its mother is important. Mother needs to feel and see her child responding to her, smiling at her, moulding his body to hers and so on. The screaming child who refuses to eat, usually in response to tensions from her, increases her anxiety. The autistic child creates coldness in his mother. Smiling develops at about six weeks. (Smiling begins later in prematurely born infants, indicating that internal growth factors are more important than environmental.) At first the smile is merely a reflex response on the part of a *satisfied* infant to a human face. Until he is four or five months old he is probably incapable of recognising anyone. Certainly the child does not begin to form his first important attachment or bond with his parents or parent substitute until about six months of age. The practical importance of this is that during these first few months it probably does not matter who, or how many people, look after the child provided his needs are satisfied. However, once memory begins to develop and the child can recognise his mother as a person who satisfies his needs, her presence does become important for his development. From five or six months onwards he may show signs of anxiety when she is away. Such anxiety is likely to be greater in a child whose early needs were not fully satisfied, either because of circumstances or because of emotional difficulties in his mother. Such a child may quickly become restless when his mother is absent and be excessively demanding of her attentions. Any lengthy separation from his mother may result in considerable and prolonged anxiety which can interfere with his development. (We discuss the effects of 'maternal deprivation' on p. 40.) It is important to realise that organic factors such as damage in utero, or some minor injury at birth insufficient to cause cerebral palsy but sufficient to cause sensory deficiencies, may also interfere with the child's development.

In general, it seems likely that the way in which a child's needs are satisfied in his early years largely determines how he will deal with his needs when he is an adult. Discomfort and anxiety resulting from continually unsatisfied needs may cause difficulties later, particularly in human relationships. However, this does not mean that the infant's every wish should be instantly met, or that his mother should subordinate completely her own feelings and needs to those of her child. Excessive spoiling of a child may cause just as much trouble later as deprivation, for it may result in the *pleasure principle* being carried on into adult life.

The *pleasure principle* describes how the new-born child expects his every need to be instantly satisfied. The infant is at first not aware of any differentiation between himself and the outside world. The breast or bottle, when he is hungry and is fed, becomes part of himself. But gradually he comes to distinguish objects and beings external to himself, and sooner or later he comes to recognise that other people also have needs. He learns that these needs sometimes conflict with his own. And he finds that it is sometimes necessary to postpone the gratification of his needs, otherwise he may incur the disapproval of his mother or other important people in his life, and thereby lose their affection. This is the beginning of the *reality principle*, and from now on the child realises increasingly that he must adapt his needs to those of others, and that he can no longer expect always to have his own way.

From about two years onwards *repression* (see p. 65) begins to operate increasingly, preventing wholly unacceptable impulses and wishes from coming into consciousness. This is the beginning of acceptable social behaviour. But the child at this stage behaves and controls his impulses because he knows he may be punished if he does what he wants. If he knows he will certainly not be caught, then he may steal a box of sweets or anything else that attracts him. A code of behaviour based on such an equilibrium of pleasure and reality will certainly cause difficulties if carried into adult life.

Most of us behave in accordance with a higher principle, that of *conscience*. This is a moral sense involving real considerations for the needs of others. A conscience develops in most children around the age of seven or eight years as a result of adopting and incorporating the attitudes, beliefs and customs of people who are loved and admired. Such people are parents, teachers, close friends. A secure, happy child who loves and admires his parents has no difficulty in *identifying* (see p. 66) himself with what he sees to be their good qualities, with modelling himself on them, for he feels that he must live up to their standards. But an insecure child, perhaps without a mother, may not be able to do this and conscience may only form much later or not at all. Defective learning of this type, due to deprivation, is probably responsible for some *psychopaths* who lack a moral sense and who are unable to control their impulses.

The formation of a conscience may also be delayed or affected if a child is excessively pampered or spoilt. Then the child or adult may continue to operate on the pleasure principle, even though such a person may himself suffer from his behaviour. It seems that there may be a *critical period* for the development of a conscience, and that if this is missed for any reason, subsequent development is very slow and perhaps always defective to some degree.

As the infant's *memory* develops, so does his *self-awareness*. He begins to distinguish himself from his outside world. Gradually he learns to recognise his hands, arms, legs and feet, and so on, as part of himself and memory adds permanence to his state of identity. As sensation and motor co-ordination grow, with maturation of the central nervous system, so self-awareness grows and is probably well developed by between two and three years old.

His growing sense of identity and his increasing agility lead, by the end of the first year of life, to his trying increasingly to assert his independence. Struggles may develop between mother and child at this time, and reach a peak around 18 months to two years. He becomes obstinate and negativistic and seems to take pleasure in refusing to co-operate or do what he is asked. Constant scenes and struggles may occur at meal-times or when he is put to bed. He refuses to use his pot, but almost immediately dirties himself or makes a puddle on the floor or wets the bed. All too easily a vicious circle may build up; his mother loses her sense of proportion and matters get completely out of hand. Some firmness and discipline is essential, but too harsh or punitive an attitude may inhibit his development and result in his becoming too conforming and docile. Provided the child is allowed a reasonable amount of self-expression and is not over-suppressed and over-protected, he gradually becomes more constructive and co-operative. This positive process is usually increased by mixing and playing with other children.

For the first three years the child's mother is usually the most important figure and influence in his life. He comes to recognise his father during the first year, but it is not until later, around the third or fourth year, that he really begins to take notice of him and imitate his ways. If the child is a boy he may begin to show signs of jealousy and try to monopolise his mother's attention. A girl, on the other hand, may try to compete with her mother for her father's affection. This family triangle was depicted by Sophocles two thousand years ago in Oedipus Rex. Freud borrowed this idea and described this 'normal' phase of development under the term *Oedipus complex*. Although many children do show some jealousy to the parent of the same sex, and openly favour the other, it is doubtful whether this situation always occurs in our present-day society, and it is certainly unknown in some cultures. Its existence probably depends to some extent on the family's attitude to childhood sexual behaviour. The more this is frowned upon, the more likely are *Oedipal* feelings to emerge.

Sibling rivalry

Much has been written about the effect on a child of a new baby in the family. So far as young children are concerned signs of jealousy towards the new baby are 'normal'. Jealousy is likely to be particularly obvious in children who had a very close relationship with their mothers; first-born children are therefore likely to be more affected than later born. The jealous child feels he will lose the affection of his parents, and it is important for parents to recognise and understand this. If the child feels particularly insecure and rejected (this will depend largely upon his earlier experiences) he may *regress* in behaviour. He then starts to behave as he did when younger. For instance, having been dry he may start to be dirty, refuse to eat properly, demand a bottle instead of a cup, or revert to 'baby talk'. A wise mother prepares the child for the new baby's arrival and lets him share in the preparations. And subsequently, within limits, she lets him help look after the baby, and is tolerant about his difficult behaviour.

The mixed feelings of a child towards his new-born brother or sister are often quite apparent. He will rock the cot or pat the baby's head, at first in play, but gradually becoming increasingly rough until he is virtually attacking the infant. He may be very friendly towards the baby as long as he gets on well with his mother, but in a moment when he is angry with his mother, he may attack the baby. With time and parental understanding these jealousies subside.

The position of a child in the family may influence his development and his personality. First-born children are often particularly close to their mothers and, perhaps because they receive more attention than those born later, they tend to be more advanced in their development. Statistically they are more intelligent in terms of IQ than those born later. Sometimes, however, the oldest of a large family may be restricted by the activities of the younger children and may be called upon to assume an excessive amount of responsibility. The youngest child – particularly if there is a large gap between him and the next child – and the only child are both liable to be spoilt and over-mothered and kept emotionally younger than their years.

Childhood habits

Certain forms of behaviour are so common in younger children that they can be regarded as normal, although they may worry parents. Almost all children, for instance, suck their thumbs at some time. They derive considerable satisfaction from this. Usually the habit stops before the age of about four years, but sometimes it persists and may occasionally give rise to orthodontic troubles, although there is no need to worry about this until the second teeth are through. Night terrors, when the child is terrified although awake, occur most often between two and three years. Head banging, hair-pulling, and masturbation may come and go. Nail-biting usually begins at about three or four years and may continue on and off for many years. Eight per cent of social class 1 and 13 per cent of social class 5 are bad nail biters still at the age of seven. Tics and habit spasms are also common and usually disappear quickly if ignored.

Neurotic disorders such as phobias, obsessions and general

unhappiness of mood are not uncommon. They do of course cause misery not only to the child but to his family, and may interfere with his progress at school, but in themselves they have no clear significance for the development of later psychiatric disorder. On the other hand, antisocial behaviour in childhood is significant. Children who are persistently antisocial in behaviour are likely to grow worse after puberty and to become delinquent. In addition, they have more marital difficulties, worse work records, poorer social relationships, more general psychiatric illness and poorer physical health.

Emotional deprivation

Emotional deprivation is all too readily equated with maternal deprivation, which is still a controversial subject. Interest in maternal deprivation developed in the mid-1930s, and in 1951 John Bowlby summarised all published works in a report to the World Health Organization. He concluded that 'maternal love in infancy is as important for mental health as are vitamins and proteins for physical health', and that 'prolonged deprivation of the young child of maternal care may have grave and far reaching effects on his character, and so on the whole of his future life'. A child needs 'a warm intimate and continuous relationship with his mother in which both find satisfaction and enjoyment'. Bowlby severely criticised the institutional care of children, including the way they were looked after in hospitals. His work has stimulated much research, both human and a variety of animal studies (which cannot easily be compared with humans as is sometimes done rather naively). Some of his conclusions were widely misinterpreted. Mothers were expected to spend 24 hours a day with their children. Mother love was elevated to almost mystical heights. Working mothers were castigated, and so were nurses and crèches.

Until the age of about six months, a child does not begin to form a bond with his mother or substitute figure. Any sizeable break in the child's relationship with his mother, particularly between the ages of six months and five years, may adversely affect his development, especially his later ability to socialise with other people. For instance, Bowlby's original study of 44 thieves suggested that psychopathy was particularly likely to be related to frequent changes of mother figures during the first two years. Certainly a *failure to form bonds* in the first three years, due to emotional deprivation is liable to lead to 'affectionless psychopathy' later. On the other hand, *disruption of bonds* already forged characteristically produces acute distress in the child. But many factors are involved, and it is as well to keep a sense of proportion and to realise that many young children are separated from their mothers for long periods at a time and do not appear to suffer damage. Constitutional factors, the child's sense of security at the time of separation, who looks after him in place of his mother, knowledge of the future, and so on, are all important in this respect. Although John Bowlby's main work has been concerned with the adverse effect of a long separation of the child from his mother, he has also pointed out that maternal deprivation can arise when the child's mother is unable to give him all the loving care he needs because of her own emotional difficulties. But the harmful effects of separation have probably been exaggerated and have led to unnecessary anxiety on the part of many parents. On the other hand, a high proportion of juvenile delinquents and people with psychopathic personalities do come from broken homes that are lacking in affection, or they have been separated from their mothers in early childhood. A child whose parents constantly row or separate is less likely to feel the security which is so important if he is to identify himself with his parents, and acquire social and moral standards. Often the child becomes a pawn in the parents' quarrels, being used by the mother or father in turn to score off the other; the child quickly learns to use this situation for his own ends for he senses a basic lack of affection for him in such parents. Mothers may encourage their daughters to fear men and to regard anything to do with sex as nasty; thus they may perpetuate their own sexual difficulties in their daughters.

Contrasting with maternal deprivation is over-mothering, which may have equally harmful effects. In the USA, overmothering is sometimes known as *momism*. The egocentric, immature, dependent personality that may result from momism is unable to adapt quickly or easily to new situations. It is essential that children should be exposed to a reasonable amount of stress from the time they are born, in order that adaptive mechanisms, both physiological and psychological, can develop.

There are many reasons for parents' abnormal attitudes towards their children. The mother's attitude to her child usually relates closely to her relationship with her husband, and on whether the child was wanted. The child may have been conceived after a long period of sterility or been born after all the other children have grown up. Or the child may have been very ill and thus aroused persistent anxiety in his parents. Both parents may over-protect or reject the child because of problems in their own childhood. Or the parents may be unhappily married and compensate for their unhappiness through the child. In some instances over-protection may in fact be a compensation for underlying guilt and rejection of the child. The father may resent bitterly the arrival of a baby and see him as a rival; not only may he reject the child but there may also be gross neglect or actual cruelty. If separated, both parents may use the child as a means of revenge through custody proceedings.

Bowlby believes the maternal bond with the child to be of special quality. This is disputed by many people and indeed there seems no good reason to suppose that it has any special quality, although it may be expected to be stronger because the mother sees most of the child.

There is evidence that women today feel a need to go out to work, and those who do so are psychologically healthier as a result, and able to be more relaxed with their children. A clear-cut relationship exists between childhood disorders and an unhappy atmosphere at home. There is a strong chance that a child whose parents are constantly bickering will develop antisocial aggressive behaviour, or become delinquent. From a forensic point of view, it is important to recognise that a child charged with some delinquent act is likely to repeat the offence if he returns to an unhappy home. It may be better to send the child to a good institution, or to foster parents, or for the family to split up and the child to be brought up by one parent, than for him to continue in this atmosphere. This has only been accepted by child care officers in the last few years. In the past, children were forced to remain in unsatisfactory homes because of child care officers' misunderstanding of Bowlby's earlier writings. On the other hand it must be said that children in institutional care are particularly likely to be disturbed psychiatrically, although this is probably because of their earlier experiences, and often frequent broken relationships.

Consistent discipline is essential for the child. It does not matter overmuch how the child is disciplined so long as discipline is consistent in its purpose. A child needs a framework in which to develop, outside which he knows he should not go. But excessive discipline may be harmful and result in later behaviour problems such as stealing, negativism, and outbursts of temper and destructiveness. It is always better to teach by example rather than by punishment. It is also important to appreciate that a child may be too young to understand why something he has done is wrong. Just as it is a waste of time to train a child to be dry before the central nervous system is developed at about 18 months, so it does more harm than good to try to instil concepts or standards that the child cannot understand.

The effect of parental illness on children

Chronic depression, psychopathy and neurosis in a parent are likely to produce psychiatric disorders in the child, especially of an antisocial nature. This is probably because neurotics tend to marry neurotics and because these disorders are associated with aggressive outbursts. On the other hand, schizophrenia in one parent does not seem to create psychiatric difficulties, mainly because the other partner is often stable and the home is not disturbed by quarrelling.

When both parents are mentally ill the family is likely to be disrupted and the chances of the child developing psychiatric disorder is high. About a third of the children seen in child guidance clinics have parents who are ill mentally.

Physical illness in a parent of a chronic or recurrent type is twice as common among psychiatric children as among control groups. Psychiatrically disturbed children who continue to be mentally ill in later life are more likely to have experienced the death of one or more parent. Children between the ages of three and five are most vulnerable and likely to show long-term damage. The death of a parent in adolescence, particularly of the opposite sex, is liable to make the adolescent vulnerable to depression later on. Many factors of course are concerned: length of time the parent was ill, whether by suicide, and particularly the reaction of the remaining partner.

Illegitimacy

The rate of illegitimate births in Britain rose steadily until the passing of the Abortion Act (1967). This, and the wider use of the contraceptive pill has reduced the number. The illegitimate child, unless adopted at an early age, may be at considerable disadvantage. He is usually the first-born child of a young mother, and is liable to be underweight at birth. When brought up by his natural parent, accommodation is likely to be poor and crowded. Compared to legitimate children the illegitimate child tends to be backward in ability and achievement at school, and to become maladjusted. The mother may choose to remain unmarried and be a one-parent family. There may be good reasons for this, but sometimes this reflects personality difficulties in making a good heterosexual relationship, difficulties which may later extend to the child.

Fostered children

Children without parents, or whose parents are unable to look after them, come under the care of the Children's Department of the local authority. Whenever possible, particularly in infancy and in the pre-school period, children are boarded out in the care of foster parents, this being preferable to institutional care. Most children who are fostered are already seriously deprived, and correspondingly disturbed emotionally. Foster parents usually require support and supervision from child care workers, responsible to the Child Care Officer.

Problems often arise in connection with the real parents. Many of them feel guilty towards their children and project hostile feelings on to the foster parents or the staff of the Children's Department. Such problems need to be met with understanding by child workers. Problems also arise when a child, fostered for his first three or four years, then returns to his natural parents, or one parent plus a step-parent. He has lost the people to whom he has become attached, and has difficulty in trusting and settling down with his new, if natural, parents.

Adopted children

Adoption is probably the best form of *substitute* care for parentless children or those lacking a suitable home. Adopted children (statistically) develop better in every way than those in residential or foster care. The Adoption Act of 1958 has made it possible to dispense with a parent's consent to adoption if that parent has failed, without reasonable cause, to discharge his parental obligations.

Between one and two per cent of children are adopted, yet adopted children make up 5–13 per cent of referrals to child psychiatric clinics. The majority of these disturbed children have been adopted after the age of six months, a finding which emphasises the adverse effect of early parental deprivation and the importance of children being placed with their adopted parents before six months.

Many of the couples who adopt are over 30 and have difficulty in adjusting to the infant's needs. Women often feel lingering shame over their inability to reproduce and this can increase their difficulties in disclosing to a child that he is adopted. Adoption societies carefully vet the reasons and personalities of couples wanting to adopt, for it is important that parents should face their conflicts and difficulties over the child honestly and frankly.

If the adopted child later becomes unhappy and disturbed, parents may refuse to see themselves as responsible, and will blame the child's heredity, his 'over-sexed' real parents, or seek other reasons.

Most of the additional stress to which an adopted child is exposed stems from unrealistic attitudes and expectations on the part of adopting parents. Large differences of intelligence between the child and his parents occasionally cause problems, although adoption societies try to avoid this by suitable placing of children. The outcome of adopting older children, often from a foreign country such as Vietnam, is not yet known.

Step-children

Step-children may encounter special difficulties. When the step-mother is insecure and uncertain of her husband's affection, she may be unable to cope with her aggressive feelings for a child, the more so if she has none of her own.

On the other side of the coin, a step-child may feel guilty and responsible for marital discords that develop. Parental quarrels over him lead to deterioration in his standards of behaviour.

Children in hospital – Regression

Any change in family stability makes some children, particularly those before five or six years old, insecure and anxious. A commonplace event such as moving house, father having to go away on a business trip, or the arrival of a new child, may cause anxiety. This may result in *regressive behaviour.* A child who has been previously dry wets the bed, speech may deteriorate, he clings to his mother and refuses to let her out of his sight, and generally becomes babyish in his behaviour. This is known as *regression.* Understanding parents see the cause of this and try to be tolerant and more openly affectionate than usual. But over-strict parents may punish this behaviour, seeing it as due to naughtiness, and thereby increase the child's insecurity and anxiety.

Separation from his mother is particularly upsetting to a young child. Mother going into hospital is not so bad if the child can remain home with the rest of the family, although her return sometimes results in some degree of regression. More disturbing to the child is his own admission to hospital, although this is now likely to be much less difficult for him than in former times, because doctors and nurses are now beginning to understand the problem. Parents can visit their children daily in nearly every hospital, and in many hospitals there are no rigid rules or times concerning visiting. Only in fever hospitals and long-stay orthopaedic hospitals, often situated some way from the child's home, are serious psychological difficulties likely to occur.

In the past nurses were sometimes more concerned with the organisation of their wards than with the mental welfare of the children. The children were expected to be quiet; the uproar that occurs when parents leave the ward encouraged the idea that visiting 'upset' the child. In fact, the child who screams when his parents leave is reacting in a healthy way to separation. The child who lies quietly in his cot, unresponsive to what is going on round him, is easier to handle but may well be seriously disturbed emotionally.

The acute distress that occurs when a child is brought into hospital and does not see his parents for some time has been well recorded in the Robertson's films. At first the child protests loudly, shaking his cot and crying for his mother (period of protest). After a day or so he shows signs of despair and grows silent, although he probably remains preoccupied with the memory of his absent mother. Finally he reaches a stage of detachment, when he appears to be distressed and to lose interest in his parents. When his parents do reappear he may pay them little or no attention, and even fail to show recognition of them.

When a child returns home after not having seen his mother for several weeks, he is likely to remain detached for some time. Then he begins to show intensely ambivalent feelings, clinging to his mother, demanding all her attention and reacting violently and angrily if she leaves him, even for a few seconds. If the period of separation has lasted for more than six months, and particularly if during this time the child has not received special attention from nurses or visitors, this stage of detachment may remain indefinitely and his affections may be permanently blunted. Of course, much individual variation in children's reactions exists, but this is typical of children between the ages of six months and four years. Below six months distress is not shown, and it diminishes after four years.

Interesting studies have been carried out on the effect of separation of infant Rhesus monkeys from their mothers. The important factor in the infant's reaction seems to be not so much his separation from his mother as the subsequent disturbance in the mother–infant interaction. When this is not disrupted and particularly when the mother is not upset, there are few ill effects.

How a child will react when he is admitted to hospital depends upon several factors:

1. *Age.* The younger the child, particularly if he is less than two years old, the more likely he is to be upset. After two years it becomes progressively easier to tell him what is going to happen to him and thus to reduce his anxiety. Some hospitals encourage the mothers of very young children to come into hospital with them, but this is not always possible, either for the hospital or the mother. However, the presence of a sibling or of some familiar person – even his teddy bear – will reduce a child's distress.

2. *Family relationships.* A child from a secure, happy home will be less upset than one from an unhappy or broken home. Over-anxious parents are liable to have anxious children and to convey their own anxiety about the admission to the child.

3. *Type of care provided in hospital.* The child's distress can be considerably reduced by the provision of toys, by the reaction of the nurses to him, and how often parents, siblings or friends are able to visit him.

Nurses become temporary mothers to the child. It is good if each child has his own special nurse. A screaming child needs to be picked up, not scolded, and the over-quiet two-year-old should not be left alone, but should be given as much attention as possible. This sometimes calls for considerable understanding on the part of the nurse, for the child may not respond emotionally to her at first. Sometimes a nurse may become too attached to a child and feel jealous and resentful towards his mother. But this is exceptional. Most nurses enjoy nursing children and get on well with the parents.

There is little doubt that such separation can have a disturbing effect on a child. On the other hand some children benefit from coming into hospital. An only child, for instance, gains from making friends and learning to play with other children. A deprived child discovers the affection and security that he previously lacked. An over-protected and anxious child may throw off his fears and learn to be more independent. Many children with such psychosomatic illnesses as asthma or eczema need to be admitted during exacerbations; not so much for specific treatment as to separate them from home tensions and thus break a vicious circle.

It is not always remembered that illness, particularly chronic forms such as diabetes or nephritis, cause anxiety and guilt in younger children and make them wonder why they have been singled out for punishment. Children may react to illness by rebelling and becoming uncooperative. Unsympathetic attitudes on the part of nurses and doctors only serve to increase the difficulties. Older children should be encouraged to talk about their fears, the unpleasantness of injections, the general problems of being ill and of being admitted to hospital. Facilities for play or schoolwork are important therapeutically, particularly when long-term hospitalisation is involved.

After returning home, and depending to a large extent on how long he has been in hospital, how much he saw of his parents, his age, and how secure his background, the child may regress in his behaviour and become demanding and difficult. Nurses can help in the child's readjustment by explaining to parents that such behaviour is only a temporary reaction to the insecurity he felt in hospital.

Handicapped children

Special problems of development arise with handicapped children. They may spend long periods in hospital or be forced to lead restricted lives at home. Any aspect of the child's development may be delayed or distorted in consequence. Unless efforts are made to correct this and help the child to compensate for his deficiencies a vicious circle can arise, leading to still further developmental disturbances.

Sick role and illness behaviour

To be ill makes a child, and an adult, 'special'. He is treated with extra sympathy. He is privileged, given treats, spoilt, allowed to stay away from school and events he dislikes or fears. His parents fuss over him. His siblings are expected to be particularly nice and helpful to him. There are, indeed, many advantages to being ill. A child soon learns this after he has had an illness – appendicitis or tonsillitis say, or even a bad cold – or has observed the effect of illness on other members of the family.

He may therefore prolong his symptoms, or develop new ones, typically headache, muscle pains, sore throat, dizziness and unsteadiness. His parents become increasingly anxious. The practitioner may then make matters worse by deciding that investigations are needed rather than looking at the child as a whole and asking himself – and the child – why he has the symptoms.

After recovery the child may try to use illness as a means of avoiding unpleasant situations, and gradually acquire a reputation for being delicate and requiring special care and attention. This is the more likely to happen when parents are anxious and insecure, or when one parent uses the child's illness for his or her own emotional ends.

School age

A child develops rapidly when he begins to go to school. He admires his teacher and tries to imitate him. He makes friends, learns to give and take, and adopts new ideas and ways of behaviour. He develops a moral sense of right and wrong; he now does this, or does not do that, because that is how those people he respects behave. At this time the child may have two quite different standards of behaviour: one for school, and one for home. Parents may be astonished to learn their son is a model child at school, tidy and helpful in the classroom and good-natured in play, while at home he is untidy and rude. Sometimes the reverse occurs and the model child becomes a destructive devil when he goes to school.

Immature parents may feel jealous of the teacher's influence and try to lower his esteem in the child's eye. This may upset the child. He may feel he must choose between parents and teacher. He may reject both or become over-dependent or hostile to one or the other. But usually he achieves some sort of compromise. He becomes reasoning and more reasonable. He learns to control his impulses and to behave in ways that are acceptable to society. Theoretically a teacher should be able to retain a more objective view of the child than the parents. But if he is a neurotic personality himself he may be unable to deal fairly with pupils who arouse his anger or anxiety. He may come under pressure from his colleagues or from parents to adopt a more authoritarian and punitive attitude towards his pupils.

By the age of seven or eight most children are reasonably well behaved. From now until just before puberty intellectual growth predominates. *Egocentric thought* gives way to *conceptual and abstract thought*. The child relates objects and ideas to one another in an increasingly complex way. He learns quickly and is constantly searching for fresh stimulation. If he is denied stimulation and is badly taught he may become bored. If he is forced to learn, or if too high a standard for his mental age is demanded, he may rebel against all forms of learning.

Puberty and adolescence

Adolescence begins with puberty and encompasses the start of independence; chronologically it covers the period from about 11 to 18 years. It is a time of upheaval in every area of life. There is acceleration of growth and a physical transformation accompanied by sex hormone changes. There is wide variation in physical development and sexual maturation. Some adolescents are sexually mature by 13 or 14, and have finished their development before others have even begun. The late developer may find himself outstripped physically and mentally by the early maturers, although since his growth continues for longer he may finally surpass them.

Increase in height and size result from several intrinsic and extrinsic factors. While growth and development normally proceed concomitantly, they are to some degree independent, under different controls. From early childhood onward, hormonal regulation plays an increasing part. In the prepubertal stage, from around eight years, gonads and breasts become more responsive to adrenal hormones and develop and grow. Growth hormone, which remains at a steady level throughout most of childhood, increases during the adolescent growth spurt, which commonly occurs between 11 to 13 in girls, and about two years later in boys.

Sexual development begins earlier in girls than boys, most noticeably in its outward manifestation. For boys, the first signs of puberty are enlargement of scrotum and testes, followed by the appearance of pubic hair. In girls breast development starts around nine years and continues over the next four or five years. The growth of pubic hair is another early sign of puberty. Development of the uterus and vagina follow. Menarche itself occurs at a relatively late stage, and usually after the growth spurt has passed its peak. The first period may occur anywhere between the ages of nine and 17; the mean age in this country is 12.9 years.

Impact of physical changes. After years of steady, undramatic, all-over growth in size, the young adolescent finds his or her body unfamiliar. Accelerating growth occurs unevenly, with hands and feet first. For a girl keen on sport, the gateway to popularity at school, breast development may be an embarrassment that makes her walk with hunched shoulders for concealment. The face of an adolescent changes, both in bone structure, fullness of lips, and increasing activity of sebaceous glands. Body image is distorted; most girls at this stage over-estimate their width, particularly of hips. The development of apocrine sweat glands, producing a distinctive body odour, together with the start of menstruation, may lead an emotionally unprepared youngster to regard her body as dirty. Menarche is an emotionally important event. Psychoanalytic theory still sometimes equates it with castration, and a recent study indicated the persistence of predominantly negative attitudes; 'the curse' is a term still commonly used. Menstruation also makes the adolescent compare herself with her mother, a comparison which may be welcome or alarming depending on the quality of the earlier child–parent relationship.

Intellectual growth. Brain size does not increase appreciably during adolescence, nor can IQ, since this is specifically related to age. But, mental ability, in absolute terms, does increase. Creativity, mathematical skill and functions reflecting biological capability, such as perceptual speed, develop rapidly at this stage, while those linked more with experience, such as verbal fluency, advance more slowly but for longer. The most important intellectual development of adolescence is the change from concrete thinking to conceptualisation. An adolescent develops the ability to think logically, to manipulate concepts rather than things. He interests himself increasingly in abstract ideas and systems. His intellectual power reaches its peak in late adolescence, in contrast to common sense and judgement, which are hampered by lack of experience.

There is increased sensitivity to things previously ignored. Beauty and ugliness are each felt more intensely. Emotional reactivity increases and is reflected in rapid swings of mood, at times distressing.

Physiological 'tasks' of adolescents. The primary task of adolescence is the attainment of an adult, durable ego-identity. A crisis of identity threatens when, at puberty, the childhood idea of self begins to lose its relevance and its effectiveness as a source of security, and the adolescent is forced to question his capabilities and goals. Self-identity is an inner awareness, the result of the continuous interplay of internal and external forces. Components of self-identity are the 'ego-ideal' and the 'super-ego'; normally they are closely inter-related, but in adolescence the demarcation is unclear. The ego-ideal embodies a person's concepts of what he wishes to be. The super-ego represents his conscience, the way in which he feels he should behave. The former defines healthy, narcissistic values, 'the kind of person I can love', the latter the kind of person who does not transgress, and can be loved by others.

The childhood ideal of a self-loving and lovable child must be replaced by adult standards. A child's super-ego mainly comprises internalised parentally-imposed values; responses to it are automatic, and are guide-lines for avoiding punishment, and more importantly, for retaining the parent's love. Guilt is felt if boundaries are overrun. The super-ego of childhood includes prohibitions that are relevant only to childhood, and others applicable to all ages. A difficult task of adolescence is to differentiate between these. For instance, a significant precept in childhood is that 'parents must be obeyed', and in some cultures this persists into adult life. In our society, self-determination is expected in adulthood. Typically, the adolescent handles this conflict by rebelling, usually on unimportant matters against his parents or other authorities.

Rebellion against an internalised value system is unnerving. Obeying the old super-ego offers safety, and earlier standards may be clung to rigidly. This is seen in the obsessional, conscientious girl who develops anorexia nervosa. She dare not go forward independently, and attempts to hold on to an earlier stage; a good child in all but 'eating up'. The danger of retaining too many old standards is that a crippling conscience may persist into adulthood. But a more likely course is rebellion against childhood values.

Dependency. Much as a toddling child learns a measure of independence by repeatedly venturing away from his mother's side and then running back, so an adolescent's confidence rises and falls. He asks his parent's advice, often on trivia, and is reassured that they are still available to help him. He may then discard whatever advice they give, demonstrating to his own satisfaction that he is, after all, independent.

Sexual drive. With increased hormone secretion the sexual drive, which has been growing steadily throughout childhood, is intensified in adolescence. For the adolescent at home, love for his parents and intensified sexual urgings may lead to reactivation of 'oedipal' feelings. Parents may complicate the conflict; a father is aroused by his daughter's budding femininity; a mother senses that her adolescent daughter is becoming a rival, and subtly conveys her disapproval. For the girl, this is a dangerous situation. She may react by denying and repressing normal affection for her father, and even refuse to have any contact with him. In some cases of anorexia nervosa for instance, the girl refuses to eat if her father is in the room.

Normally, adolescents vacillate between emotional closeness

and deliberate rejection of one or both parents. A girl may gain confidence in her femininity from her father's attitude. A close relationship with her mother gives her an opportunity to discuss her feminine problems. If the parent with whom the adolescent seeks to identify appears inadequate, or fails to reassure, this increases the adolescent's fear of failure. Men and women who lack confidence in their own sexual gender often convey their insecurity to their children.

Social changes. Social pressures play a significant part in the adolescent process; most important are the expectations of adults. The middle-class parent in particular may convey the idea that academic failure leads to failure in later life; the adolescent may come to believe that his success at school or university is a vital issue in his relationship with his family.

Social pressures from peer groups also become more insistent in adolescence, and are likely to conflict at times with adult pressures. This can produce severe conflict and strain. The expectations of parents and teachers are greater in the higher socio-economic classes, especially in the academic sphere. Social and sexual experimentation take second place to study for the 15 to 18 year olds whose next step is likely to be university.

It is virtually impossible to assess accurately the incidence of adolescent psychiatric disorders. Among university students with access to a Student Health Service, between one and two per cent develop a serious psychiatric illness at some time during their undergraduate life, a further 10–20 per cent have 'neurotic breakdowns', and about the same number experience minor transitory disturbances.

Adulthood

As the adolescent becomes more self-sufficient and independent so his relationship with his parents improves. He goes to work, enlarges his circle of acquaintances, joins groups and societies, takes on increasingly onerous responsibilities, including (for most people) marriage and a family.

Work and play

A young child's play is at first almost entirely governed by fantasy, unconcerned with solving problems in the real world. Play gradually changes in nature as the child becomes sociable and makes friends, as his intellectual powers widen, and he increasingly co-operates with others. Play gradually merges into work. Work is always directed to a specific end, and is a rational purposeful activity. To work without understanding or aim is wholly unsatisfying. In such situations a man's mental health is often only preserved by his fantasy; the alternative is to direct his interest and energies into outside activities.

Work is an important part of a person's life, not only for material reasons but psychologically. To work is to be accepted by society and to feel 'useful', to have a sense of purpose, although the present situation, with more than three million unemployed and which is likely to continue, may alter this concept. To be unemployed (or even retired) is to feel cut off from society, despised and disregarded. The type of work undertaken depends on intelligence, aptitude, personality and opportunity. Some people of both sexes follow in their parent's footsteps, wishing to emulate or outdo them, others take up entirely different work. Some nurses and doctors have felt determined to take up medicine for as long as they can remember. Fantasies, expressed initially in play, often play an important part, particularly in the professions. The contrast between fantasy and reality may result in psychological difficulties at first. But sooner or later fantasy and 'the realities of work' will intermingle and produce interest, drive and deep satisfaction. If they do not, tension and depression may develop and result in breakdown and abandonment of that particular work. Immature students tend to break down in the first nine months of their course.

Girls show maternal feelings from an early age and nursing is a good means of expressing this. Nursing and doctoring are particularly satisfying work, for not only are they highly regarded by society, but there is pride and a sense of achievement in the work. However, the work is far from easy and is associated with a good deal of anxiety and emotional strain. The psychological morbidity and mortality among doctors and nurses are high.

At the lowest level a person works solely to earn money or whatever commodity is necessary for him and his family to exist. Such a person is not able to utilise his fantasies in his work. He will take little pride or interest in his work. He will feel no sense of loyalty or of belonging. There are many reasons for unsatisfactory working conditions, including bad management and lack of communication between management and workers. Boredom and industrial fatigue grow and output falls. A good management instils loyalties in its workers, feeds them with information, makes them feel their job is valuable and that they are necessary. A bored man is a frustrated man, unable to express his feelings satisfactorily.

Accidents reflect not only physical conditions at work but also psychological and social factors. Many accidents occur because of anger, frustration or disappointment. Studies have shown that about 80 per cent of industrial accidents occur only in a small group of workers, comprising about 20 per cent of the total. These people are looked upon as *accident prone;* they tend to be tense, impulsive people who attempt to relieve their tension by physical activity.

Male and female differences

The greater part of the differences in temperament and behaviour between men and women arises from differences of upbringing. Yet there are constitutional differences present at or shortly after birth. Females sleep longer and are less irritable. There is therefore, perhaps, a tendency for mothers to pick up and hold boys more often than girls. Males tend to be heavier and taller and are physically stronger from the start, although paradoxically females are tougher and survive better. Girls sit up, crawl, walk, and learn to talk earlier than boys. They retain their superiority in verbal skills until puberty. Females are more responsive to auditory stimuli, boys have greater visual acuity and show more interest in visual patterns. This means that from birth the same stimulus will have a somewhat different significance for each sex. Females are more sensitive to pain and touch and more responsive to sweet tastes. Their sense of smell is better developed, particularly after puberty. Boys are more aggressive and competitive in common with most other mammalian species. Girls are more friendly, sympathetic, and protective towards younger children from an early age.

No one description of what constitutes characteristic male or female behaviour is likely to be universally acceptable. A woman from another culture – Indian, Chinese, Egyptian, Italian – is expected to behave very differently from an Englishwoman. But the very word Englishwoman today is misleading, for there are large differences of behaviour between social classes. A working class woman still tends to see herself as dominated by the male, her main function being to look after him and raise his children. The upper class woman is more likely to demand equality with the male. The Victorian female, certainly among the middle classes, was looked upon as the devoted custodian of her family or, if unmarried, of her aged parents; the 'angel in the house', gentle, kind, understanding, and self-sacrificing. The Victorian male was seen as a hardworking, reliable if stern husband and father, but also sexually demanding and not able to control his appetites in the way females could. Our values and beliefs have profoundly changed over the last century and inevitably so have our concepts of masculinity and femininity

Sexual development

It was Freud who developed the idea of infantile sexuality. It is important to understand what is meant by the term and to distinguish it from adult or genital sexuality. Children derive considerable pleasure from stimulation of their bodies, including their genitalia, from an early age, and orgasmic-like reactions can be observed in young children. Erection of the penis may occur shortly after birth, and is not a foretaste of superhuman virility but a reflex response to a full rectum. Infants begin to play with their genitals from around five months onwards, boys more so than girls. Ejaculation can only occur however after puberty is reached.

Sex play and self-stimulation during early childhood is not only pleasurable but comforting to the child. From three or four years onwards, sexual activities involving other children or adults are common, reflecting curiosity, pleasure and excitement. Genital exploration and display is a common feature of childhood with both sexes. Oral sex is common, but attempts at actual genital intercourse are probably uncommon in our society.

Freud pointed out the existence of erotogenic zones of the body, stimulation of which gave particular pleasure: the mouth, anus, and genital organs. He thought that in the normal process of maturation these erotogenic zones lost their sensual qualities, and sexual pleasure eventually became confined to the genital areas. He described childhood sexuality as 'polymorphus perverse', meaning that all erotic potentialities were explored by the child through his own body or through the bodies of others, directly or at a distance, by touching and watching. It is man's prolonged childhood which creates the complexities of adult sexuality. But in fact childhood sexuality is not entirely repressed. Far from it, for genital sexual satisfaction should follow on from 'polymorphus perverse' fore-play. Without that childlike love play which precedes intercourse, sexuality can be dull and unsatisfying.

By the age of seven many boys masturbate quite frequently and this proportion rises steadily, with a rapid increase just before and after puberty. Girls follow boys in this pattern, but with a lower incidence. The majority of pre-adolescent and young pubescent girls suppress their sexual feelings or project them on to some unattainable celebrity. At puberty sexual drives direct the adolescent towards his sexual object, which may or may not be attainable, and push sexual fantasies into consciousness. It is now that fears arise, often connected with underlying fantasies, and the adolescent becomes anxious, fearing that he will never be able to lead a normal sexual life. This may force him increasingly into more fantasy.

Marriage

For most people, sooner or later the question of marriage arises. Although extramarital sexual relationships are now widely recognised and accepted, few doubt that our society is still based upon marriage and the family. Russia attempted to abolish the family after the 1917 Revolution but the scheme met with failure. And even the Kibbutz system in Israel, in which the children are brought up collectively, still preserves the basis of family life; children join their parents for part of each day.

Marriage satisfies both biological and psychological needs. Women, because they mature earlier, tend to marry younger. They differ from men in that the biological need for conception and motherhood is perhaps present from an early age. This may show itself in an open desire to have babies, or alternatively in loud denials of any such wish. It is often important for a woman to invest her future husband with desirable and exaggerated qualities. This helps her to separate from her family and to accept her role as a wife. Her husband also responds to the idea of being a superman. His self-esteem and confidence increase, together with a new sense of responsibility. After marriage, of course, both become more realistic towards one another, and both have to make adjustments in their outlook and behaviour in order for the relationship to develop.

Teenage marriages are increasing. The availability of contraceptive pills, by removing the risk of pregnancy, ensures that a high proportion of teenagers of both sexes now have sexual relationships. Women tend to form more stable relationships than men and there is little doubt that a satisfying sexual relationship produces a strong 'bonding' effect. Some teenagers are mature individuals, emotionally ready for marriage. But many are emotionally unstable and may marry simply in order to escape from their parents, to gain an unrealistic security. They may invest their partners with such unrealistic qualities that they are unable to adapt to the realities of marriage.

The seriousness with which society regards marriage is exemplified in the marriage ceremony; this not only sets the approval of society on the two people living together, it also highlights the fact that society accepts them as adults and expects them to behave responsibly.

It is not always appreciated that marriage or 'living together' is a dynamic changing state, irrespective of whether or not there are children. Each partner matures, and one may sooner or later outpace the other. Dissatisfactions and resentments surface, sex suffers, the relationship fails and ends. If there are children the marriage may continue for their sake, although the benefits of this, when there is much tension between the parents, are dubious. In any case some kind of crisis in the marriage is likely to erupt when the children become independent and leave home, unless husband and wife have reached a compromise which satisfies both. One or other may have found a sexual partner outside the marriage by then. There may be considerable stresses at this point.

> John and Mary had been married 23 years. The last of their three children had left home. John had a longstanding mistress who now demanded that John leave his wife and marry her. Mary's life, without children at home, appeared empty, but she could not easily face the idea of losing her husband and 'being left with nothing'. Histrionic scenes developed and she threatened suicide. John felt guilty and remorseful, and was indecisive. His mistress issued an ultimatum: 'Divorce your wife or we finish!' At this point John collapsed and sought psychiatric help.

The divorce rate has increased enormously over the past 20 years, in line with profound changes in sexual mores, and especially the changing role of women and their expectations. It is an uneasy era, for which neither men nor women are yet well prepared psychologically. We are still orientated to the idea of a marriage for life. Perhaps we should see marriage in terms of children, and lasting only as long as they are still dependent. But irrespective of future trends, divorce today is still an upsetting event, the more so for partners who come from stable homes. It represents failure of a profound kind and is frequently followed by depression and self-recrimination.

Working wives

One woman may be thoroughly content to be a housewife and nothing else, her sense of achievement derived from the well-being of her husband and children. Another may be most reluctant to give up her work, seeing herself bored and irritated and isolated at home; the notion appals her. Both women are of course right to follow their inclinations, and should not be deviated by other people's opinions.

Some husbands object to their wives working, feeling that their own status is thereby diminished. And they may resent their wives leading lives independent of them. Such a restrictive 'old-fashioned' attitude is likely to lead eventually to considerable marital tensions.

There is now a body of evidence to suggest that working class women with young children, who do not go out to work, have a higher incidence of depression than those who do – which of course adversely affects the children, the children's behaviour, and in turn the strains on the mother. Understandably depression is most likely when the woman lacks a husband or companion to whom she can communicate her frustrations.

The single adult

There are a variety of reasons for men and women remaining single. The most obvious, although perhaps not the most common, is simply that the single state is preferred. People have freedom to come and go when and where they wish, and no one else's wishes to take into account. They may be intent on building up a career. The need to put their energies and emotional drive into this channel often excludes close relationships, especially of a sexual nature, although not necessarily ephemeral affairs. It is still more difficult for a woman, compared to a man, to reach the heights of her career. Marriage, even with a sympathetic and supportive husband, and even more so with children, can only be an obstacle in terms of career.

Both sexes may choose to remain single until middle age in order to avoid the question of children. Although most of us, and especially women, are programmed from an early age for parenthood, there are not a few who are repelled by the thought of the responsibilities, ties and demands of children.

Lastly, there is the example of one's parents' marriage. If this is viewed by the child as unhappy and destructive, then he or she may decide firmly to stay single.

There are a variety of other reasons given for avoiding marriage; unrequited love, death of an irreplaceable fiancé, illness, financial problems, a decrepit parent to look after, and so on, but these are almost invariably excuses of a kind masking deeper fears and reservations.

As the single person ages he or she may have moments of regret about marriage and a family, although how prolonged or serious such feelings are will largely depend on dissatisfactions at work and in social activities. As middle age approaches a sexual relationship may bring new emotions of such intensity to the surface that the apparently well-adjusted individual becomes increasingly upset, and even breaks down.

Middle age

Middle age can be a time of contentment and stability for many people. But it is also a potentially dangerous time. A man may feel that his ambitions can never be realised and that he is a failure. He may unexpectedly be made redundant, or lose his job for reasons beyond his control and not be able to find a comparable position. Financial problems cause mounting anxiety. He may become seriously depressed and feel that he cannot carry on living.

A woman may also encounter these problems but other factors also arise. She must adjust to the physiological and psychological changes that occur at the *menopause*. Control over emotions and impulses may be upset. She may feel that the menopause represents the end of her life as a woman and that she is no longer attractive. Difficulties may be increased for the married woman when her children grow up and leave home. For some mothers the idea of their children leaving home, or becoming engaged to marry, is extremely difficult to accept. A daughter's sexual behaviour usually has a far more profound effect on her mother than a son's. The mother's repressed sexual conflicts, resentments towards her spouse, regrets at her own lost opportunities, may suddenly erupt and create a family crisis. Loss of parents or close friends may be particularly upsetting to those who are unmarried.

Of course, many women go through the menopause without any problems. This is most likely to happen when the woman is leading a full and satisfying life, and is not largely dependent upon her family.

Sexual interest and activity will depend largely on the individual's personality and life style. Some men and women slowly lose interest and potency from middle age onwards. Others react to middle age by increased sexual activity. The cessation of menstruation need have no effect on a woman's sexual responses. In fact some women are able to respond sexually much more when their fear of pregnancy is lost. Women who have never accepted or enjoyed their sexual role may use the menopause to bring their sexual life to a close. This frequently leads to marital disturbances and sometimes results in husbands looking elsewhere for their sexual satisfaction.

Many women today are on long-term oestrogen replacement therapy, which seems to have advantages, both physically and psychologically.

There is no equivalent male menopause although psychologically there may be similar problems. Testosterone levels continue undiminished until old age, although it seems likely that the 'target organs or centres', particularly in the hypothalamus, become less sensitive to the hormones. There is no reason why people of both sexes should not continue sexual activity, relatively undiminished, until their eighties or even nineties.

Old age

Biological ageing occurs in everyone, but its effects vary widely from one person to another. Some start to age when relatively young, while others are still youthful and adaptable at eighty years old.

Retirement may be felt as a serious loss, especially if the person has no outside interests to turn to. He becomes bitterly aware of his lost status and now looks upon himself as a 'has been'. In many societies the old are respected. In our society they are all too often ignored or despised by those who are young and vigorous.

No one fully understands what happens with ageing, but there is a progressive decrease in energy and strength and ability to stand up to stress of all kinds. Physiological adaptation is impaired. A mild infection or injury is sometimes enough to kill an old person. Widespread bodily changes occur. Kidneys and the cardiovascular system are less efficient and the blood supply to the brain may be seriously diminished. Brain cells die. Sensation, including vision and hearing, become less efficient. At first these defects are compensated, but eventually their effects become prominent and the old person begins to become disorganised.

Certain mental changes characterise ageing.

1. Old people become increasingly self-centred, introspective and egocentric, and are often over-sensitive and are quick to take offence.

2. They become increasingly unadaptable. Anything new or strange is rejected at once and compared unfavourably with the

past. New skills cannot be learnt, or only slowly and reluctantly.

3. Memory for recent events fails, but incidents of long ago are remembered vividly. As a result old people come to live increasingly in the past, particularly if they lead isolated lives and lack the stimulation provided by young and more active people.

4. Depression, anxiety and a sense of isolation are common. There is increasing preoccupation with bodily functions (*hypochondriasis*), often reinforced by the death of friends or relatives, and by the bodily changes which occur with ageing. Concern over bowels is particularly common.

5. The usual sleep rhythm may be reversed, the old person asleep during the day and up at night. In the dark he may become disorientated and confused.

6. Control over appetite diminishes. Eating habits may become dirty and coarse. There may be abnormal sexual behaviour, offences against children or *exhibitionism;* all of which are extremely distressing to relatives.

Between 1951 and 1968 the pensionable population rose by 2 million to 8.5 million and the number of people over 75 increased by 700 000 to 2.5 million. The percentage of old people, particularly in the group 75 and over, will continue to increase until about the end of the century. Women greatly outnumber men. About 2 per cent of the elderly are in residential care, but many more are being cared for by devoted relatives. It has been suggested that about 10 per cent of the elderly need residential care, but this would require an enormous expansion of resources.

Grief and mourning

In every human society the death of someone who is loved causes grief. Mourning follows. Although the outward signs of mourning vary with nationality and religion, there is a characteristic reaction to the loss of a loved one.

At first there is intense distress, often accompanied by physical symptoms; shortness of breath, tightness of the throat, an almost painful emptiness in the chest and abdomen, a sense of weakness and impending collapse. Any thought or mention of the dead person heightens such feelings. Gradually these lessen, although they may recur, in milder form, at the anniversary of death.

The mourner becomes preoccupied with memories of the deceased; in extreme grief he feels totally cut off from other people, and virtually in a world of his own. He may even deny for a time that the loved one is dead, and continues to speak of him as though he were still alive. Visual hallucinations are common; the face, or the complete person may be seen. Auditory hallucinations are less usual; most of these occur as the mourner is waking up or dropping off to sleep, but sometimes the dead person is heard calling. He searches his conscience for instances of how badly he behaved to the dead person when alive, and is consumed with a sense of guilt for his failings and insensitivity to the other's needs. Occasionally he blames someone else for the death: a doctor, a nurse, a relative, or a friend is selected as the scapegoat. But gradually a sense of reality returns and the mourner comes to accept his loss, helped by sharing his sorrow with friends and relatives.

He continues to think and speak of the dead person. But gradually his feelings become less painful and he comes to interest himself again in other people. He may adopt some of the qualities of the dead person that he particularly admired, or take on some of his responsibilities. Sometimes mourning lasts as long as a year, but eventually it is complete. He can now think realistically and with reasonable detachment about the dead person.

Occasionally grief continues indefinitely. The smallest reference to the dead person causes an emotional outburst. People who react in this way may rebuild their lives around the dead person, even going so far as to preserve the dead person's possessions or rooms exactly as they were in life. They are unable to enjoy their life in any way. Nearly always in such cases anger is to blame; anger against the dead person which cannot be openly expressed.

> Joan's husband died suddenly of a heart attack when she was 48. Her marriage had been 'a wonderful one' although in the last year she had been uneasy about the nature of his relationship with a female colleague at work. After his death she became increasingly sensitive to any reference to her husband, and withdrew from her friends into an unrealistic world of the past.

Natural grief can be severe for up to six months but then begins to decline. However it may continue for much longer if there is unacknowledged resentment towards the dead person. The loss of a spouse is associated with an increased risk of suicide. In the year following death this is about 2½ times greater than normal. But mortality is also increased among the bereaved from other causes. During the first 4 years of bereavement there is a greatly increased risk, for widowers in particular, of coronary thrombosis and arteriosclerotic heart disease; the risk is especially high during the first six months following bereavement.

The effect of the death of a parent on children is difficult to predict, and depends on various factors. However, it seems that they are more prone to psychiatric disorders, particularly depression and phobic anxiety, both as children and later as adults. Children most at risk are those bereaved between the ages of three and five, and in early adolescence. Girls seem to be more vulnerable, especially if they are under 11 years of age, to the loss of mother; father's death has a more profound effect on adolescent girls. A child's position in the family is important, and the presence of an older sibling of the same sex as the dead parent lessens the impact. Much of course depends on the reaction of the surviving parent, financial circumstances, the need to move home and school, and so on.

5
Mental Mechanisms and the Unconscious

Although the concept of unconscious mental processes had long been considered by philosophers and psychologists, it is to Freud that we owe the idea of a dynamic unconscious. The unconscious (sometimes called the preconscious) can be compared to an underground vault wherein are stored memories, fantasies, ideas, events and emotional experiences which are no longer remembered and cannot normally be recalled. Freud believed that these experiences were so terrifying and unacceptable to the individual at the time that their remembrance was suppressed and pushed into the unconscious. The mechanism, which Freud saw as a protective device, is known as repression.

Repression ensures that the forbidden material lies below conscious recall, but nonetheless it is still influential. It is in no way inert. It exerts a profound, although often unsuspected influence on virtually every aspect of thought and life; out of sight it may be but certainly not out of mind. Freud compared the mind to an iceberg; consciousness is the visible tip, and the unconscious the huge area below the surface.

Freud postulated three aspects of mind; a conscious Ego which deals with reality and directs thought and behaviour into realistic channels; a submerged Id, made up of primitive instinctive forces (unacceptable to the socialised individual); and a Superego, a form of conscience which is concerned with moral attitudes and behaviour; it is partly outside consciousness. These three aspects of mind are in constant interplay, and all behaviour can be seen and understood in terms of these forces. The ego has to adapt constantly to the pressures from the Id, the superego, and external reality.

A number of defence mechanisms are employed by the ego to create acceptable adaptation. The same mechanisms are used by normal, neurotic and psychotic individuals, but clearly a greater distortion of reality accompanies psychotic illness.

Repression underlies all the defence mechanisms. Through repression the ego prevents all unbearable wishes, feelings and impulses from reaching consciousness. A simple example of repression is 'forgetting' an unpleasant appointment, or an embarrassing slip of the tongue. Repression needs to be distinguished from *suppression*, which is a conscious attempt to control undesirable ideas or impulses, and denial. A man dying of terminal carcinoma may deny he is ill and plan his holiday for next year. A wife, suddenly bereaved, will deny her husband is dead.

Reaction formation. An unacceptable attitude is prevented from becoming conscious by the adoption of the opposite attitude. A man with strong homosexual leanings becomes vitriolic and intolerant of homosexuals.

Displacement. This is a common mechanism in everyday life. Feelings are displaced from some person who is desired or feared on to someone or something else less dangerous. The ward sister, criticised by her superior, may displace her aggressive feelings on to one of her nurses and give her a severe dressing down. The nurse in turn perhaps vents her anger on her boy friend.

Transference, the relationship which springs up between doctor and patient and nurse and patient, is based upon displacement, the patient displacing unconscious emotions and attitudes of earlier childhood relationships onto the doctor or nurse. Similar displacement mechanisms are involved in *counter transference*, the unconscious emotional attitude of the doctor and nurse towards their patient. Psychoanalysis, and the more interpretative type of psychotherapy are particularly concerned with the examination of transference feelings and their relationship to child–parent bonds.

Identification or introjection. Through this mechanism a person identifies with, and models himself upon, another person. It is regarded as an important factor in the development of a child's personality, and psychosexual identity. It is made use of in behaviour therapy (modelling). Identification is also a means by which unacceptable impulses are made acceptable. For instance, a man with strong sadistic wishes identifies with the actions and style of a sadistic, powerful person.

Projection. Unacceptable feelings are not only repressed but attributed to, i.e. projected onto, someone else and then seen to come from that person. A woman projects her sexual feelings for another man onto him, and believes that he is constantly trying to seduce her. Although common enough in children, adult projection usually entails considerable distortion of reality.

Substitution. Unacceptable impulses are switched into acceptable activities. Murderous rage is used up in punching a pillow or chopping down a tree.

Sublimation. Unacceptable sexual and aggressive drives are, by this mechanism, directed into socially acceptable channels. Freud considered that civilizations arose through the sublimation of sexual instincts.

The well balanced person is one who has managed (as a result of his early experiences and perhaps inherited constitution) to integrate his unconscious instincts into his personality in such a way that they can emerge in acceptable and useful forms. If they continue to lead a life of their own, it is as though a civil war were being waged within the individual, and his personality ravaged and depleted, allowing neurotic or psychotic behaviour to develop.

6
Consciousness, Hypnosis, Sleep

Consciousness, from the point of view of clinical psychiatry, refers to a person's state of wakefulness, his awareness of the world around him, and the part he plays in it, his ability to think and reason rationally. The less conscious he is, the less can he understand events, judge them properly and make reasonable decisions.

Most adults are considered to be in a normal state of consciousness when awake, and responsible for their actions (so are most children, after the age of 7 or 8. But legally, children under the age of 10 are not considered responsible for their actions). Intelligence itself is not directly related to consciousness, although a low intelligence obviously does influence rationality and judgement.

Consciousness can be impaired by a number of substances; alcohol, large doses of depressant and stimulant drugs, hallucinogenic drugs, disease of, or injury to the brain, epilepsy, toxic states, dementia, and certain psychiatric conditions. Awareness can be heightened – in a limited sense – by excitement and emotional arousal.

We are never fully conscious of everything that happens around us. Certain objects and events receive full attention, others are ignored or only partially noticed. It is this characteristic of conscious perception which causes truthful witnesses to give such varied and sometimes differing accounts of what they simultaneously see; not only are they liable to focus their attention on different aspects of the event, but they are also likely subconsciously and unwittingly to fill in details missing from the whole picture (see Gestalt psychology, p. 17). Consciousness can conveniently be pictured as three concentric circles, as in Fig. 6.1.

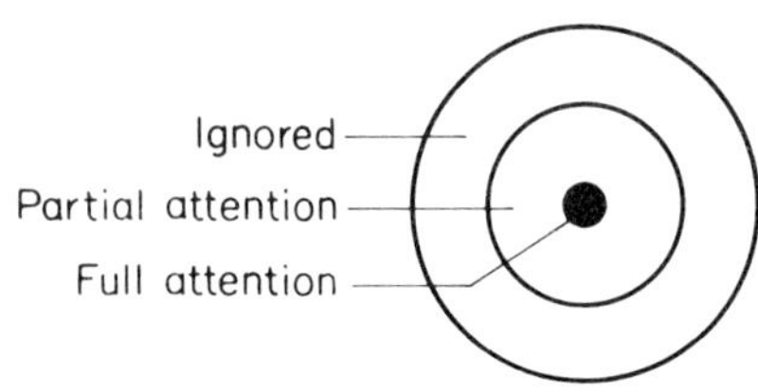

Fig. 6.1 The three levels of consciousness

The term *subconscious* is used here to include all mental activity outside consciousness at any moment. You may be engrossed in a book when suddenly you remember that you must telephone your mother at a certain number. Until that moment the thought and the telephone number were held in the subconscious part of the mind, although readily available.

Many of our mental processes go on subconsciously. You may have a difficult problem to solve or a decision to make. Having thought about it fruitlessly all day you eventually go to bed in despair. Next morning you wake up with the problem solved.

The term *unconscious* is used here to refer to that part of the mind which contains memories inaccessible to consciousness by ordinary means. (The psychoanalytic view of the dynamic unconscious is described on p. 65.) An unpleasant event that occurred in the past may be 'forgotten' (repression). No amount of trying on the part of the person concerned can recall it. But under *hypnosis*, or the influence of certain drugs, forgotten memories and feelings may be brought into consciousness. During deep hypnosis, a subject may be instructed to perform some action after waking. At the same time he is told that he will not remember the instruction. When the time comes he automatically carries out the order, although with no recollection then or later of having been told to so. Unconscious material can, in this way, influence conscious behaviour.

Hypnosis, both individual and mass, has probably been used since before recorded history. Mesmerism and animal magnetism, which are clearly allied to hypnosis in their mode of action and effect, were widely used from the 17th century onwards. During the 19th century, before the introduction of chloroform, hypnosis was used in surgery, although it never became a popular way of inducing anaesthesia. Scientific interest in the subject developed towards the end of the 19th century. Charcot, in Paris, took this further and concluded that the hypnotic state was nothing but a manifestation of hysteria. Freud, after studying hypnosis under Charcot, went back to Vienna and, together with a medical friend, Joseph Breuer, proceeded to abreact by hypnosis a number of women with hysterical symptoms. They improved after revealing forgotten early emotional traumas, usually of a sexual nature and involving their fathers (and incidentally, falling in love with the therapist). Subsequently Freud came to believe that the memories abreacted were largely fantasy and not real events. He and his colleagues came to see the hypnotic state as a particular kind of loving relationship, a child–parent relationship, the patient obeying the therapist as he would have done his parent in his childhood. But Freud gradually abandoned hypnosis in favour of free association and dream interpretation.

In the last 20 years or so hypnosis has aroused increasing interest, both in its application and its nature. The hypnotic state is not related to sleep, although changes in electrical activity do occur in the hypnotised brain. It can alter a person's awareness in the widest sense, but the neurophysiological mechanisms responsible for this remain hidden. There may well be a common link between hypnosis and acupuncture, transcendental meditation and other esoteric techniques. Certainly, in all instances, there is reduced arousal and awareness.

Sleep

Our understanding of sleeping and dreaming has been greatly increased by the application of the electro-encephalogram to human sleep. Sleep is of two kinds: (1) Rapid eye movement (REM), or paradoxical sleep, which takes up to 25 per cent of the night's sleep, and (2) Non-rapid eye movement (NREM), or orthodox sleep, which is subdivided into four stages, the fourth stage producing the slowest waves on the electro-encephalogram.

REM and NREM sleep alternate with each other every 60–90 minutes during normal sleep. REM sleep always follows stage two of NREM. REM sleep is accompanied by eye movements, increased blood flow to the brain, fluctuations of pulse, blood pressure and respiration, and erection of the penis. On waking from REM sleep dreams are clearly remembered and reported. But mental activity occurs at all stages of sleep, and in orthodox sleep has a conscious thoughtlike content. For instance, on waking from orthodox sleep a man will often report that he has been thinking of the day's events.

Patients with coronary insufficiency sometimes develop angina at night. This is most likely to occur during REM sleep, and least during stage four of deep sleep. Duodenal ulcer patients frequently waken with pain after two or three hours sleep. They tend to secrete large amounts of gastric juice at night, and it is now known that maximum secretion occurs during REM sleep. Sleepwalking and night terrors are related to deep sleep, which is why they are not remembered. Nightmares, on the other hand, occur during paradoxical sleep. Depressive illness is associated with reduction of stage four orthodox sleep.

Many drugs upset the normal balance between these two stages of sleep. Barbiturates suppress paradoxical sleep. If they are continued for any length of time tolerance builds up. Stopping the drug results in REM rebound, with insomnia, or restless sleep, and vivid unpleasant nightmares. It is because of this rebound phenomenon that so many people become habituated to their hypnotic. Indeed it seems likely that REM rebound may be related to the addictiveness of any drug; it occurs with amphetamines, alcohol and most hypnotics.

Both kinds of sleep are necessary, and deprivation of either or both can cause perceptual and mood disturbances, and be followed later by rebound. It is now known that the large nocturnal output of growth hormone, which is concerned in the synthesis of ribonucleic acid, is dependent on orthodox sleep. It may well be that orthodox sleep helps to restore body tissues, while paradoxical sleep is linked with synthetic and restorative functions in the brain. (See p. 99 for Sleep Disorders.)

7
The Physical Background to Psychology

So far we have been mainly discussing mental processes and functions. Now we must briefly describe the physical structures upon which these mental processes depend.

Neurones and nerve impulse

Neurones are the structural units of the nervous system (Fig. 7.1). They are made up of a cell body, with protoplasmic outgrowths known as *axons* and *dendrites*. When the cell body is stimulated an electric signal, the *nerve impulse*, is transmitted along the axon. The axon ends at a *synaptic junction*, separated by a short gap from dendrites of neighbouring neurones. The nerve impulse does not

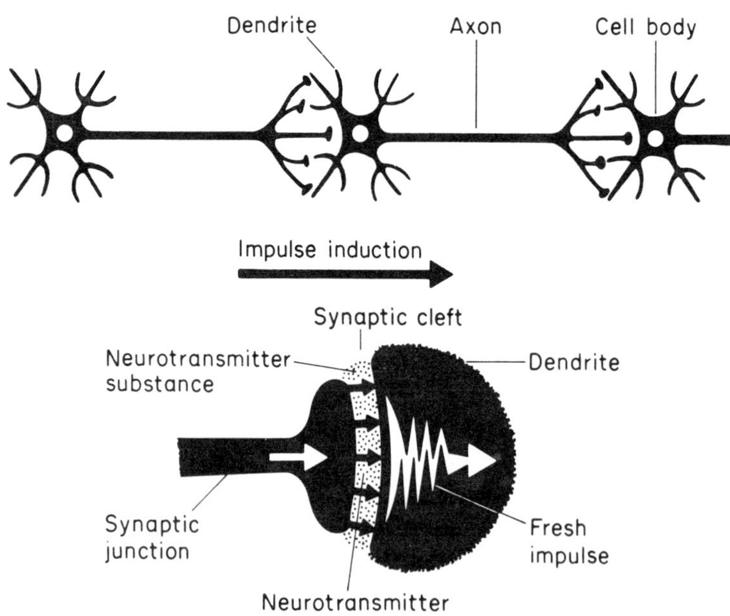

Fig. 7.1 Structure of neurones and transmission of nerve impulses

jump this gap. Its arrival at a synaptic cleft releases a neurotransmitter substance from vesicles in which it is stored at the end of the axon. This diffuses across the synaptic cleft to the neighbouring dendrites. Depending upon its nature, the neurotransmitter may produce excitation, causing a new impulse to be set up in the next neurone, or it will set up a state of inhibition, reducing the excitability of the neurone. The action of the neurotransmitter is shortlived. Most of it is rapidly taken up again into the end of the axon, the rest being destroyed by enzymic activity.

That acetylcholine and noradrenaline are neurotransmitters in the peripheral nervous system has long been known. Our knowledge of neurotransmitters within the brain itself is much less clear. Noradrenaline, serotonin, dopamine, acetylcholine and gamma butyric acid (GABA), have been identified among others. Noradrenaline exists in the hypothalamus and midbrain areas and seems to be concerned with mood and reward signalling systems. Serotonin is scattered through the midbrain and perhaps influences mood, perception and sleep. The action of antidepressant drugs is believed to be related to their ability either to prevent the re-uptake of a neurotransmitter or to prevent its destruction (see p. 355).

Brain

The anatomical pathways and physiological mechanisms of emotion and thought are only just beginning to be understood. Not so long ago the *brain* was believed to be made up of ascending layers with the *cerebral cortex* at the top and in control. It is true that we owe our superior intelligence to the development and differentiation of the cerebral cortex. But we now realise that there are continual interactions between parts of the brain (Fig. 7.2). Not only does the cortex influence subcortical structures, but these in turn affect the cortex.

The cortex can be divided from the point of view of its evolutionary development, into an old *visceral cortex*, and a comparatively new *neocortex*. In lower animals the visceral cortex is related to smell and emotional expression. In man the relationship of the visceral cortex to emotional expression has been retained. The neocortex seems to be mainly concerned with intelligence. It is significant that the visceral cortex and subcortical structures of man have not evolved to anything like the same extent as the neocortex. These probably provide the emotional background against which man functions intellectually.

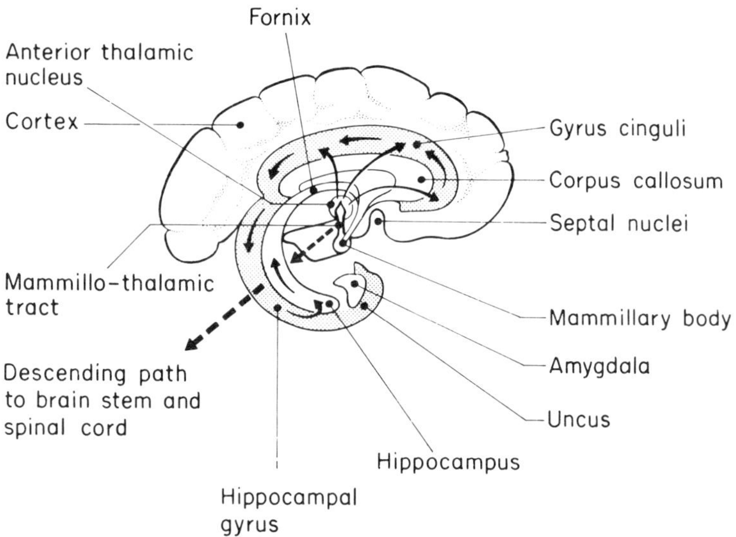

Fig. 7.2 Main connections between the hypothalamus and the cerebral cortex. The limbic lobe is shaded. Solid arrows show the hypothetical circulation of impulses during the experiencing of emotion. The thick dotted arrow indicates the descending path to the brain stem and spinal cord for expressing emotion. Olfactory afferent fibres are lightly dotted. (After Gatz, A. J. 1970 *Manters Essentials of Clinical Neuroanatomy and Neurophysiology*. Philadelphia: F. A. Davis)

Below the cortex are the *hypothalamus* and the *thalamus*.

The most interesting (in terms of current knowledge) subcortical structures are the hypothalamus, ascending reticular activating system and the limbic system. The ascending reticular system stretches from the bulbar region to the medial thalamus. It is concerned with wakefulness, alertness and attention. Wakefulness demands a constant inflow of sensory stimuli, and this is relayed through the reticular system. Damage or destruction to the ascending reticular system causes sleepiness, inattention and general lack of interest.

The *limbic system* is a complex of structures lying around the intraventricular foramina in the cerebral hemispheres, intimately linked to the temporal lobes. It includes the hippocampus, amygdala, cingulate and dentate gyri. The main connections of the system are with the reticular formation and the frontal lobes.

The limbic system is concerned with emotional experience, expression and behaviour. Removal of both temporal lobes in monkeys, including the amygdala and most of the hippocampus, produces what is known as the Kluver – Bucy syndrome: increased and often perverse sexual activity, over-eating, visual agnosia and lack of fear. Bilateral amygdalectomy alone results in hypersexuality and over-eating. It seems that the amygdala exerts an inhibitory controlling influence within the system. In cats, hypersexuality following amygdalectomy can be abolished by destroying the ventral nuclei of the hypothalamus. Similar operations have been carried out on humans with uncontrollable antisocial sexual perversions, with some degree of success (but these are still highly experimental and controversial).

Bilateral removal of the hippocampus upsets memory and learning of the type which requires comparison of one stimulus with another. Suppose, for instance, two stimuli separated by a short gap are presented to an animal. The animal responds in one way when the stimuli are identical, in another when different, and is rewarded (or not punished) when successful. In order to learn this the animal must be able to retain the memory of the first stimulus and compare it to the second. Hippocampus-deprived animals cannot do this. *Korsakov syndrome*, a complication of alcoholism, is associated with damage to the hippocampus.

The hypothalamus, lying in the diencephalon, plays a major role in homeostasis, controlling the body's internal needs, and maintaining a fine balance between input and output. Its influence extends over body temperature, need for food and water and sex, cardiovascular and gastro-intestinal functioning.

The hypothalamus contains large collections of neurones (nuclei) which control and integrate endocrine and autonomic nervous system activities. It exerts a direct influence on posterior pituitary hormones. For instance, antidiuretic hormone is produced in the hypothalamus and travels via nerve trunks to the pituitary to release vasopressin. Anterior pituitary hormones such as growth hormone and gonadotrophins are controlled by hypothalamic substances which travel to the pituitary via the portal blood vessel system. A sensitive feedback system allows a very fine control to be maintained.

There are well-defined 'centres' within the hypothalamus. Thus (in rats) stimulation of part of the medial hypothalamus decreases the amount of food eaten. Destruction of this area results in over-eating. Stimulation of the lateral part produces over-eating. Anorexia follows its destruction. In the normal state a balance seems to exist between these two centres. Hypothalamic disturbances are common in psychiatric disorders. In anorexia nervosa for instance, the onset of amenorrhoea is almost certainly due to the influence of the hypothalamus.

The *autonomic nervous system* controls internal organs, such as the heart, bowels, and secretory glands, which cannot be voluntarily controlled. The system is composed of *sympathetic* and *parasympathetic* divisions. Although these two divisions have opposing actions, they normally co-operate and so produce a delicate regulating system. *Sympathetic activity* dilates the pupil, increases the heart rate, dries the mouth, blanches the skin and brings on a cold sweat, raises blood pressure, inhibits peristalsis and causes muscle sphincters to contract. In addition, the adrenal medulla is stimulated to secrete *adrenaline*. *Adrenaline* not only reinforces sympathetic activity, but releases sugar into the blood from the liver. Erection of the penis depends upon sympathetic activity.

Parasympathetic activity slows the heart, constricts bronchioles, increases the flow of saliva and peristaltic movement, and causes muscle sphincters to relax. Insulin secretion from the pancreas is stimulated, leading to a fall of blood sugar.

The autonomic system prepares the body for fight or flight when danger arises. At such times sympathetic activity predominates. But the autonomic system also serves to maintain homeostasis through its control of respiration, temperature regulation, digestion and excretion, blood distribution and so on. For this purpose the parasympathetic system predominates.

The physical basis of emotion

What happens within the brain when we experience fear or anger?

1. The hypothalamus is alerted from the thalamus and by direct branches from the reticular system. From the hypothalamus there occur *simultaneously:*

(a) An upward discharge of nerve impulses to the old visceral cortex; particularly important is the limbic system. This results in emotional feeling and the need for some kind of action.

(b) A downward discharge through the sympathetic and parasympathetic centres and the pituitary gland. *This results in appropriate bodily changes.*

2. The neocortex is alerted to the danger through its associations with the limbic lobe and the reticular system. *The action required to meet the situation is rapidly decided on and begun.*

In emotional states, such as fear, sympathetic activity predominates. In others, such as grief, parasympathetic activity is more marked. But individual differences are great; sympathetic or parasympathetic activity always predominate in certain people's reactions. One student always has frequency or diarrhoea (parasympathetic effects) before an important exam, another develops sympathetic overactivity with tachycardia, a dry mouth, and restlessness.

The general adaptation syndrome (GAS)

Hans Selye believes that when someone is put under a stress two kinds of reaction occur in the body. The first is a local reaction, which depends on the nature of the stress, such as a burn or a cut. The second is a general reaction of the body, which is always the same no matter what the stress may be. This general reaction he calls the *general adaptation syndrome* (GAS).

He describes three stages in its development. The first stage is the *alarm reaction*, which is comparatively short. The autonomic nervous system becomes active, *adrenaline* is discharged into the blood stream, and *adrenocorticotrophic hormone* (ACTH) is secreted by the pituitary gland. This stimulates the adrenal cortex to produce its hormones.

If it survives this stage the body adapts to the stress, and the *stage of resistance* begins. This may last for years, but if the stress continues for long enough eventually the *stage of exhaustion occurs.* Physiological mechanisms begin to fail and symptoms of illness appear. When homeostasis can no longer be maintained death results.

Selye has called those illnesses showing the symptoms of this last stage *diseases of adaptation.* It is questionable how far this theory can be applied to mental disease. But analogous stages are apparent in fighting men during battle. Efficiency and alertness increase rapidly to a peak, which is maintained for a variable time. Sooner or later exhaustion occurs, alertness diminishes, and men begin to break down.

8
Mental Disorders

Historical

Mental disorders have existed throughout recorded history. The Greeks and Romans treated their own mentally ill members (but not their slaves) with reasonable tolerance and understanding. With the arrival of Christianity attitudes towards the mentally ill began to change. Mental illness came to be equated with the Devil and his works. This came to a head during the Middle Ages, and for three centuries the mentally ill, particularly female, were persecuted and burnt as witches.

During the 18th century a more humane and enlightened attitude towards the mentally ill began to spread through Europe. People were repelled by the way the insane were treated. At the end of the 18th century the Frenchman Pinel freed patients in the Bicêtre from their chains. In England, William Tuke founded The Retreat at York. He forbade the use of chains and manacles and patients were treated with respect and kindness. This 'moral treatment' of the insane created widespread interest and concern. Eventually an investigation into conditions in madhouses was set up in 1815, which revealed a horrifying state of affairs. But already in 1808 a bill to provide for the better treatment of the insane had been introduced: Amending bills eventually led to the creation of the Lunacy Commission.

Mental hospitals now began to be built throughout the country. These were often very large, with 2000 or more beds, situated well away from the large towns from which they drew their patients. The enlightened views of the early reformers gradually gave way to indifference and apathy among the staff. Patients were herded together in locked wards, often heavily sedated, and given little or no opportunity to develop self respect and initiative. They were in a sense social outcasts, segregated from normal people and herded together like animals. By the Lunacy Act of 1890 *only certified* patients could be admitted to a mental hospital, and this remained so until the Act of 1930. This Act allowed mental hospitals to admit patients on a voluntary basis. In 1948 the National Health Service was created and overnight all hospitals, general and mental, were taken over by the State and given equal status and financial help. Morale among the staff of mental hospitals rose and spread to their patients. New forms of management were introduced and efforts made to counteract the deadening effects of institutionalism. Doors were unlocked and the concept of a *therapeutic community* put into practice. Patients were treated as dignified human beings, allowed freedom and independence. All this was enormously helped by the introduction in the early 1950s of the phenothiazine group of tranquillisers and, a few years later, the antidepressants. The 1959 Mental Health Act completed the process of abolishing the statutory distinction between mental and physical illness. From now on any hospital might admit the mentally ill, whether on a compulsory section order or informal basis. The 1959 Act has been replaced by the 1983 Act (see p. 382).

Meanwhile the old mental hospitals were proving to be too large, dilapidated and unwieldy for modern psychiatric needs. Because of improved treatment, the setting up of Day Hospitals, the more enlightened and tolerant attitude of people to mental illness, and the provisions of the 1959 Act authorising local health authorities to provide residential accommodation and care for the mentally disabled – alas, far from satisfactory – the rate of discharge from mental hospitals increased. A survey carried out in 1961 suggested that the need for psychiatric hospital beds would fall steadily. It was decided therefore that part or all of many of the old mental hospitals could be closed, and indeed dates for their closure were decided upon, prematurely it now seems. It is heartless to discharge chronic psychotics into the community when facilities for their care and further treatment are so often limited. The chronic mentally sick are likely to be a problem for the foreseeable future.

The Department of Health and Social Security sees the needs of specific populations being served by District General Hospitals, within which are Departments for the mentally ill. Such Departments will include day-patient and out-patient services, and facilities for psycho-geriatric assessment. It is hoped that ultimately they will be able to replace totally the large mental hospitals, provided they are backed up by adequate community services, which must include hostels, therapeutic social clubs, industrial therapy, and adequate staff, with nurses and social workers for home visits. The key to the successful development of such a comprehensive service lies in the concept of the 'therapeutic team', and adequate accommodation and community resources. A team consists of a consultant psychiatrist and a staff of nurses, occupational therapists and social workers, responsible for a population of about 60 000. The aim is to provide a flexible service, and whenever possible to treat the patient in the community. A good relationship between members of the team, family doctors, district nurses, health visitors, and local authority social workers is essential. The concept is an exciting one which will call for new skills and initiative from nurses, particularly the community psychiatric nurse. Indeed, psychiatric care is going to depend increasingly on nurses, and they will have to accept responsibilities unthinkable a few decades ago.

Traditionally, psychiatry is intimately linked to medicine; mental disorders are studied, investigated, treated and classified along the same lines as other medical diseases. This application of the medical model to psychiatric disorders has been challenged by 'anti-psychiatrists' like Laing and Szaz. They maintain that the idea of mental illness is a misnomer; rather a patient is labelled 'deviant' because his family or society disapproves of some aspect of his behaviour. Once labelled, a vicious circle arises; he is expected by society to behave abnormally; and he learns sooner or later to behave as expected. Schizophrenia is seen by Laing as a reaction to intolerable emotional pressures within the deviant's family, which he cannot face; schizophrenia is his way of protecting himself from such pressures. While this concept may sometimes be usefully applied in neurotic and psychopathic disorders, it is highly misleading to do so in psychotic illness. Nonetheless, it has led to greater awareness of the interactions that go on between a patient and his relatives, and the fact that he is often forced into the role of scapegoat. It is certainly erroneous to suppose that traditional psychiatrists do not take social pressures into consideration when searching to understand the reasons for psychiatric illness. No one breaks down in a vacuum; mental disorders always arise from the interaction of a patient's constitution and personality with his environment.

Crisis Intervention

Crisis intervention is now a fashionable concept. A psychiatric team, or an individual from the team, intervenes in a human situation where anxiety is high and a crisis is imminent. The arrival of the team rapidly lowers the tension and leads to a plan of management being agreed upon by all involved. Crisis intervention has the additional advantage, compared to seeing the patient for the first time in an out-patient department, of showing the team what the patient's home background is really like.

Alice lives with her husband and two teenage sons. Three years ago she was admitted to a psychiatric unit for a week, after an overdose of 60 paracetamol tablets. This time she had rung her general practitioner saying that she was 'fed up' and was going to kill herself if nothing was done to help her. A community psychiatric nurse arrived at the home within an hour to find Alice screaming at her husband over his alleged infidelities, the frightened younger son bleeding from his nose, and a good deal of broken crockery in an otherwise well kept flat. The situation gradually calmed down as the nurse listened to both sides of the problem. A plan of treatment was agreed upon. Alice was asked to come to the out-patient department next day. Arrangements were made for husband and wife to be seen together for 'marital counselling'.

Mental illness

Mental illness can be considered from a subjective or objective point of view. The patient himself can say that he is ill, that he suffers from intolerable anxiety and fears which seriously interfere with his life. Another patient may believe himself to be sane and rational yet his friends consider him to be mad. For instance, a man was sure that he was being watched, followed, talked about in newspapers, television and radio. The man was a manual worker, holding no special position of importance in the community. Had he been a leading political or business figure, or a member of the Royal family, his beliefs might have been accepted by many people as perhaps reasonable. As it was, because his ideas were so bizarre, given his background, he was considered to need psychiatric treatment.

It is impossible to evaluate a patient fully without understanding his social and cultural background. But extreme forms of mental illness, schizophrenia and psychotic depression, severe mental impairment and dementia, are recognisable in any culture, even though we may not understand how or why they develop, and what social stresses are responsible. Schizophrenic illnesses occur throughout the world, as much in backward as in developed countries. Information collected by the International Pilot Study of Schizophrenia suggests that the main symptoms of schizophrenia are recognisable whatever a patient's race and nationality.

In a developing country such as, say, Nigeria, where psychiatric facilities are limited, particularly in rural areas, only severely ill patients whose behaviour can no longer be tolerated by the community, are admitted to mental hospitals and treated. In the UK nearly all new cases of schizophrenia are admitted initially to a psychiatric hospital or unit.

Psychiatry is concerned with the study and treatment of mental illness and disordered mental processes; these in turn may produce physical disorders. Increasingly, as social conditions and the overall physical health of the population have improved, so paradoxically has the demand for medical treatment risen. Symptoms which 50 years ago would have been accepted stoically, helped by support from an 'extended' family, are now brought to the doctor to investigate and treat. The number of prescriptions for psychotropic drugs rises steadily, as does the amount of sickness and absence from work from psychoneurosis.

Medicine, of which psychiatry is a part, has reached a crossroad. No longer is it possible to ignore a patient's social problems and psychiatric state. Epidemiological studies suggest that at least 20 per cent of patients present with 'conspicuous psychiatric morbidity', although this is not infrequently overlooked by doctors. This is largely because the patient expresses his symptoms in strictly physical terms, physical illness still having greater social acceptance and respectability. In addition, many psychosomatic conditions such as asthma, dermatitis, colitis, are strongly influenced by emotional states.

It is essential to understand that psychiatric patients are ill, not simply 'lacking in moral fibre', and that they need and can benefit from treatment. Some people find this difficult to accept and are resentful, hostile and frightened when they first come into contact with psychiatric disorders.

Psychiatric disorders are widespread. Mentally ill patients occupy nearly half the National Health Service hospital beds in the country. It is estimated that about one woman in 15 and one man in 20 are likely to need psychiatric treatment in hospital at some time in their lives, and that one family out of every five will contain someone with psychiatric illness.

Causes of mental illness

Mental illness is the result of the interplay of a number of factors, some of which are intrinsic to the patient – part of his constitutional make up – while others are external. There is never a single cause. To understand why a patient has broken down and how, it is necessary to look not only at the stresses in his life, but his personality, his cultural and family background and, so far as this is possible, his genetic constitution.

It is important to recognise that external stress is not necessarily bad and to be avoided. We require continual stimulation from our environment to function efficiently. Freud saw the ideal state of mind as a lack of tension, but this is only possible with death. It is impossible to have life without stress, which is only another way of saying that everyone has to adapt continually. Without stress there would be no stimulation and probably no development. Young children go out of their way to seek stimulation. Watch how a small child continually explores and experiments with his environment. This is essential for the growth of his mental abilities; children who are overmothered and protected from stress are less able to fend for themselves in later life.

But on the other hand stress can be overwhelming and destructive. In a young child severe stress can retard one or more aspects of his mental development. What and when it is overwhelming depends partly on constitutional factors and on previous experiences. There are probably critical ages for the development of different functions, and whether or not a stressful situation has adverse effects may depend on the age of the child at the time. For instance, there is evidence that the stress caused by separating a child of under five from his mother for more than three months may, in some cases, upset his emotional development and warp his personality.

It may be helpful to think of stress in terms of physics. Stress there refers to any force exerting pressure on an object. The internal reaction of the body to the stress is known as *strain*. The nature and extent of the strain depends on the material of the body and on the way in which it is constructed. Thus different bodies show strain in different degrees and in different ways. Stress is tolerated up to a certain level. Beyond that level there is a danger that the stress will prove too much for the body to withstand. Consider, for example, a boiler which can only function efficiently above a certain pressure of steam. But if the safety valve sticks and the pressure goes on increasing inside, sooner or later the boiler explodes.

People vary enormously in their reaction to stress; one man breaks down when his wife leaves him, and needs psychiatric treatment; while another one is comparatively unaffected and reacts to his loss by working harder. Each of us have our own way of dealing with stressful situations, our own type of mental defence mechanism which develops during early life.

Certain events are shocking for most people, for example a bad road accident or rail crash. Others affect one person much more than another. The sudden death of an old mother understandably causes grief in all her children; but the unmarried daughter who lived with her may become increasingly depressed, attempt suicide and require psychiatric treatment. An examination failure may have little effect on one nurse, whereas in another it may precipitate a breakdown because her self-esteem depends on her doing well and gaining acclaim. The death of a cat is not likely to be a serious tragedy in a happy family, but a lonely old lady may collapse when her cat dies.

Stress can also occur on a physical level. Starvation, thirst, injury, physical illness, and extremes of heat and cold may directly damage the body, or bring about changes which interfere with its efficient functioning. If the stress is too great the homeostatic mechanisms break down altogether and death may follow.

Overwhelming stress disrupts the normal activity of the central nervous system; maladaptive and inappropriate behaviour results. The man who was previously decisive and calm breaks down and becomes indecisive, emotional and fearful. The soldier under attack who cracks and panics runs straight towards the enemy tanks instead of taking cover. The wife who has just seen her husband killed laughs and jokes as though nothing has happened. The girl who is assaulted and raped tries to shout but loses her voice. Removal from the stressful situation, rest and sedation, in many instances quickly restore normal behaviour. But in some people the abnormal reactions persist and require prolonged psychiatric treatment.

The possible relationship between stressful life changes and life events and the development of physical and mental disease has aroused much interest in recent years. Studies have shown that bereavement is followed by increased mortality and both psychiatric and somatic morbidity (see p. 63). The onset of acute schizophrenia may be immediately preceded by considerable emotional stress. Bereavement, or an important loss, is a frequent event in the year or so before depressive illness develops. During a war or revolution, psychiatric morbidity among the combatants is directly related to the physical casualty rate and presumably therefore, the dangers encountered.

Sometimes it seems that psychiatric disorders follow immediately from the stressful event, for instance after childbirth or hysterectomy. In other instances psychiatric disorder emerges into the open only after months or even years have passed. We still do not know how stress brings about mental and physical disease, although Selye's general adaptation syndrome may provide a partial explanation. Nor do we know whether the stress acts merely as a non-specific precipitant to the illness, or has a more specific effect by linking up with and bringing forward earlier conflicts and disturbances.

The more common stresses today stem from loss and disappointment.

1. *Loss of family or social cohesion.* Bereavement has already been discussed. Loss of a parent, particularly a mother, in early childhood, predisposes to depression in later life. Bereavement in middle age is liable to be followed by depressive illness and increased risk of coronary thrombosis. Divorce and separation, the break up of a family, or loss of a job, or retirement from work, may all be followed by severe depression and even suicide. Until their mid-fifties, single women are more prone to commit suicide than married women or men, presumably because of feeling isolated and having less opportunity for closeness and emotional outlet.

A marriage which to an outsider may appear to be an unhappy one is not necessarily stressful. An aggressive husband with a 'masochistic' wife who seeks punishment compulsively, may have frequent quarrels but these may well be necessary to keep the marriage together. On the other hand, frequent and violent quarrelling is known to be very stressful to the children. With the passage of time the original psychological needs of one partner for the other are liable to change. The arrival of a child often alters the quality of relationship between husband and wife. One or other of the partners may become involved in an extra-marital affair.

Suppressed resentments over a long period can bring about intolerable tensions and depression. A woman trapped in an unwanted marriage by a child whose birth is resented, an unmarried daughter supporting and living with a cantankerous old mother, may both eventually break down and require psychiatric treatment.

Bad housing and overcrowding have adverse effects on physical and mental health. But moving to a new and more satisfactory home is not necessarily advantageous. Strange surroundings, unfriendly neighbours, create an increasing sense of isolation which can be extremely stressful. The concept of 'suburban neurosis' among people, especially women, who move from the central city area to a peripheral housing estate, was described in 1938. This was then attributed to the loss of familiar surroundings, social isolation, distance from employment and high expenses. Although the relationship between the social conditions of new housing estates and neurotic disorders has recently been questioned, such a situation is undoubtedly stressful to some people.

For a long time it has been recognised that immigrants other than political refugees have a considerably higher than average risk of developing psychiatric disorders. Immigrants to this country, particularly when coloured, have to contend with considerable stresses, although these are often cushioned by the presence of their families and friends. Bad housing is an additional stress for the immigrant, but many will not seek help for psychiatric symptoms until severely ill.

2. *Stress related to finances and work.* A man may run into financial difficulties because of circumstances beyond his control, or because he is unable to adapt his way of life to reality. He may spend far in excess of his income in order to keep up appearances and bolster his weak ego; run a large house, drive a Rolls Royce, maintain his children at expensive schools, because without such trappings he feels destitute. Sooner or later of course, he is likely to become so. The resulting stress for such a man is considerable, and he is likely to break down.

Most people are upset if they lose their job or their business collapses, the more so when they have worked hard and loyally, and feel they have been treated unfairly and inconsiderately. Not only may financial stresses follow, but self-esteem suffers especially if the family has to move to a less prestigious house or sell treasured possessions.

Work itself is sometimes damagingly stressful. A man who is conscientious and hardworking, but limited, may reach a position of responsibility – particularly in a large organisation – beyond his capability. Sooner or later the strain makes itself felt and eventually he collapses.

Another type of patient has great drive and ability. At first fantasy and reality interwine. Success follows success and suddenly he finds himself in charge of a large organisation and there seems no reason why he should not continue to expand. But he is unable to delegate responsibility, cannot trust anyone else to do a job properly. Bogged down by detail, he becomes increasingly exhausted. Anxiety mounts and suddenly explodes into panic attacks.

A *life event* scale has been devised, based on the severity of the event; that is, how much the individual's social adjustment and equilibrium was threatened and how long it lasted. For instance, the death of a spouse rated 100, birth of a child 39, loss of a job 47. The scale is of course used in research, where numbers of people are being looked at, and should not be taken too seriously in individual cases. For interest see figures illustrating the rate of life

Event	*Scale*
Death of spouse	100
Divorce	73
Jail sentence	63
Death of close family member	63
Personal injury or illness	53
Marriage	50
Loss of job	47
Reconciliation	45
Retirement	45
Birth of child	39
Death of close friend	37
Beginning or finishing school	26
Change of habit	24
Moving house	20
Vacation	13
Minor violations of the law	11

Fig. 8.1 Life event scale

events in 16 three week periods before the onset of depression in 114 women, compared to 382 'normal' women (from Brown and Cooper, in *Handbook of Psychiatry*, Ch. 4, 1983, ed. G Russell L Hersov. Cambridge: CUP).

Psychiatric Classification

A really adequate classification of diseases requires a reasonable understanding of its causes. Pneumonia a century ago was a syndrome, a group of symptoms indicating disease of the lung. Today the pneumonias are clearly classified on an aetiological basis. Psychiatry, unfortunately, is still in the syndrome stage. Our understanding of the aetiology of psychiatric disorders is rudimentary, although growing. The classification of psychiatric disorders is bound therefore to be unsatisfactory. Yet a classification is necessary for psychiatrists to be able to predict the outcome of any illness, and to research and communicate with one another. The International Classification of Disease (ICD), now in its 9th revision, is used by most countries today, thanks to the efforts of the World Health Organisation.

A syndrome is made up of a number of symptoms which, when grouped together, form a recognisable pattern and often follow a characteristic course. Not all symptoms necessarily have to be present for a diagnosis to be made. It is important to understand that a disorder such as schizophrenia is a syndrome and not an aetiological entity. Schizophrenia was first identified as a syndrome by Emil Kraepelin (1856–1926) under the name 'dementia praecox'. Just over a decade later, Eugene Bleuler (1857–1939) suggested the term schizophrenia. Unlike Kraepelin he believed that the disease might remit and did not invariably cause serious deterioration of the personality. Today, in an attempt to narrow the syndrome of schizophrenia and to gain greater diagnostic agreement among psychiatrists, Kurt Schneider's concept of 'first rank' symptoms is often used. But only when a neurochemical basis for schizophrenia is discovered is their classification likely to become satisfactory.

Neurosis and psychosis

It is still customary to use these terms, although it is sometimes difficult to make a clear distinction. A patient with a neurosis recognises that he is ill, although he may not connect his symptoms with an obvious emotional conflict. Only *part* of his personality is involved and he remains in contact with reality, able to recognise the subjective quality of his symptoms and to distinguish between 'me' and 'not me'. The psychotic patient on the other hand has his entire personality distorted by his illness. He accepts his symptoms as real, and out of them he reconstructs his environment, recreates a world which only he can recognise; he is followed by strangers, rays are directed at him, women are secretly having intercourse with him, unknown voices criticise him, and so on. No amount of talk will persuade him to change his mind.

While most neurotics can continue to adapt socially, the psychotic cannot and ultimately is no longer capable of continuing his work or even of living with his family. Indeed, his sense of self-preservation is seriously disturbed. An acute schizophrenic or severely depressed patient can be seen to be psychotic and in need of treatment. But such a patient in the early stages of his illness may occasionally retain insight to some degree, recognise that he is ill and seek treatment himself. On the other side of the coin, a neurotic patient sometimes appears to be incapable of distinguishing between his fantasy world and what is real, and is as incapable of adapting to society as a psychotic patient.

The neuroses are usually separated from *personality disorders*. Again the distinction is in many ways an artificial one since the neuroses often overlap or co-exist with a disordered personality. A neurotic patient suffers from his symptoms, while the patient with a personality disorder is more likely to make other people suffer. The term *vulnerable* personality implies that a patient overreacts or breaks down under quite mild stress. The expression '*borderline state*' is used increasingly today, in place of the older *pseudoneurotic* or *latent* state, to describe patients who do not fit easily into either schizophrenia or neurotic or personality disorders.

Organic and functional psychoses

Anything which interferes with the normal functioning of the brain is likely to cause changes in behaviour. Acute confusional states (delirium) and chronic organic states (dementia) have many causes. The term *functional* psychoses refers to manic depression and schizophrenia, the causes of which are still unknown.

The psychiatric examination

The psychiatric examination aims at collecting as much information as possible about the patient, in order that the various factors contributing to his breakdown can be evaluated.

It is important to put the patient at his ease, and gain his confidence and co-operation. It is best to let him tell his own story at first, without unnecessary interruption. Good interviewing is probably an art, but something of it can certainly be learnt. The good interviewer must know what information he seeks to draw from his patient. He must not be over-anxious himself, and above all he must have the capacity to listen and observe, for good interviewing involves both verbal and non-verbal communication. The way a patient behaves during his history, when and where he pauses or avoids certain topics, when he blushes or shows strong emotions, are important clues to the patient's problems. The first psychiatric interview is not only of diagnostic value but is often highly therapeutic, particularly if the patient feels himself accepted and understood by the interviewer.

Whenever possible, the patient's account should be verified from a close relative or friend. This is sometimes done by a psychiatric social worker (PSW) or community nurse, who may visit the patient's home, or may already have done so as a member of a crisis intervention team.

Family history

It is important to find out whether any blood relative, on either side of the family has had any form of breakdown, killed himself, drunk excessively, been in prison or in a mental institution. Patients are sometimes reluctant to reveal family skeletons. Thumb-nail sketches of parents and the childhood home atmosphere should be obtained.

A *predisposition* to functional psychoses such as manic depression and schizophrenia is inherited. The risk of the child of one schizophrenic parent developing schizophrenia is around 10 per cent compared to just under 1 per cent in the general population. If both parents have had schizophrenia, the chances rise to 40 per cent. It is important to remember that it is *predisposition* to the disease which is inherited. Certain environmental stresses must also play some part before signs and symptoms of disease appear. Even when one of a pair of identical twins develops schizophrenia, the other escapes in at least 20 per cent or more of cases. As they have similar genes the differences must be in their environments. The incidence of depressive illness for first degree relatives depends on whether it is of the unipolar or bipolar (manic depressive) form; unipolar illness carries a risk of between 11 – 16 per cent, bipolar of up to 25 per cent. When one parent has schizophrenia, and the other manic depression, both conditions appear with equal frequency among the offspring.

There is less evidence about the way *neurotic illnesses* are inherited, although they are certainly more common in some families than in others. The relative roles of nature and nurture in psychiatric illness are still disputed. There is no convincing evidence for assortive matings in married neurotics. The husbands of agoraphobic housewives, for instance, seem to be stable men, unaffected by their wives' behaviour. On the other hand, when a husband develops a neurotic illness, his wife is more vulnerable and liable herself to develop symptoms. Clearly, if the behaviour of both parents is maladaptive, this is liable to be transmitted to their children through learning processes. A parent with a personality disorder is particularly likely to upset his children. Broken homes, continual parental quarrels, desertion or absence of a parent are common findings in the history of neurotic patients, and need always to be explored. The death of a parent during early childhood may predispose a patient to depressive illness in later life.

The birth order of a patient may have significance, particularly in the formation of his personality. Each child has a special individual role in the family. Often, without suspecting, parents treat each child slightly differently. First and last born, and only children, tend to have particularly close relationships with their mothers. The larger the family the less attention each child receives. This is more than compensated for by the sense of security which exists in large families. Neurotic reactions are less common in their members. There is no evidence that birth position influences the development of psychotic illness. Adopted and one parent children are liable to encounter particular difficulties (see p. 43).

The patient's past history

Birth weight and delivery, infancy

Prematurity, a history of fetal distress, birth injury or jaundice may be factors in mental impairment (see p. 288).

Information about breast-feeding usually has to be obtained from the patient's mother. Whether he has been fed with breast or artificial milk is probably of no importance in itself. But breast-fed babies tend to be handled more than bottle fed babies and tactile stimulation seems to influence the emotional development of infants. The mother's own emotional state and attitude during the patient's infancy may be glimpsed by her account of the child's feeding habits. A mother who satisfactorily breast-fed for six months or more is unlikely to have been rejecting or over-anxious.

Feeding difficulties, severe constipation or constant bouts of sickness in the child's early years, suggest that his mother was anxious and uncertain of herself. Sometimes everything seems to have gone well for the first three or four years. Then the mother again becomes pregnant, or she or the child has to spend some weeks in hospital, away from home. After this the child's behaviour becomes difficult.

Many so called '*neurotic traits*', such as nail-biting, tics, food fads, tantrums and sleep-walking, are so common in children as to mean nothing except in relation to total behaviour. Bed-wetting, in boys especially, may go on until seven or eight or even later. There is however a strong relationship between persistent antisocial behaviour in childhood and later delinquency and criminal conduct.

Progress at school

This is a rough guide to the patient's level of intelligence. Arithmetic is particularly difficult for anyone of below average intelligence. A few children have great difficulty in learning to read and spell, a condition known as *dyslexia*. In some of them emotional factors may be responsible for the backwardness. But often physical and psychological facts are both responsible, a vicious circle readily arises, and emotional disturbances eventually come to assume major importance. It is useful to enquire about events at home at the time the work of a child, who was previously doing well at school, falls off markedly.

Serious reading retardation is present in about four per cent of seven year old children in the UK, excluding those with severe mental impairment. There is a strong link between backwardness in reading and delinquency. Childhood ambitions are sometimes revealing. Children who lack self-confidence may set themselves unrealistically high targets; others aim too low in order not to have to admit failure.

Occupation

A person's work record often indicates his stability and perseverance. After leaving school young people may change jobs frequently before finding what they want. But the person who goes on changing his job, never staying anywhere for longer than a year or so, usually has little ability to withstand every day tensions and frustrations, and has a poor grasp of his own identity and needs. The significance of this may be altered to some extent by the unemployment situation today, but the basic principle remains.

Puberty calls for changes in attachments and childhood values (see p. 50). How a patient deals with his conflicts at this time influences the development of his personality and his ability to cope with future stresses. He may still be tied by strong emotional bonds to his parents, unable to stand freely on his own feet, to make decisions and develop attachments uninfluenced by neurotic guilt. How he now sees his parents, the way in which he discusses them, particularly vis-a-vis himself and his siblings, is revealing in this respect. Sexual attitudes and behaviour need to be explored in some depth, but with sensitivity and tact at the beginning; signs of embarrassment, indicating areas of conflict and guilt, should be noted, but only explored later and if relevant to the patient's current problems. Much harm can be done by unnecessary, perhaps prurient, questioning.

The characteristics of his sexual partners often indicate his fantasies and some of the reasons for difficulties in relationships. Love and sexual needs may be at variance, due to persisting childhood conflicts, and sometimes cause sexual difficulties later. It is not uncommon for a man to be potent with his mistress and lose his libido and potency with her from the day he marries her – or for a woman to become frigid – because of such underlying problems.

Expectations from marriage may be unrealistic and childlike, the spouse being pushed into the role of parent—which he or she then accepts, because of their own personality. Attitudes to pregnancy, childbirth and children at their different stages of development are fruitful areas of exploration, for the acceptance of a new role of mother or father, inevitably brings to the surface identification conflicts; strongly hostile or ambivalent feelings for a parent which were ignored or suppressed before, may now create anxiety and depression, unrealistic attitudes to the child, and demands on the husband.

The menopause can bring out depression and abnormal behaviour in dissatisfied women, who have perhaps hidden their conflicts behind their families; by being 'good mothers' they have preserved their self-esteem. But when their children reach adolescence and proceed to act out the very conflicts these women did not resolve during their own adolescence, psychiatric symptoms emerge. Inevitably psychological problems of adolescent children of such women are increased; it is a useful axiom that the psychiatric difficulties of adolescents reflect their parents unresolved conflicts.

A study of *past health* should include not only major illnesses, but minor symptoms which have led to time off school and work. In childhood, long periods of absence from school for minor illness may reflect an overprotective, anxious mother. In adult life, frequent absenteesim is often a sign of emotional disturbance. If there have been previous psychiatric breakdowns, knowledge of their duration, and response to treatment may suggest how long the present symptoms are likely to last.

Personality before the onset of symptoms must be carefully assessed. A patient's account of himself when ill may be misleading. A depressed man may describe himself as a monster of depravity; an inadequate psychopath may paint a grandiose picture of himself. Neither account will tally with what each has done with his life, or what friends and relatives say about him.

Questions of the following sort are helpful in the assessment of the patient's personality:

Cyclothymia

Do you swing easily and for minor reasons from happiness to the depths of despair and vice versa?

Anxiety

Do you always tend to anticipate and fear the worse? Do you worry for days or weeks beforehand over an important test or encounter? Does failure loom large?

Schizoid

Do you usually prefer your own company to that of others?

Do you feel that you do not need friends?

Obsessive

Do you have to check and recheck to an unnecessary degree your work, that you have locked doors, switched off taps and put out lights?

Are you more irritated than your colleague by an unexpected change of routine at work?

Paranoid

Are people jealous of your talents?

Do you feel that people are always trying to do you down?

Are you treated unjustly at work?

Hysterical

Do you feel that everyone eventually fails you, and that no one comes up to your standards?

Do you need to be the centre of attention at any gathering, and if not, fail to enjoy yourself?

Hypochondriacal

Do you worry continuously about bodily health in spite of medical reassurance? Do you take pains to keep fit; jog regularly and eat health foods?

History of the present illness

Ask the patient when he last felt really well. This may give you the approximate time of onset of the present illness. Then enquire about possible precipitating factors and life changes over the past two years.

Not all patients are co-operative. Some may insist that there is nothing wrong with them, that they have been made to attend under false pretences. Some will say that it is their spouse who is ill. On occasions husband and wife may accuse one another, and it then becomes apparent that both are mentally ill. Some degree of *folie à deux* is not at all uncommon; the dominant partner is usually the sick one, the other following.

A history cannot be obtained from a patient whose consciousness is seriously disturbed, or who is stuporous or grossly overactive and distractible. All that can then be done, and it is important that this is extremely thorough, is to record appearance, behaviour, and talk.

Physical examination should be done as soon as possible. Cerebral neoplasms, endocrine disorders, renal and liver failure, disseminated sclerosis, and such like may present with psychiatric symptoms. The patient's behaviour during the examination may be revealing.

It is worth recording *the body build*. There is a rough correlation between a patient's build and the form of mental illness he develops. *Manic depressive* illness tends to occur in *pyknic* or *endormorphic* people, *schizophrenia* in those of *asthenic* or *ectomorphic* build. If schizophrenia develops in someone of pyknic build the chances of recovery are increased. Conversely, depression in an asthenic individual sometimes has a schizophrenic colouring.

Examination of the mental state

Appearance and behaviour

Facial expression, neatness of dress, speed of movement and tone of speech, and attitude towards other people are quickly noticed. A hypomanic patient is over-active, over-talkative, constantly interrupting, impatient, sometimes threatening and aggressive, and often amusing. Obsessional patients try to control the interview and may clearly reveal their conflicts between obedience and defiance; they repeat the examiner's questions, perhaps treat the most banal remark as a pearl of wisdom, ask him to define his questions more clearly, glance at their watches, produce long written lists of symptoms and questions; characteristically they arouse both boredom and irritation in the interviewer. The patient with a hysterical type of personality is at the opposite pole to the obsessive; difficult and child-like in behaviour as the hysteric may at times be, he is never dull. A depressed patient may be dressed carelessly, his movements and speech slow and his face fixed in a mask-like expression of misery. This slowness is known as *retardation*. A dementing patient may or may not be untidy, depending on the care of others; he is often slow, inattentive or puzzled. If pressed he may collapse like a child, in what is known as a 'catastrophic reaction'. A schizophrenic may smile fatuously and make strange gestures and grimacings; or advance cautiously into the room, looking suspiciously about him before sitting down; he may be negativistic, refusing to respond or speak to the interviewer, appearing to be in a world of his own, perhaps listening to voices.

Disorders of mood and emotion

(*Affect* is often used in place of mood.) Some anxiety is shown by most patients at the first interview, particularly neurotic patients. Tense muscles, constantly fidgeting hands, and clammy skin are easily recognised. Total absence of anxiety is one of the hallmarks of hysteria; some schizophrenics also show noticeable lack of concern; and a severely depressed patient is too wrapped up in his own worries to feel anxious.

Agitation occurs when anxiety overflows into motor activity. The patient cannot keep still. He continually paces the floor, wringing his hands and muttering aloud to himself. Agitation is particularly likely to occur in states of *depression*.

Depression is usually obvious from the patient's air of gloom and despondence, although 'smiling depression' is seen from time to time. There is a marked contrast between depression and the infectious gaiety and over-activity of *mania*. Suicidal ideas should always be asked about openly.

Flattening of affect occurs in schizophrenia, resulting in apathy and lack of emotional response. *Rapport*, that indefinable feeling of being 'on the same wavelength', is absent. Talking to a schizophrenic is sometimes likened to having a pane of glass inserted between you and the patient.

Splitting of affect is also characteristic of schizophrenia and describes the divergence between mood and thought. This causes *incongruity of affect*. For instance, a patient giggled most of the time as he described how his beloved mother had died of cancer. Ecstatic states are sometimes experienced by schizophrenics, and the patient feels a sense of exaltation, of mystical possession and rapture. It differs from the elation of hypomania in that it is not associated with over-activity and flight of ideas, and rapport is absent.

Depersonalisation and *derealisation* describe feelings that everything has altered and become shadowy and unfamiliar, as though seen in a dream. *Depersonalisation* affects the individual. He himself has changed and this is why the world looks different. He has become a robot, an observer of himself and his thoughts rather than concerned in them. He has no role, just 'nothingness'. In *derealisation* the world itself changes, not the observer. A depersonalised patient said, 'This is not my body,' although she knew rationally that it was. Her everyday feelings of familiarity had been lost. These conditions can occur in various disorders, but are particularly common in depression, phobic anxiety and obsessional illness. They may also be experienced by normal people, when tired.

Déjà vu is an inexplicable feeling of familiarity, of having 'been here before', of knowing what is about to happen. It is a common phenomenon and should not be regarded as abnormal unless associated with other pathological features.

Disorders of perception

What we perceive is influenced by our interests, needs and emotions. A man in the desert who is parched with thirst sees water in place of the sun's reflection off the sand. A shipwrecked sailor mistakes the crest of a wave for land. Misinterpretation is known as an *illusion*. *Illusions* are conspicuous during states of confusion and fear. A *delirious* patient mistakes fluff on her bed for insects. A frightened man sees the post at the foot of his bed as a menacing shape looming out of the darkness.

Hallucinations differ from illusions in that no external stimuli are necessary. Mental images arise spontaneously within the brain and are projected to the outside world as though real.

Hallucinations need to be distinguished from dreams. Hypnogogic and hypnopompic hallucinations are experienced by many people as they are about to fall asleep or when waking up. The commonest hallucinations are auditory, usually hearing your name called; then come visual hallucinations. They are of no significance on their own. In schizophrenia the characteristic hallucinations are auditory, repeating a patient's thoughts, or criticising and abusing him. Visual hallucinations are more typical of acute organic and confusional states. Visual hallucinations occur in schizophrenia but are not of primary diagnostic value in that condition. They occur in hysteria and epilepsy, particularly involving the temporal lobe. Lilliputian hallucinations, the patient seeing tiny people (*micropsia*), occur in temporal lobe epilepsy. Tactile hallucinations are experienced in confusional states and sometimes by drug addicts. A cocaine addict may feel animals crawling under his skin (*formication*). Schizophrenics sometimes report hallucinations of touch, and some middle-aged female depressives complain of bizarre sensations around their genitalia. Hallucinations of smell occur in organic conditions, particularly temporal lobe epilepsy, schizophrenia and psychotic depression. So also with hallucinations of taste.

Disorders of thinking

Thought processes, as well as bodily movements, become slow in depression. This is known as *retardation*. Retardation may be so pronounced as to amount to *stupor*. All activity is reduced to a minimum, but consciousness is not affected. Remarks made near a stuporous patient are remembered by him and may later prove embarrassing. Stupor also occurs in catatonic and atypical schizophrenia.

Thought processes become accelerated during *mania*. One idea rapidly suggests another, and the stream of continuous talk changes frequently (*flight of ideas*). But there is always some connection between the changes, unlike the sometimes rapid but disconnected talk of the schizophrenic. Manic patients are *distractible* and rarely stick to one idea for long. Sometimes the flow of thoughts is so great that speech becomes incoherent. *Pressure of thought* amounting to incoherence can also occur in schizophrenia. The schizophrenic may be unable to maintain his train of thoughts because of *thought blocking*. Mental processes are split and fragmented, with the result that thoughts suddenly stop and the schizophrenic's mind goes blank. Association of one idea with another may be impossible for the observer to follow, resulting in the (chess) knight's move type of thinking. A characteristic of most schizophrenics is over-inclusion of thought and talking past the point. This produces a curious 'woolliness' and vagueness of talk, so that although the patient appears at any one time to talk sense, at the end of the interview the therapist may be left feeling curiously mystified about what has actually been said.

Ideas of reference are *delusional beliefs* that certain external events are specifically concerned with the patient. Atomic bomb tests, broadcasts, road repairs, a change of postman, may be felt to have some special and personal significance. Delusions may arise from attempts on the part of the patient to rationalise his abnormal sensations. He may come to believe that his neighbour is interfering with his thoughts and preventing him from thinking, blowing gas through the wall into his bedroom, or directing laser beams through the ceiling. These are known as *secondary delusions*. *Primary* or *autochthonous* delusions arise from 'out of the blue'. They are invariably a sign of *schizophrenia*. The start of a schizophrenic illness was a sudden 'blinding revelation' to the patient that he had a divine mission. All *delusions* are false beliefs, absurd in the light of the patient's intelligence and background, which fail to respond to reason. They occur in organic and psychotic disorders.

Delusions are not uncommon in psychotic depression. Such patients have delusions of guilt, that they are wicked sinners and have ruined their family; that they are fit only to be arrested and put into prison; because of this they are being followed, watched and their houses are bugged. Nihilistic delusions also develop, the patient believing that his mind or even his body has ceased to exist. Delusions of poverty and of ill health are common. However, hypochondriacal delusions can arise in almost any condition.

Certain thoughts may preoccupy the mind to the exclusion of everything else. When such preoccupations are recognised by the patient to be unreasonable, but persist in spite of every effort to suppress them, they are known as *obsessions*. The realisation that the thought, or its persistence, is absurd indicates that the patient has *insight*; contrast this with the lack of insight of patients holding delusional beliefs.

Perseveration is most characteristic of organic brain disease. The patient's pattern of behaviour and thought continues far longer than is necessary. Some perseveration sometimes occurs in normal people when tired. Perseveration needs to be distinguished from stereotypy, which occurs in catatonic schizophrenia and may be associated with verbal perseveration. *Echolalia* is the repetition of a word or phrase spoken to the patient. *Echopraxia* is the imitation of someone's actions or part of them. They occur in catatonic schizophrenia, and are often associated with automatic obedience and *waxy flexibility*. Echolalia and echopraxia also occur in dementia.

Disorders of sleep

Disorders of sleep are common at all ages. Sleep disorders arise in children when they are anxious, or when family sleeping habits are erratic. Among young people anxiety is the most likely cause of difficulty in falling asleep (initial insomnia). Once asleep the individual may then sleep soundly until daybreak, but if anxiety is severe he is liable to waken repeatedly. The obsessional individual in particular may become preoccupied by initial insomnia and start to agonise within a few minutes of turning out the light that he is still awake. This of course ensures that he does not fall asleep.

Depression frequently upsets the sleep pattern. Typically, the patient with endogenous depression rapidly gets to sleep but wakens after 3 or 4 hours, depressed and worried, unable to relax and go back to sleep. The reactive depressive is more likely to have initial insomnia, or to waken after a few hours and then sleep only fitfully, perhaps falling into deep sleep just before he is due to rise. Among this group is the middle aged woman who gets up and gorges herself – the night eating syndrome.

Demented patients are liable to have broken sleep, and to wander during the night. Reversal of the usual pattern, sleeping by day and activity at night, is not uncommon, and very tiresome for relatives or others looking after the patient.

It is always necessary to exclude obvious causes of insomnia: organic illness such as heart failure, emphysema, and painful conditions; excessive intake of stimulants at night time like coffee and certain drugs; and alcoholism. The alcoholic gets to sleep quickly but wakens after 3 or 4 hours because of withdrawal symptoms.

Less commonly a patient complains of *hypersomnia*. This may be a symptom of narcolepsy, but this is a rare condition. It is more likely to be associated with neurotic depression and responds to treatment of that condition.

Disorder of memory

Memory is made up of *learning*, which requires the patient's *attention*, *retention*, *recall* and *recognition*. Memory may be affected at any or all of these stages:

(a) Any disturbance of the level of consciousness, marked distractibility and inattention will obviously interfere with memory. Sudden transitory disturbances of memory occur in epileptic seizures and post-concussional states.

(b) *Retention* is impaired in the *Korsakov syndrome*. The patient cannot retain recent happenings, although events long past may be clearly recalled. Patients sometimes compensate for this type of memory deficiency by *confabulation*, filling in the gaps with fabrications.

(c) *Recall* of past memories may be affected by strong emotion. Overwhelming anxiety may result in a patient developing an hysterical *amnesia*, or loss of memory. A *fugue* is loss of memory in a patient who has wandered off. That retention is unaffected is shown by the ease with which memory can be restored in such cases (see p. 119).

Tests of memory from a practical point of view are divided into relatively recent and later events. Recent memory is particularly likely to be impaired in the early stages of dementia and brain damage. In progressive states of dementia loss of memory extends increasingly far back.

Disorders of consciousness and intelligence

A patient may be disorientated and unable to say where he is or what he has been doing recently. This may be due to delirium or dementia or hysteria.

Delirium is a state of confusion, usually of sudden or sub-acute onset, with full or varying degrees of recovery. Delirium tremens for instance may terminate with full recovery of memory and mental functions, but may be succeeded by the Korsakov syndrome.

Dementia is a state of permanent and often progressive intellectual impairment. Memory is always affected. Emotions become unstable and the finer aspects of a patient's personality give way to selfishness and egocentricity.

Mental impairment (previously subnormality) means that the person has, and always has had, an intelligence well below average. This term has been introduced by the 1983 Mental Health Act and is explained on p. 382.

Some simple tests, taking the patient's social and intellectual background into consideration, will provide further information.

Tests of orientation

Ask the patient his name, address, where he is and where he came from, how long he has been in hospital, time of day and date.

Tests of immediate memory

(a) Test the memory span for digits, i.e. ask him to repeat 791368. The average adult can retain at least six digits forwards, four digits backwards.

(b) Ascertain whether the patient can retain a telephone number for at least three minutes. Make sure he understands the question by asking him to repeat at once the number you give him. Carry on with the examination and then ask him for the telephone number three minutes later.

(c) Can he learn the *Babcock sentence?* 'One thing a nation must have to become rich and great, is a large supply of wood'. Adults of average intelligence can usually reproduce this sentence after one or two repetitions unless very anxious or lacking motivation. A dementing patient may require ten or more tries.

(d) Test ability to reproduce the gist of a short story with a moral. A simple one is of the donkey and the sponges. 'A donkey, laden with bags of salt, stumbled and fell as he was crossing a river. He lay in the cool water for several minutes and when he got up was surprised to find that his load was much lighter. Next day he repeated the journey, this time laden with sacks of sponges. Thinking to lighten his load, he lay down in the river but when he tried to rise the load was so heavy that his back was broken and he drowned.' After the patient has been asked to reproduce the story he should then say what it signifies. He may give a literal (concrete) interpretation, suggesting mental impairment, dementia or schizophrenia. This tests concentration and conceptual thought, as well as memory.

Another test of attention and concentration is 'serial sevens'; subtracting 7 serially from 100, i.e. 93, 86, 79, . . . , 2. A similar but simple test is to repeat backwards the days of the week.

General knowledge

General knowledge questions are useful as tests of memory, and occasionally cause a patient to reveal delusional ideas; current events that have featured in the newspapers within the last few weeks; the present Prime Minister and predecessors; names of members of the Royal family; the capitals of various countries.

Tests of abstract thought

The short story with a moral has already been described above. Ask a patient what he understands by a proverb such as 'a rolling stone gathers no moss', or 'people who live in glass houses should not throw stones'; a dement or the mentally impaired patient gives concrete interpretations; so also may a schizophrenic, or the interpretation may be extraordinarily bizarre. It may also be helpful to ask the patient to describe differences or similarities between objects like apple and orange, horse and donkey, man and monkey. Ask him to define an abstract concept such as goodness, beauty; all these require conceptual thought, which is frequently disturbed in mental illness and dementia.

In dementia, conceptual and abstract thought is replaced by literal, concrete thinking. The patient's vocabulary, however, remains intact until late. A man's IQ roughly corresponds to the size of his vocabulary, and it is therefore sometimes possible, by comparing vocabulary IQ, with IQ derived from other tests, to determine the degree of dementia.

Tests of arithmetical ability

These may show up mental impairment, dementia, confusion and inattention. They obviously need to be adjusted for age and background. It is useful to recognise that subtraction is harder than addition, and division more difficult than multiplication.

Finally, it is useful for the interviewer to sum up his general impressions of the patient, the consistency of the history, feelings aroused in the interviewer, negative and positive, the likely diagnosis and further investigations needed.

The present state examination (PSE) is a systematic recording of most relevant symptoms, and is claimed to be diagnostically reliable. We believe that the state of psychiatry is such that intuition and subjective feelings on the part of the examiner are still of great importance in coming to a diagnosis. This does not exclude the use of diagnostic scales or other tests, but they must be used alongside clinical skills.

Psychological tests

Psychological tests of a quick paper and pencil type which can be administered by anyone can be of ancillary use. For a general assessment of intelligence Raven's Progressive Matrices or the Mill Hill Vocabulary Scale are useful. When the result is of considerable diagnostic importance, as in mental impairment or early dementia it is advisable to send the patient to a competent psychologist for formal testing.

The Eysenck Personality Test provides a personality profile. It measures psychoticism, neuroticism, and extraversion/introversion. No psychological test result should ever be accepted on its own. It is often extremely helpful, but it cannot replace a full clinical assessment of a patient.

9
Neurotic Disorders

Anxiety states

Definition

Most people feel anxious before an important event, or when faced with grave danger. Anxiety or fear are natural reactions at such times and serve a useful purpose; they disappear when the cause is removed. An *anxiety state,* on the other hand, is a continual and irrational feeling of anxiety, in the absence of any justifiable cause. The anxiety may amount to panic and interfere with mental and social functioning. There is no qualitative difference between normal and pathological anxiety.

Incidence

Anxiety states are among the most common psychiatric disorders encountered today. About 25 per cent of patients attending a psychiatric outpatient clinic have an anxiety state; and at least that proportion of patients visit their general practitioner. Anxiety states occur about equally in both sexes, and most develop either between adolescence and 30, or in old age. Transitory anxiety symptoms are common in childhood. There is no evidence linking social class with anxiety states in this country, although in the USA anxiety states are said to be more prevalent in the upper social groups.

'Suburban neurosis', anxiety states brought about by loneliness and lack of interests and outlets, among women in suburbia, was described in 1938. A similar kind of anxiety neurosis has been described in women living in high rise flats; but doubt has recently been cast upon both these as common causes of anxiety.

The physiological changes of anxiety

Sympathetic and parasympathetic activities increase, although the sympathetic predominates. The adrenal cortex and medulla are both stimulated. As a result the levels of corticosteroids, and of adrenaline and noradrenaline in the plasma are increased. Adrenaline, which is more potent than noradrenaline in producing the sympathomimetic effects of anxiety, is secreted in greater quantities. Anxiety symptoms can be produced in anyone by giving them intravenous adrenaline.

Free fatty acids are released from fatty tissues by the action of adrenaline, and probably increase the risk of myocardial infarction in those with already diseased hearts. There is a redistribution of blood to the periphery, which perhaps accounts for the symptoms of faintness and dizziness so common in anxiety states. The increased flow of blood in the forearms of patients with anxiety states can be measured by means of a plethysmograph, and provides a useful measure of anxiety. Conductance of the skin to an electrical current depends upon sweat gland activity. Anxiety neurotics tend to have sweaty palms, and therefore lower skin conductance levels (increased psychogalvanic reflexes).

There is no consistent change in the EEG, although alpha activity is often reduced in chronic anxiety.

Symptoms

Anxiety states tend to be long lasting and to fluctuate widely in severity.

Patients may complain mainly of feeling anxious and irritable. But more often they are troubled by bodily symptoms and discomfort resulting from increased adrenergic activity. Symptoms vary widely from patient to patient, although each patient tends to keep to a similar pattern over a long time. Exacerbations of anxiety may progress to attacks of panic, when the patient fears his last moment has come, or that he is about to go berserk, mad, lose control of his actions, and disgrace himself in public. The sense of unsteadiness and vertigo that often accompanies anxiety may increase to such a degree that the patient collapses and is hurried to hospital as a suspected medical emergency.

Anxiety is often accompanied by restlessness and irritability. Concentration becomes difficult, short term memory is upset, and patients tire easily.

Sleep is frequently disturbed, particularly getting to sleep. Patients sometimes become preoccupied with insomnia, and work themselves into a state of near panic at bedtime at the prospect of not falling asleep. Hypnotics, or large nightcaps, are not infrequently taken to excess. When the patient does eventually fall asleep he may be woken by unpleasant dreams. Eventually, when it is time to rise, he feels exhausted and sleepy. Occasionally this picture is reversed, and sleep is increased, both in depth and duration; to such an extent that narcolepsy is suspected.

Sexual interest and activity are likely to diminish; men may become impotent, women frigid. On the other hand, anxiety sometimes increases sexual tension, and there is increased activity, in masturbation and intercourse.

Appetite for food is similarly affected, but is rarely seriously reduced; weight loss, when it occurs, only involves a few pounds. But a considerable increase of weight can occur when anxiety leads to compulsive eating. This is particularly liable to affect women, and is an occasional cause of obesity.

Cardiovascular symptoms are common; palpitations, tachycardia, and pains over the heart often lead a patient to fear a heart attack. *Cardiac neurosis* or effort syndrome, an anxiety state associated with cardiovascular symptoms, pain over the heart, hyperventilation capable of producing tetany, and lightheadedness, is a not uncommon and often intractable condition.

Muscle tension is increased, and is responsible for headache, and pains around the shoulders, neck and spine. Headache characteristically affects the fronto-temporal region, and is sharp and painful, unlike the dull, heavy or 'inflamed' quality of depressive headache.

Gastrointestinal symptoms include difficulty in swallowing, nausea and vomiting, bouts of diarrhoea and/or constipation, distension and abdominal pain from spasm of the colon, usually above the epigastrium or right iliac fossa. Gynaecological and genito-urinary symptoms may predominate: menorrhagia, occasionally amenorrhoea, frequency, dysuria; premenstrual tension is usually marked.

Fatigue is sometimes the main symptom. Any exertion brings on a remarkable sense of exhaustion, which may be accompanied by palpitations, dizziness, and fear of collapse. Depression of mood may also become prominent; at times it may be difficult to decide whether anxiety is the primary condition, or is secondary to depressive illness.

Aetiology

Genetic factors. People vary enormously in their threshold for experiencing anxiety; differences in autonomic reactivity and temperament are noticeable from birth, suggesting that genetic factors play a part. It is always difficult to separate heredity from childhood experience and learning, but the fact that monozygotic twins show a higher concordance for anxiety states than dizygotic twins favours genetic influences. Temperamentally, people who develop anxiety states are likely to have high scores for intraversion and neuroticism on the EPI.

Learning. However learning clearly plays an important role in addition to constitutional differences. Situations or objects which are seen by a child to be threatening are likely to arouse, and become associated with, anxiety. The most obvious examples are the monosymptomatic phobias; a mother who screams with terror and calls for help every time a large spider runs across the floor, or a thunderstorm breaks, or a wasp approaches her, is likely, through modelling, to transmit her fears to her child.

A child reared in an atmosphere of insecurity and quarrelling, forever fearing separation, is readily provoked to strong anxiety when threatened with the loss of an important relationship in later life.

> Mary presented with feelings of anxiety, at times verging on panic. She was irritable, almost intolerably so the week before menstruation, and suffered constant headaches and pains across the shoulders. She came from an unhappy home, her parents having finally separated when she was 15. She had been married for 7 years, and for the five months before being seen had been emotionally involved with another man, a local Casonova. Mary's sense of guilt grew and she became increasingly apprehensive that her marriage was threatened. Yet without her husband's help she felt she was unable to break off the affair. Through psychotherapy she was able to untangle the more important problems, and eventually, through marital therapy, was able to come to terms with herself and her husband.

Situations which precipitate anxiety states range from severely stressful to apparently trivial, and depend on constitutional vulnerability, prior conditioning, and the amount of support he or she has; an appalling accident, a 'bad trip' with a hallucinogenic drug, a quarrel with a close friend, the birth of a first child, any of these may be followed by severe anxiety.

Psychodynamic theories

Subconscious conflicts, between forbidden inner impulses, particularly those of a sexual nature, and inhibitions, are seen by Freudian psychoanalysts as the source of chronic anxiety. If such conflicts can be brought to light, it is suggested, anxiety disappears.

However, as we have pointed out, conscious conflicts can frequently be identified in patients with anxiety states; an extramarital affair, yet strong dependence on a spouse; ambition, greater than a patient's abilities; resentment amounting to hatred for a dependant, contrasting with a strong need to look after her. If these can be discussed anxiety often improves quickly.

Differential diagnosis

Anxiety may be the result of organic disease rather than the cause of physical symptoms. Thyrotoxicosis, or hypoglycaemia, are readily mistaken by the unwary for anxiety. Anxiety may be felt before a serious illness reveals itself. Anxiety is absent in essential hypertension until the patient is informed about the condition. Anxiety itself raises blood pressure, especially systolic, and not a few anxious patients are regrettably 'treated' with hypotensive drugs, often to their psychiatric detriment.

Depression is nearly always accompanied by anxiety and should always be suspected in the middle aged. Schizophrenia is often ushered in by anxiety symptoms. A patient in the early stages of dementia, before insight is lost, understandably feels anxiety and depression.

The diagnosis of an anxiety state should rest on positive evidence of an anxious and predisposed personality, and/or understandably severe stress in the recent past.

Treatment

1. *Acute anxiety* (following a traumatic incident), needs heavy and immediate sedation. The longer it is allowed to persist the more difficult symptoms are to remove. Continuous narcosis, 72 hours or so, may be necessary at times. Barbiturates are still invaluable for acute anxiety.

2. *Psychotherapy* at some level is required in all anxiety states. Simple explanation and reassurance about somatic symptoms can bring about considerable improvement. Underlying conflicts and problems need to be explored and related to anxiety and resolved. Psychoanalytic methods are rarely indicated. It is wise not to probe too deeply into the background of inadequate patients, for fear of breaking down still more their weak psychological defences. Both individual and group psychotherapy are at times needed. Often it is helpful to see a patient and his or her partner together.

3. *Behaviour therapy* can be effective, both on its own or in conjunction with drugs or psychotherapy. '*Anxiety management training*' consists of coming to recognise anxiety symptoms for what they are, and their relationship to anxiety provoking situations; learning about body mechanisms through which anxiety creates its effects; and the way in which anxiety symptoms create yet more anxiety; and learning to relax and substitute in his mind's eye some pleasant relaxing scene for the anxiety situation.

The patient can be taught this by an individual therapist or by a tape recording of instructions.

4. *Physical treatment*. Minor tranquillisers, such as diazepam, are helpful; they may be required continuously for a time – between 6 – 20 mg diazepam a day – or when a specific need arises, before an important meeting say; some caution is then needed, in case of side effects, and it is advisable to try out the drug beforehand; an obvious time is shortly before going to bed. Patients must always be warned of the potentiating effect of alcohol.

Many severe anxiety states, particularly when somatic symptoms or phobic anxiety are prominent features, respond particularly well to a monoamine oxidase inhibitor such as phenelzine, usually combined with a tranquilliser. When there is a strong depressive component present, a tricyclic or quadricyclic antidepressant is sometimes helpful; however, patients with anxiety states are often unable to tolerate the side effects of such drugs. Occasionally, in cases of longstanding, incapacitating anxiety, ECT may be helpful, provided it is given with heavy sedation. Great care is needed, as ECT is liable to make the average primary anxiety state worse.

Very occasionally, when all else fails, and the patient's life is a misery, prefrontal leucotomy can be considered. In carefully selected patients, stereotactic methods give good results.

Prognosis

This is, by and large, good, although relapses are likely. Much depends on a patient's constitutional vulnerability, and his ability to adapt his life so that what for him are serious stresses can be minimised. With age patients become more stable; their autonomic systems react less readily, and most of them develop a protected way of life. When anxiety states persist in spite of treatment, it means that the underlying conflict continues; although when saying this the patient's personality must be taken into account.

Phobic Anxiety

Anxiety rarely remains 'free floating' for long. Frequently it attaches itself to objects or situations, which are then avoided, or to physical symptoms, which results in hypochondriasis. Specific fears of this nature are known as *phobias*. A phobic situation or object is always feared and avoided, in contrast to obsessional fears (see p. 127).

1. *Agoraphobia* was first described in 1871. Although the name implies fear of being in open spaces and streets, anxiety is also commonly aroused by crowded shops, public transport, cinemas and theatres, and lifts. The patient becomes increasingly anxious that she is about to collapse and 'make a fool of herself', or is on the brink of dying. (It is the state of *dying* rather than death that the agoraphobic fears.) The more crowded the place, the more isolated and the further from home she is, the greater her panic. Three-quarters of the sufferers are women.

Agoraphobia commonly starts somewhere between the late teens and early thirties. The individual suddenly experiences terrifying panic while shopping or travelling. Sometimes she even faints or collapses, and is then taken to a nearby hospital, when no physical cause is found. Terror may now prevent her from leaving her home at all without her husband or trusted friend or relative. Or she may be able to walk a short distance alone to a local shop. Some are able to drive or bicycle on their own. Other can go out alone – or with a companion – only at night when no one can observe them. Some can walk in daylight but only by clinging to walls and buildings as they stagger uncertainly along the pavement. Back at home they feel secure, but usually features of anxiety and depression of mood are present.

The agoraphobic's life and that of her family are considerably disrupted. Her husband has to take the children to school, do the shopping, accompany his wife everywhere. Some protest, but others not only take this in their stride but seem to encourage their wives to ever greater dependence. Indeed a few even seem hostile to treatment and almost go out of their way to sabotage it.

Although agoraphobia can be secondary to depressive illness, and is sometimes found with obsessional symptoms, it is generally agreed that agoraphobia exists as a specific entity.

> Joan was 24. When travelling by train to work she felt so panicky that she left the train at the next stop. She sat on the station for almost 2 hours, and was then calm enough to catch an empty train home. She has been unable to travel at all, except when driven by her husband, for over 3 years, and has given up all work.
>
> Joan is an inhibited woman, still very attached to her mother. Her marriage is outwardly a reasonable one, for the couple never row, although she is sexually frigid. Her husband is keen to start a family but she is ambivalent towards the idea. The night before the initial panic attack he had upset her by his

criticisms that she had never grown up and that her mother was 'a pain in the neck'. Joan, as usual, felt unable to answer back, slept little that night, and was still brooding angrily over the incident when she left for work next morning.

Simmering resentment in an immature inhibited individual is often the basis for the start of agoraphobia. Secondary factors and habits then strengthen the phobia, and cause anxiety to spread. In this case agoraphobia served as a punishment, a means of binding her husband to her, and perhaps a maladaptive means of avoiding the question of children.

2. *Social phobias.* These are centred on a fear of meeting other people and drawing attention to oneself. They include phobias of eating in public places – or even with anyone outside the family. There is intense fear of vomiting or collapsing in public. Remarkably common is phobic anxiety connected with drinking in public; a dread that in lifting a glass or cup to drink the hand will start to shake and draw attention to the sufferer. Some patients have a similar dread of writing a cheque or receipt in front of people. Fear of blushing may be so intense as to bring social intercourse virtually to an end.

Social phobias are likely to develop in late adolescence and early twenties, at a time when self-confidence is low; often after the loss of a supportive companion. About 60 per cent of patients are female. Generalised anxiety is not usually as strong as with agoraphobia, unless the condition is seriously interfering with social life.

A woman of 19 went with her parents and her fiancé and his family to a restaurant to celebrate their engagement. The room was hot and she felt mildly unwell soon after arriving. During the main course she became increasingly queasy and unable to swallow. Anxiety grew and she became terrified of being sick. Eventually, in a state of panic, she rushed from the restaurant. Since then she has not been able to eat away from her own home. She has begun to abuse alcohol and tranquillisers prescribed by her general practitioner.

3. *Hypochondriacal phobias* are extremely common. They may arise episodically, associated with anxiety, and move from one system of the body to another, or remain of permanent concern. The hypochondriac sometimes goes to considerable lengths to 'avoid' his symptoms; exercising to keep fit, special diets, ensuring his bowels move daily. He is preoccupied by his symptoms, is

likely to talk about them at every opportunity, and constantly to seek medical reassurance (which may be short-lived). The hypochondriac is fearful that he is about to 'lose control' of himself. He cannot run away from his symptoms, but he can run panic stricken from one doctor or cure to another repetitively, but of course without avail. It is important to differentiate hypochondriacal phobias from hypochondriasis secondary to depression, anxiety or obsessional states, and when bizarre, schizophrenia.

4. The fourth group, the *monosymptomatic phobias* are not associated with anxiety feelings when the phobic object is absent. Phobias of animals, such as spiders, cats, etc. are commonly learned in childhood.

Most children grow out of them, but in a few, mostly females, the phobias persist into adult life. They make up only about one per cent of phobic states, and are rarely more than a nuisance. Phobias of the dark, flying, heights, water, thunder, and so on, are often acquired later in life, as a result of some frightening experience. Fear of flying, however, is often part of an agoraphobic syndrome.

Causes

1. *Genetic factors* are only likely to be concerned in so far as they influence the degree of stability or lability of the autonomic system.
2. *Learning* from parents and other people important to the child is certainly a major factor in monosymptomatic phobias, and probably in agoraphobia and social phobias.
3. *Agoraphobic* female patients are likely to be sexually frigid, still emotionally tied to parents, and inhibited people, rarely able to express readily and openly their stronger, especially aggressive, feelings.
4. *Conflicts,* often subtle rather than obvious, can usually be discerned. The phobia, excluding the monosymptomatic, frequently represents a way, albeit maladaptive and inconvenient to the patient, of removing or bypassing the conflict.

Treatment of Phobias

1. *Behaviour therapy.* Some form of behaviour therapy is usually necessary. Ideally, exposure to the feared situation – getting the agoraphobic to return to a crowded shop, or the social phobic to a restaurant – is most effective, but not always possible, although it

may be so with the temporary help of a tranquilliser. The therapist must often accompany her for the first few outings, but if she becomes too dependent on the therapist this is self-defeating. Relaxation exercises are important, following the same lines as described on p. 368.

2. *Psychotherapy* is needed to give support, sift out and deal with relevant conflicts, and to focus on the immediate future and what the patient expects when she loses her symptoms. She must think in positive terms in this respect. Husband or parents may need counselling, and marital therapy is often necessary.

3. *Drugs* are useful but are often abused both by doctors and patients. A tranquilliser, say Lorazepam, taken 45 minutes or so before the anxiety-provoking situation, will reduce fear and help the patient to face the situation. Regular long term usage of tranquillisers is not without dependency problems, and withdrawal effects can increase phobic symptoms and liability to panic.

Beta-adrenoceptor blockers like propranolol – up to 120 mg a day – are most likely to help when autonomic symptoms, especially cardiac, are prominent. They can be combined with a tranquilliser. Antidepressant drugs, both tricyclic and MAOI, have good effects at first on many phobic patients. However, their effects sometimes wear off. But more of a problem is their need to be taken for long periods, often years, and relapse occurs if they are prematurely stopped.

Hysteria and hysterical reactions

The term *hysteria* is used in a number of different, although related ways.

Hysterical personality (and see Personality Disorders, p. 131) describes an excitable, flamboyant, suggestible person, always wanting the limelight, who remains childlike in his or her emotional relationships and needs. Hysterical personalities are dependent on and demanding of those people involved in their lives; when they fail, they are considered to be useless, weak, or villainous; when they do what is asked of them they are heroic, wonderfully reliable. Sexual relationships are inevitably tempestuous. Frequently frigid, at times demanding, the hysterical personality expects to be both lovingly cared for and protected, yet also treated roughly sexually, even brutally. When her problems, which are all too often created by her own behaviour, become too difficult for her to manage, as she ages and loses her attraction and power, she may escape into illness, take to her bed and (like Florence Nightingale) dominate her world from there.

Hysterical personalities rarely develop dissociative states. They are often highly intelligent and attractive people, but never easy to live or work with.

Hysterical behaviour and '*hysterical overlay*', implies that a patient's emotional reaction to pain or illness is greatly exaggerated, distorts his physical condition, and prolongs his disability beyond the time of natural recovery. Thus, a small peptic ulcer causes such an expression of pain that the surgeon feels impelled to operate. Afterwards, although the patient's postoperative recovery is uneventful, his agonising discomfort continues. Such behaviour is designed, although not consciously, to draw attention to the patient, to indicate that he or she needs help. It is, of course, common to see hysterical behaviour in children and in old people, particularly when they are lonely, with little to look forward to after leaving hospital. It is not unusual for doctors and nurses to be irritated by hysterical behaviour, with the understandable result that such behaviour worsens. Of course, a painful chronic illness may well dispose the sufferer to behave in a childlike fashion and to regress into hysterical behaviour.

Hysteria (which cannot easily be separated from the last) is used to embrace a huge amorphous group of symptoms and conditions, such as headache, low back pain, colitis, rheumatism, repeated upper respiratory infections, frequent vomiting, for which no reasonable organic cause can be found. Hysterical personalities make up many of these patients. But it is better to describe the condition in terms of the underlying psychiatric state, like anxiety or depression, which is primarily responsible for the symptoms.

Hysterical dissociative and conversion symptoms. An apparently healthy person may suddenly lose the use or sensation of some part of his body, memory may vanish or a personality change dramatically. Yet the paralysed limb can be shown to work when the patient's attention is distracted, and memory loss is of a different quality from that due to organic disease. A striking feature of hysterical conversion is the way in which the loss or change of function corresponds to what the patient believes it should be, rather than corresponding to interruption of actual anatomical nerve pathways; a paralysed arm say, is not found on testing to be associated with signs of an appropriate nerve lesion.

Hysterical conversion symptoms develop out of emotional conflicts. According to Freud, conversion symptoms solve a conflict for the patient. A psychosexually immature young female music student was playing a duet with a male student. The man reached out to touch her thigh, she moved her hand to stop him, but before she could do so her arm became paralysed. The primary conflict was between her sexual inhibition and attraction for the man, and the primary gain was (because her arm was helpless) to 'allow' sexual contact. A secondary gain later became apparent when the paralysis persisted; she had to give up music, something she had long wanted to do but had not previously dared to go against the will of her domineering father. Such primary and secondary gains are usually, although not invariably, apparent.

Conversion symptoms often symbolise underlying conflicts. Thus, a woman who wanted to tell her bullying husband that she hated and meant to leave him for another man suddenly, during a heated quarrel with him, lost her voice.

Freud recognised that patients unconsciously converted their conflicts into somatic or mental symptoms from his work with Breuer on hypnosis. Emotional feelings became dissociated from the symptom and as long as this persisted the patient remained free of anxiety. This lack of concern, or *belle indifference*, is apparent in most patients with hysterical conversion.

Hysteria derives its name from the ancient belief that the disorder is due to the 'wanderings' of the uterus. But men as well as women can develop hysteria. A sexual causation has long been attributed to hysteria. Galen, who first proposed the idea of male hysteria, thought it came about from retained semen, due to sexual abstinence.

Incidence

Short-lived hysterical conversions are not uncommon in childhood; blindness, paralysis of a limb, inability to speak or swallow. They occur in response to stress and nearly always resolve themselves completely and quickly without treatment the more so when they do not arouse concern in adults. Only if hysterical symptoms persist or appear frequently in childhood need they cause concern.

Hysteria has occurred throughout recorded history. It was common in the latter half of the 19th century, partly because of medical interest in the condition at that time. Today, hysterical conversion states still occur. But gross symptoms, total paralysis of a limb and bizarre gait and posture, mostly only develop in patients with low intelligence. Medical ignorance, isolation and fear, all increase the incidence, which is greater in primitive societies.

Clinical symptoms

Symptoms are most easily considered under separate headings: motor, sensory and mental. But all types of symptoms can be seen in the same patient.

Paralysis, spasm or *contracture* of any *voluntary* muscle can occur. But typically, movements rather than individual muscles are affected. Testing shows inconsistencies. Reflexes are normal. Passive movement often meets with undue resistance, which can be seen to affect a wide range of musculature. When, as rarely happens, hysterical paralysis lasts for several years muscle tone and reflexes diminish, there is disuse muscle atrophy and the overlying skin is cold and cyanotic.

Tremor is usually gross, often varies and may cease if the patient's attention is drawn to something else. Abnormalities of *gait* vary from a drunken stagger to extraordinary contortions. Speech may be affected. Aphonia is rarely complete and the patient is able to whisper, sing and cough loudly. *Stammering* is a common symptom.

Hysterical fits may be difficult to distinguish from *epileptic fits*. They are most likely to be seen in epileptics or in patients who have an epileptic relative. In fact some epileptics may bring on true fits by overbreathing. Hysterical fits do not have the tonic/clonic phases of epilepsy. They invariably occur before an audience and may continue for half an hour or more. Attempts to restrain the patient's excessive movements lead to redoubled activity. Foaming at the mouth, wild cries and facial contortions produce a dramatic scene. Such patients rarely harm themselves during fits.

Anaesthesia, blindness, deafness and loss of taste may be presenting symptoms. Hysterical anaesthesia is typically of a 'glove and stocking' type of distribution corresponding to the patient's ideas rather than to any known nerve distribution. Examination often induces changes in the area of anaesthesia.

A patient may complain of blindness, yet be able to find his way to the door across a room full of obstacles. Occasionally he complains of 'funnel' vision.

Amnesia and fugue have long been known. Rarely, a patient splits into two or more separate and apparently integrated personalities, like Dr. Jekyll and Mr. Hyde. Hysterical splitting bears no relationship to schizophrenic splitting. In the former, each personality appears outwardly to be complete. In the latter, the schizophrenic's personality is split in all aspects, which produces disintegration of character and function, and a virtual loss of the former individuality.

Amnesia, or loss of memory, occurs after a terrifying event which overwhelms the patient. A respectable young man fell in love with a good-time girl and stole from the petty cash in order to entertain her. He was subsequently accused of theft by his manager. Panic-stricken he ran into the street. Suddenly all memory of what he had done disappeared from consciousness and was replaced by unconcern. But so great was the *repressing force* needed to do this that other memories were also affected. In this example the young man was unable to recall his name or anything to do with his past life. He was admitted to hospital with total amnesia.

Sometimes a patient who has developed amnesia wanders far away. This is known as a *fugue state*.

Hysterical *stupor* is rare and usually only occurs after intense and prolonged stress. Patients become motionless and have to be hand fed. Similar baby-like behaviour, without stupor, occurs in hysterical *puerilism*. Such patients behave as though aged three or four years. Occasionally a hysteric may behave like a dement. During this state of *pseudo-dementia* he answers questions in such an absurd way as to make it obvious that he knows the real answer, i.e. '2 + 2 = 5, a cow has 3 legs, 2 cows have 6 legs.' This tendency to give approximate answers often fluctuates. There is too, some variable clouding of consciousness (in the so-called Ganser state), which raises doubts about the diagnosis of hysteria. Some patients recover suddenly and fully, but others go on to develop florid dementia or schizophrenia.

Hysteria and malingering

By definition, hysterical conversion symptoms occur through *unconscious* mechanisms. But it is often impossible to say where unconscious mechanisms end and conscious deception or *malingering* begins. When the gain is very great, malingering frequently replaces hysteria. Probably, whenever hysterical amnesia lasts for more than a few weeks there is some degree of malingering; as, for instance, in the example of the young female music student above.

Doctors are sometimes called upon to distinguish between hysteria and malingering in cases of *compensation or accident neurosis*. Patients with this condition complain of disabling nervous symptoms, headache, dizziness, inability to concentrate, insomnia, loss of libido and so on, after an accidental and often trivial injury. Invariably the patient must believe the accident to have been the fault of someone else, and that he is entitled to financial compensation. Many of these patients have been exceptionally healthy before the accident, and given no signs of hysterical tendencies. Compensation neurosis is rare after injury at sport, where compensation is not expected. It is more common in minor than severe injuries, perhaps because the question of compensation is in doubt. And so far as industrial injuries are concerned, compensation neurosis is most common among the lowest socio-economic groups.

Psychiatric treatment is rarely effective while compensation is pending. After compensation the majority recover spontaneously and return to their old jobs. But in a few cases symptoms continue. It seems probable that cases of compensation neurosis range from 'gross conversion hysteria at one end of the scale to frank malingering at the other'.

Munchausen's syndrome (after the fictitious Baron von Munchausen) is a curious condition describing those people who repeatedly seek hospital admission and treatment. They have often had laparotomies. Many have curious clinical signs, unequal pupils, papilloedema-like optic discs, abnormal reflexes which, together with their complaints, lead to their admission. These patients are sometimes dependent on opiate drugs, are often psychopathic personalities, and very rarely accept psychiatric help. It is debatable whether or not they are fully conscious of their actions. Nonetheless, when detected they immediately discharge themselves from hospital.

In conditions such as *dermatitis artefacta*, the patient is aware of what he is doing from the start. Patients may mutilate their faces and bodies in a horrible and seemingly compulsive manner. One women, over the course of ten years, gradually lost an arm by dipping it in phenol and causing gangrene.

Causes

Hysterical reactions can occur in many people under severe and prolonged stress. But the majority of hysterical disorders seen today occur after relatively minor stress. The nervous systems of these patients seem unable to tolerate much tension and *dissociation* occurs readily.

Genetic and early environmental factors both play a part. Hysteria usually occurs in a characteristic type of personality, obsessional, anxious, and psychosexually immature. Patients with gross symptoms are likely to be of below average intelligence, or come from an unsophisticated foreign culture, and are peculiarly suggestible in a roundabout way. In terms of Eysenck's personality scale, hysterics show extroversion and neuroticism. Many symptoms are the result of suggestion. Aphonia develops after laryngitis, paralysis follows a mild attack of poliomyelitis, amnesia grows out of a blow on the head, aided perhaps by a tactless remark from a doctor or nurse.

Hysteria is particularly liable to occur during an organic illness such as *multiple sclerosis* or a *cerebral tumour* or in the early stages of dementia. Hysterical reactions are also liable to be released by mental illness, especially depression or schizophrenia. Loss of weight, such as occurs in *anorexia nervosa*, may also bring out hysterical tendencies.

Diagnosis. This must always be based on positive as well as negative findings. There should be positive evidence of an immature personality, of past hysterical episodes, of emotional conflict and gain. *Hysteria occurring for the first time in middle age, in the absence of organic or depressive illness, is rare*; an underlying cause should always be sought.

Treatment

It is usually easy to uncover conflicts and gains underlying hysterical symptoms. Sympathetic discussion in calm surroundings with plenty of time may be sufficient to relax the patient and allow him to disclose his problem. If this fails, or speed is essential, intravenous Sodium Amytal or Pentothal can be used (see Abreaction, p. 10). Hypnosis is also effective. Hysterical symptoms then disappear, and are usually replaced by those of anxiety.

However, to prevent relapse it is essential to help the patient to deal with his problems and relieve his anxiety. This is best achieved through psychotherapy, sometimes combined with minor tranquillisers. Physical factors, like loss of weight, must also be treated.

Martin Johnson

It can be seen from Martin's care plan that he has only *one main problem* that is affecting his activities of daily living. In such a situation it is frequently appropriate to plan a behavioural regime that tackles the root cause. In turn the other problems are likely to resolve themselves.

Naturally the behavioural regime needs to be planned together with the patient by a therapist who is skilled in this field. This may be a nurse, doctor, psychologist or occupational therapist.

The ward nurse's role in the initial stages of admission is that of accurate observer. Together with Martin she should record his observable behaviour over twenty-four hours. Martin could also be asked to rate his anxiety about feeling dirty or germ ridden on a scale of a 1–10.

After a complete assessment an individual behavioural programme can be planned. The principles of this work are detailed in Chapter 27. In addition the nurse's role is to reinforce the patient's self-esteem. She should try to ensure that the patient's stay in hospital is as near to everyday life as is feasible. At all times an individual like Martin should be encouraged to be independent – thus the suggestion on his care plan that he might go out in the evenings.

Nursing Information Sheet

Hospital no: 7999 77 Wards: / / / Date of Admission: 7.9.1984

Surname JOHNSON
Forename Martin Howard
Address 7, Clapton Road, London, S.E.11.

Likes to be known as: Martin
Date of birth: 3.5.1948 Age: 36 Sex: M
Marital status:
Religion: R/C Nationality: British

Relevant Psychiatric and General Medical History
Martin has been treated as an outpatient for excessive cleansing over the last year without success

---

Is patient formal or informal?
Informal
Section

Occupation and Past Work History:
Sub-manager in a bank

Source of finance:

Next of kin: Mrs Nicola Johnson
Address: As above

Tel. no.: 761 9999
Person to contact in case of emergency:
(if different from above)
Address: work
Masters Bank
London S.E.11.
Tel. no.: 761 0000

Home conditions
Materially-excellent four bedroomed detached house

Community resources (CPNS voluntary agencies)
Community psychiatric nurse

Significant persons in life
Wife and two children. Angus 11 years and Sarah 6 years

Special nursing observation

Patient's profile
Height 6 feet
Weight 75 kgs
Build Medium
Complexion White
Hair-Colour Brown
Eyes-Colour Blue
Marks and Scars

Reason for admission:
Excessive cleansing ritual which is interfering with job and home life.

Waiting List Admission

Referred by: Accepted by:
Consultant Psychiatrist Outpatients

T.P.R. T36°C P 95 R17
B.P. 130/90
Urine Nothing abnormal detected

G.P. Tel No.:

Dr J Alison
The Penge
Clapton High Road
London S.E.11.

Present Situation	Actual and Potential Problems (Level of independence/ dependence)
1. Maintaining a safe environment Martin is fully independent in that he is mobile and has been managing to go to work prior to admission. He says he is not depressed.	Independent
2. Personal hygiene Martin has been using two bars of soap and six large boxes of tissues a day in order to keep his hands clean, they are red, swollen and sore. In addition he has been washing his hair and bathing three times a day. He says he believes he spends 4 hours a day cleansing because of the germs which may contaminate him.	Red hands. Excessive cleansing due to anxiety regarding germs
3. Special factors Sore, red hands	Sore, red hands
4. Care of clothing Meticulous with regard to his clothes. Changes underpants, socks, shirt three times a day. Washes these things himself at home in washing machine. Dry cleaning bills for suits, etc. approx. £7.50 a week.	Changes clothes 3 times a day - due to fear of germs. Cleaning bills large
5. Co-operation in ward life He still feels rather strange being in hospital and wishes he had managed to be treated at home (this was tried but failed). He is pleasant to other patients when spoken to and rigidly conforms to mealtimes - at 12.30 pm he sat at the table - having been told this was the time.	Independent - conforms to routine rigidly. Upset that he didn't manage to be treated at home
6. Attitude toward medication No medication prescribed at present. Martin would like something to reduce his anxiety which he says has increased due to admission.	Martin would like some medication to reduce his anxiety
7. Working and playing – social mixing Martin's work has been affected by his cleanliness - he has been arriving late in the morning and taking two hours for lunch in order to bathe. He used to go out to a darts evening once a week but this has stopped due to washing at night.	Late for work. Reduction in social life due to excessive cleansing

Aim of Nursing Intervention	Plan of Care
That Martin retains his independence	Allow Martin to leave the ward but ask him to inform staff when he is going to. Explain this merely so that if he is wanted we know where he is
Accurately assess Martin's washing over 24 hours. Reduce time and cost of cleansing	Together with Martin, chart his washing over 24 hours. Rating anxiety on scale 1-10 prior and after washing. Then review and plan behavioural programme
Reduction of inflammation of Martin's hands	First 24 hours encourage Martin to use lanolin handcream. Review daily and report to doctor if they get worse. Behavioural programme after 24 hours assessment
Reduce changing of clothes and thus cleaning bills	See 2. After 24 hours when behavioural programme organised review
Reinforce independence Reassuring that in-patient treatment does not mean ill for life	Talk with Martin explaining that many people are only admitted to hospital once and never return with psychiatric problems. Listen to him about his feelings and respond positively pointing out he still has a job and family, etc.
To get Martin to accurately describe his anxiety regarding admission and find its cause	Talk with Martin about his anxiety. Observe physiological state when anxious i.e. pulse, blood pressure. Ask Martin to tell the doctor he would like medication. Inform doctor of physiological response in order that a proper assessment (i.e. medication) can be made
Maintain Martin's self-esteem and social relationships	Encourage Martin to join in ward activities particularly darts. Remind him that despite his problems he has maintained his job. Ask him how he feels about friends visiting him. Point out he can leave the ward in the evenings if he wants

Present Situation	Actual and Potential Problems (Level of independence/ dependence)
8. Communicating	
Martin is articulate and well able to discuss his situation. His speech is 'clipped and precise' - gets faster when he is talking about washing. He looks anxious and taps his foot	Well able to communicate speech rapid when talking about cleansing
9. Perception	
Martin says that he is aware that his hand washing has become a problem. He is shocked at having to come into hospital because he always thought a mental hospital was for 'real cases' and he is surprised that he can relate to some of the other patients	Aware of problem. Shocked at need for hospital admission
10. Finance and budgeting	
Martin says he has been spending £20 a week on cleansing materials. His wife believes it to be about £35. There is no immediate financial problem as both of them work	Cleansing bill £20 - £35 a week
11. Mobility	
Fully mobile. He says that sometimes he takes a long time to get from A to B because he tries to avoid dirty areas i.e. tubes, public lavatories	Fully mobile. Sometimes takes a long route to avoid dirty areas which delays him
12. Eating and drinking	
Eats with his family - his wife prepares all the meals. Does not go out to pubs to drink or eat at work all due to fear of contamination. Occasional sherry at home in the evenings	Normal diet. No longer goes out for a drink at pub due to washing
13. Eliminating	
Normal elimination pattern. Bowels open daily in the morning after which Martin bathes	Independent Potential problem - diarrhoea due to anxiety. Washes after each time bowels open
14. Expressing sexuality	
Martin says that he feels that he is behaving like an 'old woman' but that he cannot stop all his washing due to anxiety. His wife has started sleeping in the spare room because if she doesn't have a bath at night Martin can't share a bed with her due to anxiety	Feels he is like an 'old woman' Physical separation from wife due to cleansing
15. Sleeping	
Martin says 'I'm so exhausted by the time I go to bed I sleep soundly'. Sets alarm to wake about 6 a.m. in order to complete washing rituals and get to work	Sleeps soundly - due to exhaustion

Aim of Nursing Intervention	Plan of Care
Reduce discussion about cleansing after initial assessment	After 24 hours assessment period explain to Martin that other than at times when he is wishing to wash/clean himself these subjects are to be avoided in conversation
Increase self-esteem	Tell Martin that he is respected for recognising his problem and being admitted as this is often more difficult than ignoring it. Ask his wife to reinforce this
Reduce cost of cleansing	When 'behavioural plan' organised after assessment period cost should become reduced
Reduce need to take long routes to avoid dirty areas	As 10
Long term - that Martin can start to eat and drink outside the home	As 10. Observe whether he eats and drinks hospital fare
Prevention of diarrhoea	If Martin suspects diarrhoea or develops it due to anxiety - inform doctor and see that Martin receives appropriate medication
Reinforce Martin's masculinity	Ask Martin's wife to discuss this with him and reassure him that she sees him in a masculine vein. See 9. In addition as 10
To assess that he sleeps well in hospital	Observe Martin's sleep pattern on first night in hospital

10

Obsessional and Compulsive Neurosis

The obsessional personality is in many ways the opposite to the hysterical. The obsessional loves order and routine, sameness and reliability. He is conscientious and rather unadaptable. He does not easily lose his temper or openly show strong feelings. Unlike the hysterical personality, who concerns herself with sweeping ideals and grand designs, the obsessional is likely to become bogged down in detail and trivia. The strongly obsessional personality is liable to be a bore. Yet he is a valuable, reliable member of society. Some degree of obsessionality is necessary for anyone wishing to succeed at work or play.

Definition

An obsession is a thought, image, feeling, impulse, or movement which an individual feels compelled to carry out, usually repetitively, in spite of a strong urge to resist. He recognises that this thought or behaviour is absurd, but he cannot dispel it. *Compulsion* describes the impulse to act, and the action itself. Obsession and compulsion frequently accompany one another.

Obsessions must be distinguished from (1) *delusions*, where the idea or impulse is accepted as reasonable and is not resisted, and (2) *overvalued ideas*, like superstitions, which fall midway between the two. Obsessional compulsive states have much in common, and often co-exist with phobias. Thus the obsession of a woman that she might kill her child resulted in phobic avoidance of knives.

Incidence

Obsessional behaviour is common in children, and again in old age as people become less adaptable. *Obsessional neurosis* occurs most frequently in adolescence and early childhood. Single and transitory obsessions occur from time to time in many people. These include catchy tunes, absurd phrases, impulses to jump off high places or step in front of approaching trains.

Symptoms

Symptoms can be described under three headings:

1. *Obsessional thoughts.* These are usually of an unpleasant

nature. Blasphemous, aggressive or sexual thoughts continuously run through the mind. Fears concerning dirt, germs, and venereal disease may arise in response to guilt aroused by masturbation or some sexual incident. These sometimes become linked to religious obsessions and lead to every action being analyzed for fear it be a mortal sin.

Patients ruminate on unanswerable problems, such as 'Why are we here?'; 'Is there a God?'; 'Am I really alive?' Students feel compelled to check back to original sources for every statement, and to write an essay or read a chapter of a book may take weeks. Clerks have to check and recheck their work and are only able to keep up to date by working late into the night. Patients may become so slow and indecisive from endless questioning of the pros and cons of their actions, that everyday life comes to a halt. This is known as *folie de doute*.

2. *Impulses.* Obsessional impulses are frequently of an aggressive or suicidal nature. A patient feels an impulse to strangle her child, knife her husband, shout obscene words in church, or misbehave in public. Such feelings, which are often directed against those whom patients love most, cause intense anxiety and distress. However, it is excessively rare for patients to give way to such impulses (in the absence of serious depression), and they can usually be safely reassured.

3. *Compulsions.* Compulsions may arise on their own or as a defence against an obsession. For example, an obsessional fear of germs or dirt may lead to compulsive washing rituals. This secondary compulsion is not resisted as much as the obsessional fears of dirt, and tension is not so marked. But it is often crippling in its effects.

> A woman developed an obsessional thought that her hands were dirty and that she was in consequence likely to contaminate anyone she encountered. She formed a ritual of washing and drying her hands seven times in a row, using a clean towel for each wash. This was repeated every two hours throughout the day. Her hands became rough and sore. She had to give up her work. Social life virtually came to a halt.

Compulsions may be concerned with sexual or destructive obsessions.

> A girl of twenty was obsessed wth the idea that she would become pregnant if seminal fluid was present on anything she touched or sat on. Before she sat down she wiped the seat

> fourteen times. She changed her underclothes seven times a day, and dressed and undressed seven times on each occasion. If interrupted, she had to start all over again.
>
> A man became obsessed with the thought that he had caused a piece of glass to be chipped off his milk bottle and left inside. This he thought would be overlooked in the dairy and the customer who later received that bottle of milk would die. He therefore washed each bottle in a special way twenty-five times, five times a day, before returning it to the milkman.

All these patients realised that what they were doing was absurd, but were unable to stop themselves thinking and behaving in this way.

Resistance to such compulsions results in increasing tension until eventually they are carried out. This gives a short-lived feeling of dull relief until the compulsion returns again. Many patients become depressed by their symptoms, and this in turn causes obsessional and compulsive symptoms to increase.

Unreality and depersonalisation are quite common symptoms in obsessional neuroses. Symptoms usually begin suddenly and strongly.

Medico-legal

Although obsessional impulses and thoughts are frequently of an aggressive nature, they rarely result in harm to others. But sometimes sexual offences and cases of arson seem to be compulsive. Possibly the personality of this type of obsessional patient is less rigid than most. Resistance to the compulsion builds up tension to a level at which consciousness becomes clouded, so that fantasy is 'acted out', and the crime is then committed.

Causes

1. Heredity and early environmental influences are obviously important, but are difficult to separate. Obsessional parents not only pass on their genes, but are likely to bring up their children in an obsessional way. Over three-quarters of the patients who develop obsessional neuroses show, prior to the onset of symptoms, obsessional personality features. And over a third of the parents of these patients have had obsessional, anxiety or depressive illnesses.

2. An obsessional personality who becomes depressed is likely to develop obsessional symptoms. The presence of obsessional symptoms in depressive illness militates against suicide.

3. Schizophrenia may be ushered in by what appears at first to

be an obsessional neurosis. Usually such obsessions have a bizarre quality and the patient may not be altogether sure of their absurdity. Their presence in schizophrenia lessens the chance of serious personality deterioration.

4. Obsessional symptoms may be caused by organic conditions, such as encephalitis lethargica and brain damage.

5. Psychoanalytic theory postulates fixation at the anal level (see p. 132) – a time when a child is believed to derive sensual pleasure from his faeces; passing or retaining them, looking at and smearing himself with them. Obsessional/compulsive symptoms develop as a defence against the reactivation of such unconcious sexual and aggressive conflicts. Obsessional fear of dirt and compulsive washing, for instance, can readily be seen in such terms.

Treatment and prognosis

When severe and prolonged symptoms occur in childhood the outlook is ominous. Most obsessional illness develops slowly between the ages of 15 and 25. Many recover spontaneously within six to twelve months and some of these have no further trouble. However symptoms tend to recur, and after each episode the prognosis is less good. Symptoms generally become less troublesome in middle age. About two-thirds of patients seen by psychiatrists improve or recover fully. If symptoms have persisted unabated for more than five years the prognosis becomes poor. Increased responsibility at work or in the home is likely to cause obsessional symptoms to worsen. On the other hand danger and excitement results in improvement, as many patients discovered during wartime.

1. Psychotherapeutic support and help in avoiding or reducing anxiety are valuable, and may be all that is required in mild cases. Analysis and interpretative psychotherapy should be avoided for, in general, these do more harm than good in such cases.

2. Tranquillising drugs, especially small doses of phenothiazines, are useful in reducing anxiety. Particularly where phobias co-exist, a combination of phenelzine with a tranquilliser is helpful.

3. In recurring obsessional states, and where obsessional symptoms are coloured by depression, anti-depressive therapy with drugs, particularly clomipramine, or even *electro-convulsive therapy* may be effective. But anti-depressive treatment will not help pure obsessional states.

4. Behaviour therapy, particularly flooding, modelling (imitation learning), or methods which prevent a patient from carrying

out his compulsive acts (response-prevention, see p. 374) (astropetic therapy) provide the most promising types of treatment available.

5. Severe long-standing obsessional states, crippling in their effects, can sometimes be improved by prefrontal leucotomy, particularly when there is a marked affective component.

11
Personality and Personality Disorders

Personality is categorised in terms of types or traits. The ancient Greeks divided people into four types, depending on which of the four 'humours' predominated. Fifty years ago personality was equated with an individual's 'dominating' endocrine gland: i.e. the thyroid personality, highly strung and excitable. While hormones can certainly influence behaviour and mood their use in the classification of personality, like humours, is outmoded.

A tenuous relationship between a man's physique and personality has long been recognised. The German psychiatrist Ernst Kretschmer (1888–1964) linked schizophrenia and a schizoid personality (see below) with an asthenic build – lean, flat chested, narrow shouldered- and manic depression and a cyclothymic personality with a pyknic build – broad and thickset. Sheldon carried this work further and photographed and measured bodies from three angles. He created three somatotypes, the strength of each ranging from 1–7. An extreme endomorph (expressed as 711) he believed to be linked to a viscerotonic personality, while the contrasting ectomorph (117), goes with a cerebrotonic personality. These correspond to Kretschmer's pyknic and asthenic types respectively.

The terms *introvert* and *extravert* were first used by Carl Jung (1875–1961) to describe personality. An extravert is sociable, outgoing, a man of action rather than thought, a 'feely' rather than a 'thinky'. The introvert, on the other hand, is more concerned with his inner world. In practice there is no clear dividing line, but a continuous dimension of extraversion and introversion; most people being a variable mix of these traits (Fig. 11.1).

Jung's ideas received support from Eysenck's studies. Studying a large number of healthy and neurotic soldiers, and submitting his data to factorial analysis, he found two orthogonal bipolar dimensions of personality; these he named extraversion/introversion, and neuroticism/stability. The introvert was unsociable and cautious, and if neurotic he developed anxiety or reactive depression. The extravert, on the other hand, was outgoing, and when neurotic was liable to develop hysterical symptoms. Eysenck later claimed a third dimension, psychoticism. Eysenck went on to link his work with that of Pavlov, and suggested that extraversion was characterised by cortical in-

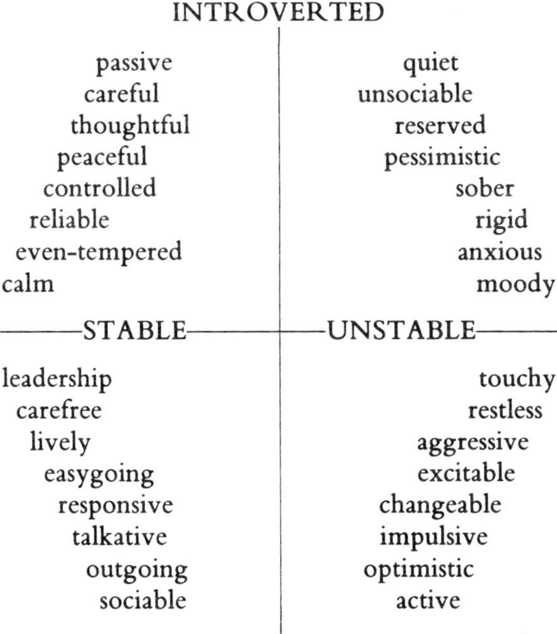

Fig. 11.1 Continuum of extraversion and introversion

hibition, introversion by excitation. There is some experimental evidence to support this.

A rather different type of classification originated with Freud. Freud remarked that young children respond pleasurably when their bodies are stimulated, sometimes intensely so. He postulated the existence of specific erotogenic zones or areas, which were readily aroused during certain specific stages of development: the mouth in the first 18 months, the anus during the next two years, and later the phallic or genital area. The development of a normal personality occurred while and as a result of the child passing successfully through these phases. Disappointments and frustrations might cause the child to become 'fixated' at any of these levels of development, and this would determine the nature of his personality. Thus the oral character is a dependent type, expecting to be cared for and looked after. The anal character is orderly, parsimonious and obstinate. Overemphasis on toilet training is given much credit for producing this type of character, although this idea seems simplistic. Those fixated at the phallic stage are likely to be rather narcissistic, ambitious and exhibitionistic.

Personality traits should ideally be measurable by objective tests.

In the USA Cattell, using factor analysis, has searched for source traits which he regards as the fundamental structure of personality. He sees a trait as a 'mental structure' which is regularly and consistently present. He claims to have isolated 16 traits, including outgoing/reserved, tense/relaxed, selfsufficient/group dependent, venturesome/shy, and so on.

None of these classifications and descriptions is entirely satisfactory, either for research or clinical work; all of them, even those claiming to be scientific, have a 'blunderbuss' quality, and lack really well defined meaning. For instance, the term *obsessional* may imply a tight control of every aspect of a man's life: neat and tidy, always on time, an unvarying routine. But many people labelled obsessional are so only in certain aspects of their lives; they work obsessionally at the office, but at home may be almost the reverse.

In practice most clinicians employ a simple descriptive classification. Many people show a mixture of personality traits, and may therefore be described in mixed terms; 'an immature hysterical personality, with obsessional features', or 'a depressive paranoid personality'. The following brief descriptions are all of an extreme type.

Hysterical personality. (Although seemingly more often applied to women, there is in fact no shortage of male hysterical personalities.)

> Maggie has always needed to be the centre of everyone's attention. No sooner is one drama over, and peace and affability restored, than another erupts. She seems continually to be playing a part. Her moods are so mercurial and changeable that those around her are rarely able to relax for long. In many ways she is like a small child, making excessive demands and exhausting her companions. She falls in love, but the lover never consistently lives up to her ideals, and always fails her in the end. Her passions appear terrifyingly strong, but they never persist for long, and she cannot understand how others cannot forget and forgive as quickly and easily as she can. A destructive scene which leaves the other person drained and on the verge of collapse is immediately followed by a vivid declaration of undying love and trust; bewildering to all but Maggie. A small slight or careless remark is sudden evidence that she is despised, and may be stored away and brought out much later during a scene, to the bewilderment of friends, who have probably long forgotten the incident.

Yet difficult and childlike as hysterical personalities frequently are, he or she is never dull, and is capable of giving a great deal of themselves to those they like and trust.

Obsessional Personality.

Harry is excessively conscientious no matter how trivial or important the task; the result is invariably good, but it takes him four times as long as anyone else. He is tidy in his dress, and frequently critical of his wife if his shirts are not perfectly ironed. He is always punctual himself, and very irritated by unpunctuality in others. In his conversation he is pedantic, and in order to be sure that he is fully understood, inclined to be repetitive. Only very occasionally is there a gleam of humour. He does not like change and is upset by any alteration in his routine. He likes to feel he is in complete control of himself and his world. He keeps his emotions well under control, and rarely loses his temper.

Interview of a patient with a strongly obsessional personality often arouses irritation in the interviewer. This comes from the resentment felt by the obsessional at the interviewer's attempts to penetrate his defensive control. The strict obsessional cannot express angry feelings openly and has to fall back on indirect outlets. He tries to control the interview by giving overdetailed answers to questions, constantly checking dates by referring to a diary, reading out notes he has made, frequently glancing at his watch, repeating unexceptional comments of the interviewer as though they are of immense profundity. Such behaviour is likely to make the inexperienced interviewer uncomfortable.

The schizoid personality lacks emotional warmth and friendliness. He is socially isolated out of choice, because he prefers his own company. He is not interested in other people and prefers to follow his own thoughts and ideas and interests, which are likely to be of an intellectual and impracticable, even bizarre, nature. For the most part he leads a quiet, uneventful life, unaggressive and unambitious (although in a job that suits his personality and intelligence he may rise high, i.e. a computer programmer or a research scientist).

The paranoid personality is likely to have few friends, not because he wants to be left alone but because he is liable, sooner or later, to perceive them as unfriendly and threatening. He is touchy, oversensitive, generally humourless – certainly lacking any sense of the ridiculous – and incapable of accepting criticism, however well meant. An inflated sense of his own worth gives him a one-sided view of his world. Everyone is out of step with him.

Inevitably he is difficult, if not impossible, to work and live with. When of outstanding intellect and drive he can, under suitable social conditions, become the leader of a new sect or political group; for instance, as Hitler did.

Depressive personality. All of us react with depression to the loss of someone we love, through death or the ending of a relationship; to failure in an important exam or interview; to loss of a job; in fact to anything that lowers our self-esteem and emotional security. In someone of a depressive type of personality this natural reaction to loss is exaggerated. Those he loves must continually reassure him that he is lovable. At work he needs a steady flow of success and praise in order to feel secure. The smallest hint of failure results in misery and despair. Pessimism and a sense of inadequacy are never far from the surface of his mind.

The cyclothymic personality also reacts with emotional excess, not only to what he perceives as failure but also to success. Like the depressive personality he is plunged into deepest gloom by loss or failure. But instead of the latter's mere pleasurable reaction to success, he reacts with wild joy and emotional abandonment. He fluctuates between depression and elation, joy and despair, between pessimism and euphoria.

The anxious personality is always apprehensive, expecting disaster to fall. And when all aspects of his life appear to be under control and going well he anticipates misfortune and trouble, and anxiously scrutinises the future. In fact, when faced with real difficulties the anxious personality is often competent and decisive, not at all prone to 'flap'. It is when he is not under pressure, when his natural apprehensions are not engaged by worrying events, that he is most likely to feel anxiety.

Narcissistic personality. (Narcissus, as a punishment by the gods, was made to fall in love with his own reflection. He died of a broken heart – and was turned into a flower.) This describes the person who is unable to separate clearly his feelings and needs from the people and events he encounters. In this sense he is like a small child. His needs are paramount. The loved one reflects his own emotional wants and feelings, and the other's requirements and satisfactions very much take second place to his. His love for anyone directly reflects that person's ability to make him feel admired and perfect. There is of course some of this quality in the relationship of most lovers, but then it is a two way process. The loved one is, in a sense, the narcissistic personality's mirror image, giving back to him all that he desires to see and feel about himself.

Work satisfies him only in so far as it enhances his self esteem. His egocentricity ensures that he is quickly disenchanted with working in a team. He needs to bask in the limelight. Not surprisingly therefore many stage celebrities have this type of personality.

When people break down they do so in characteristic ways, reflecting their predominant personality traits; the anxious personality develops an anxiety or phobic anxiety state; the obsessional personality increasingly loses his spontaneity and becomes more and more bound by routine habit as his uncertainty and distrust of himself increase; the paranoid personality's suspicions grow; the hysterical personality is more demanding and histrionic; depression overwhelms the depressive personality and so on.

Personality disorders

The term *personality disorder* is used to describe a large mixed bag of patients, whose symptoms and/or obnoxious behaviour arise from their abnormal personalities. Such abnormalities are not the result of psychosis or other illness, but arise because the development of that personality has been markedly uneven. Some aspect of the personality has failed to grow, so that in that particular area of his life the adult is still emotionally a child. He perceives and reacts in a childlike manner. His expectations are childlike. His ability to respond realistically to strains and tensions, to adapt, to learn from mistakes are limited. The result is that men and women with personality disorders create their own stresses from which they, and those with whom they are concerned, suffer in varying degree. In other arenas, people with personality disorders may well be highly responsible, successful, satisfied individuals, well thought of by their friends. Inevitably, however, if the tensions created by this disorder are great enough, they will sooner or later affect most aspects of life.

It is particularly in the area of personal relationships that personality disorders manifest themselves. Patients continually seek emotional satisfaction by ways and means which, while appropriate enough for a 5 year old, are no longer so for the adult. Their behaviour mirrors a child's conflicts, desires and anxieties, a bottomless need for love and security, a clash between longing for dependence and the urge to break away and become free and independent. Friendships and marriage come and go, each one remarkably like the last, each accompanied by emotional strains, never a lesson for the next time. Patients may be able to continue at work, unaffected by the storms outside. Sometimes the reverse occurs, a patient being unable to come to terms with authority. Resentment continually surges up and leads to repeated clashes with the boss. What was perceived as tedious, but just tolerable behaviour at school and university, becomes unacceptable at work. He is considered to be a misfit and asked to leave. Resentment mounts to bursting point, for such a patient is never in the wrong; the fault invariably lies in the boss's intractableness.

Sexual disorders of all types are related to personality disorders (these are discussed later in Chapter 12), as are many cases of drug dependence and addictive habits such as gambling. Criticism is sometimes made that anyone deviating from the social norm is liable to be labelled 'personality disorder', and by implication mentally ill. The dangers and consequences – social, political, and moral – of equating social deviance with mental illness is all too apparent. In an effort to give more precision to the term, which is essentially descriptive, the predominant personality trait of the patient is often used to qualify the disorder. Short case histories are given below:

Hysterical personality disorder. Referred by her G.P. because of depression (query a suicide risk?).

> Joan is an intelligent, attractive, well educated woman of 39. After a good degree in History she joined an advertising firm and achieved success and promotion. She then married her boss, 15 years older than herself. The marriage was disastrous from the start. The husband was 'unkind, selfish, and more interested in his work than in me'. There were violent scenes, several separations, several overdoses, and eventually a divorce. She had custody of her two children whom she looked after meticulously well. After a few years she met her present husband, 14 years older, a widower with grown-up children. He was a quiet, rather obsessional man, looking for warmth and companionship, attracted by her vivacity, capable nature, and apparent joie de vivre. The engagement was a pleasurable time and they seemed outwardly an ideal couple, complementing each other's natures. Things began to go wrong immediately after the marriage. She became jealous and possessive, making increasingly preposterous accusations and demands. On the way home from an enjoyable outing she would accuse her husband of ignoring her, paying undue attention to other women, and insulting her in public. The more the unhappy man protested his innocence, the more angry and abusive her behaviour. On occasions she physically attacked him. Once she caused him to

lose control of the car and run off the road. At another time she jumped out of a moving car and badly bruised herself. Scenes at home were accompanied by destruction of furniture. She took to rushing out of the house, screaming, vowing to kill herself. On at least two occasions she took overdoses of tranquillisers, and had to have a stomach washout in Casualty. At first these dramatic scenes, which left her husband upset and drained of energy, were followed by demonstrative reconciliations. But eventually her husband found their life together unbearable. He felt that he was living with two women in one; one a loving, still marvellous, wife; the other a malicious witch determined to destroy him. After much misery and soul searching he eventually divorced her.

Obsessional personality disorder. Referred because of recurring tension and depression.

John is 28. He joined the civil service after leaving school. He has never been able to express his feelings openly. His work dissatisfies him, understandably since the heads of the various departments he has served have arranged a transfer for him as quickly as possible. He is meticulous and very slow. The smallest decision is delayed by soul searching questions, and eventually made by an irate senior. John seethes with frustration over his indecisiveness and resentment at the cavalier manner of his boss. He has no one to whom he can let out his anger. He is regarded by most people as a dull bore. He is vaguely aware of all this, yet he seems trapped within a narrow circle of his own making, unable to escape.

Depressive personality disorder. Referred because of alcoholism and depression.

David is in his 40s. He has spent his life alternating between feeling that one moment he is a success, the next a failure. He is intelligent, hardworking and likeable and unobtrusively obsequious to his superiors at work. On the other hand he is loyal, almost paternal-like to his juniors. Tension is never far from the surface of his mind. He needs recognised success and appreciation of his ability. Even the threat of failure, however unimportant the matter, is enough to cause a black mood and heavy drinking. Beneath his outward confidence and ability lies a sense of inadequacy and failure. The more responsibility he has, the greater his apprehension and anxiety, the more difficult it is for him to delegate. No one can do the job so well as him, and he does not enjoy shared success. He is clearly on a downward path of self-destruction.

Paranoid personality disorder. Referred because of increasingly difficult behaviour at work.

Eric is 46, an efficient motor mechanic. He resents that he has never become the foreman of his section. The work of this post is well within his capacity. But Eric has always had difficulty with his work mates. He constantly complains to the management that their work is unsatisfactory, and that this inevitably upsets and reflects on his own working. He accuses them from time to time of being jealous of his careful work and timekeeping and even of deliberately sabotaging his efforts. Dislike of Eric has built up on the factory floor to a serious level, with demands for his removal from the factory.

All these four patients were unhappy, angry and anxious in varying degree. But they were not suffering from endogenous depressión, in spite of intense depression of mood and even thoughts or threats of suicide. None of them was 'mad' in the sense of totally lacking insight, although at times they may have become so tense and disturbed as to behave for a time in a psychotic manner. Their behaviour was, in certain circumscribed aspects of their lives, childlike and repetitive. It is as though a frightened child has taken control of the adult. Joan, Case 1, suddenly feels unloved, demands impossible proof that she is loveable, and in the process makes herself just that. John, Case 2, the obsessional, resembles the child who picks his way carefully over the pavement stones for fear of stepping on a crack and bringing harm to those he loves. He mistrusts himself to such a degree that any assertion of himself, any decision he makes, is fraught with danger; it is safest to do nothing. David, Case 3, seems to require repeated reassurance that he is good and therefore lovable. Eric, Case 4, deals with an innate sense of 'badness' by projecting that badness on to other people, and seeing them as threatening and hateful.

What distinguishes these patients from actual children is that most of the latter are able to learn from experience, and gradually adapt their behaviour towards realism as they grow. These patients all have an Achilles heel, some aspect of their personalities which never develops, which causes them to remain forever vulnerable; which leads them into recurrent neurotic behaviour, causing both them and others to suffer unhappiness.

The ideal treatment aims to allow the patient to become aware of the neurotic unadaptable nature of his behaviour, to help him understand how his depression and undesirable behaviour have come about, and to encourage him to accept responsibility for much of what has happened.

Psychotherapy is essential here, although how deeply the therapist probes and how subtle his interpretations will depend to some extent on the patient's intelligence and cultural background. These patients are often extremely difficult to treat, even though it may be comparatively easy to lift depression and restore calm at home and at work. It is another matter to bring about significant changes in the patient so that he can avoid repeating his unhappy past. Patients seem to understand their problems, yet fail to alter their neurotic patterns of behaviour. However, there are some who can come to recognise their apparent helplessness in this respect, and concentrate on trying to avoid those situations likely to trigger off neurotic behaviour, an advance of sorts.

Sometimes the spouse or close friend of the patient needs to be involved in treatment, perhaps individually but more likely with the patient. One objective is to expose unrecognised 'collusion' that may exist between husband and wife. For a patient's outbursts and misery will sometimes, on a subconscious level satisfy neurotic needs in the spouse.

Drugs may be helpful; an antidepressant, tranquilliser or a small dose of a neuroleptic. Ideally these drugs should be given for short periods only, to enable a patient to return to work quickly or function efficiently again at home. But all too often both therapist and patient come to rely on drugs to maintain a somewhat precarious status quo, aware that without them depression and increasing chaos will return.

Psychopathic or sociopathic disorders

Definition

A psychopathic personality is selfish and lacks foresight and feeling for others. He is unable to profit from past experience, however much this is pointed out to him. He cannot plan ahead realistically or understand the consequences of his actions. He is impulsive, like a small child, and cannot control his whims as most other people do. He feels little or no sense of responsibility, of right and wrong, or remorse for what he does. Neither punishment nor kindly treatment appear to alter him. He is impulsive and liable to explosive outbursts of violence. With other people he is continually demanding, rarely giving anything in return. He seems to be incapable of any deep warm feelings for others. Not unexpectedly, the psychopath may come into conflict with society. Perhaps because female psychopathic personalities are less likely to act aggressively, break the law and draw attention to themselves, psychopathy is considered, mistakenly, to be more common among men.

> Jane was expelled from school when she was 16 for stealing from her friends. Her parents arranged for her successively to attend a secretarial course, cookery school, flower arranging classes, and found her openings for various jobs. She either gave up or, more usual, was asked to leave within a few weeks. She stole from her parents, and was eventually thrown out by her father after selling the silver cutlery when her parents were away: 'I had run out of cigarettes,' was her excuse. Since then she has drifted in and out of prison, convicted of a variety of petty crimes, mostly shop lifting, and prostituting. She has lived with a number of men, but never stays with anyone for long. She is unhappy, unsettled and aimless, constantly appealing for help to her parents, yet making no effort to accept any responsibility for herself and her actions. Many people have tried to help her, but without success. She takes whatever she can, giving little in return.

History

In this country the concept of psychopathy was first used by the Englishman Pritchard in 1835 in connection with *moral insanity*. As a result, psychopathy became linked with the term *moral imbecile* in the *Mental Deficiency Act* of 1913. In fact there is no relationship between intelligence and psychopathy, although mental impairment and psychopathic personality can coexist in one individual.

The *Mental Health Act* of 1959 separated the two conditions. In the 1959 Act, *psychopathic personality* is defined as 'a persistent disorder or disability of mind (whether or not including significant impairment of intelligence) which results in abnormally aggressive or seriously irresponsible conduct on the part of the patient and requires or is susceptible to medical treatment'. In the 1983 Act the definition is unchanged (see p. 383).

Types of psychopath

Psychopaths are described as *inadequate* or *aggressive* on the basis of their behaviour. They are also sometimes categorised in terms of their main personality features.

The *inadequate psychopath* lacks persistence and cannot stand on his own. He never stays in a job for long, and becomes bored and depressed by routine. Everyone else is held to blame for his misfortunes, never himself. Sometimes he possesses considerable charm and is able to enlist sympathy and help from those he meets. But anyone trying to help him is likely to find himself drained dry of money and emotion. Women are sexually promiscuous and incapable of forming stable relationships. Swindlers and pathological liars are frequently inadequate psychopaths. They lie habitually, often without reason (*pseudologia fantastica*), living more in a world of fantasy than reality, unable to distinguish clearly one from the other. A number of them compensate for their inadequacies by drinking excessively or taking drugs.

The *aggressive psychopath* acts out his impulses. Explosive outbursts of anger occur, often for little or no reason. Anger may be so intense that *clouding of consciousness* develops, and what little self-control there was is lost. Brutal assaults and murders have been committed at these times. Such an outburst clears the air and for a time the psychopath feels relaxed and cheerful, but sooner or later tension returns. Sexual assaults and serious offences may occur. The psychopath's lack of social sense ensures that he is a disruptive influence in any group; he is excluded and regarded as an outsider. In consequence, he and society come to regard each other as enemies.

There is no absolute distinction between these two types. The inadequate psychopath may have explosive outbursts. The aggressive psychopath may attempt to cling to others for support. Both are childlike in their responses and this has given rise to the idea that psychopaths are immature. There is some objective evidence for this view. Electro-encephalographic patterns are often of an immature kind, particularly when there is much aggressiveness.

Diagnosis

No one should be labelled psychopathic or sociopathic without good evidence. It is unwise to diagnose a child or young adolescent as a psychopath. Such a diagnosis should never be made readily and rarely under the age of 20. Many young people occasionally react to difficulties by behaving psychopathically. Depression and psychotic illness may release psychopathic behaviour. Psychopathic behaviour may be the first sign of impending senility.

Diagnosis must depend on a good knowledge of the patient's life, his consistent inability to form close relationships and to work with other people, failture to hold down jobs, an unrealistic view of himself and his problems, and that everyone but himself is to blame for his misfortunes. It is important (but often difficult) to distinguish criminal from psychopathic behaviour; and the two obviously merge at times. The bankrobber who repeatedly goes to prison may be happily married and have many close friends; he is in no way psychopathic (whatever the reasons behind his robbing banks). The psychopath does not have the emotional ability to become a member of a robber gang (although occasionally, when talented, he may assume leadership of a gang, with horrendous consequences: for instance, Charles Manson).

Promiscuity and other immoral conduct, sexual deviance, and dependence on alcohol or drugs are not reasons, on their own, for diagnosing psychopathy and mental disorder.

Causes

Genetic. Psychopathic disorders tend to run in families. Genetic factors may predispose the personality to develop towards psychopathy, given certain types of upbringing. Alternatively, genetic factors may interfere in some as yet unknown way with the maturation of the central nervous system, so that the normal learning and development of conscience and social restraints and interactions are impaired.

Brain damage. There is an increase of brain damage and epilepsy among psychopaths, as borne out by EEG studies.

Environmental factors. These probably play a major role in the sense of providing faulty training. Many psychopaths come from unhappy homes, deprived of affection and emotional security as children. There is a strong correlation between consistent parental quarrelling and violence, and childhood antisocial behaviour and delinquency. Follow-up studies show clearly a link between childhood behaviour disorders and later psychopathic disorders. But many psychopaths come from homes that are far from unhappy, and with siblings who have developed into normal adults. It seems clear that no *one* factor can be accepted as wholly responsible for psychopathy.

Prognosis

Psychopaths are most commonly met in early adult life. Although people frequently declare that psychopathy is incurable, the fact remains that this condition often does improve with age. As instinctive urges become less strong with age, particularly from middle age onwards, so the aggressive psychopath in particular is likely to begin to mellow, and therefore adapt better to his environment. Individual psychopaths may suddenly mature and become responsible beings with the help of some devoted friend. But there is an increased mortality from suicide and accidents, and not a few spend many years in prison or special hospitals such as Broadmoor.

Treatment

Treatment is difficult and regarded by some as impossible. A patient may refuse treatment, saying that he is not ill. When admitted to a conventional psychiatric hospital or unit he is all too often a disruptive influence through his habit of 'acting out' with the other patients or staff.

1. Special hospitals, such as Henderson Hospital at Belmont, Surrey and psychiatric prisons like Grendon Underwood, specialise in treating psychopaths. Treatment is based on the concept of the therapeutic community, and on 'teaching' the psychopath to behave in a more responsible way to others. He is subjected to social pressures, of approval and disapproval from his fellow patients. Through such criticism and interaction he is encouraged to develop greater self control and toleration.
2. When psychopathy is due predominantly to brain damage, neurosurgery can be considered, i.e. temporal lobectomy (see also section 57 of the 1983 Mental Health Act, p. 388).
3. Drugs are occasionally useful. Minor tranquillisers lessen explosive outbursts – although sometimes they can, by reducing what little inhibition there is, make matters worse – undesirable sexual behaviour can sometimes be controlled with stilboestrol, benperidol, or cyproterone acetate. But the psychopathic patient is not a reliable pill taker. However he may accept injections of a longacting neuroleptic such as fluphenazine decanoate, which

lessens impulsive outbursts and thereby increases the patient's self control.

Nursing care

These patients are frequently difficult to nurse; they may resent the nurse because of the authority she represents. At one moment they appear charming and rational, and for a time young nurses may feel warm towards them. But they are persuasive and manipulative and are particularly liable to play one nurse off against another. Psychopaths also demand a great deal of the nurse's time. Much of their disruptive behaviour arises from wanting to draw attention to themselves. It is not uncommon for these patients to inflict injuries on themselves for this reason.

In order to nurse psychopathic patients with any degree of success, it is essential that nurses are aware of the nature of psychopathy, especially the childlike behaviour and difficulty in self control, even when patients are at their most charming. If a nurse knows that her patient feels little responsibility for his actions, she need not feel unduly discouraged when his behaviour becomes disruptive. If she recognises that he is manipulative, she can be on her guard.

The best attitude to adopt from a nurse's point of view, and of her patients, is one of friendly firmness. If a nurse becomes angry when she feels her patient has misbehaved and let her down in some way, she will have reacted in the way the patient intended. Ideally she should make it clear to the patient that this behaviour is unacceptable to her as a person. Although psychopathic patients find the equable nurse infuriating at times, it is usually this type of nurse who succeeds most in re-educating the patient to a limited degree and helping him to mature.

Medico–legal

A psychopath can, under the 1983 Mental Health Act, be compulsorily detained for treatment, provided such treatment is likely to alleviate or prevent a deterioration of his condition (see p. 383).

12
Sexual Development

Human sexual identity arises under the influence of several interacting components. Abnormalities can occur at any stage, resulting in sexual problems later.

Chromosomes contain the genes which initiate and control sexual development; the normal male genotype is XY, the female is XX. The basic state of 'resting tissue' is female. Differentiation to male and the development of male organs occurs only under the influence of androgen hormones. If hormonal influences fail there may be ambiguity about the individual's sex, and in extreme cases, hermaphroditism. Androgens are also of vital importance in sensitising the brain to develop towards maleness. There is a critical period of foetal growth, probably before 20 weeks, when this occurs. If androgen effects are insufficient, it seems that the brain develops among 'feminine' lines. Variations in this respect may be responsible in part for the weakness or strength of an individual's sex drive, and the nature of his sexual preferences, for instance whether he is homosexual.

But although the foundations of sex are laid down *in utero*, social learning subsequently plays a major role in equating maleness with masculinity and femaleness with feminity. As soon as the infant is recognised from the appearance of external genitalia, he or she is treated as such. Imprinting and conditioning result in the child behaving 'like a boy or girl', and what is perhaps more important, seeing himself as one. Intrapsychic factors, for instance the resolution of oedipal conflicts (see p. 38) also probably play an important role in early childhood, although the evidence for this is not well grounded. There do seem some grounds however for thinking that some individuals fail to resolve satisfactorily their oedipal conflicts, or become fixated at anal or oral levels of development, and that this may at least influence their sexual choice and behaviour later.

However the relative importance of each of these various processes is still more dependent on dogma than scientific evidence. We do not yet know precisely why most people at puberty are sexually drawn to someone of the opposite sex, or why a minority is attracted to their own sex. Is the brain conditioned *in utero* to learn more readily heterosexual – or homosexual – preferences after birth? Or is learning, especially that related to early intrapsychic struggles, more important? All we can at present say is that, from the point of view of treatment of sexual disorders, all three need to be taken into account.

Sexual Disorders

Sexual disorders are common, although it is likely that only a small proportion of dissatisfied men and women seek help. *Men* complain mostly of failing to obtain or maintain penile erection for a reasonable time, or of ejaculating far too quickly for their partner's satisfaction. They have, in other words, varying degrees of *impotence*. *Women* are more likely to complain of 'lack of enjoyment' or 'loss of interest' in sex. In spite of media emphasis on orgasm, comparatively few women complain of difficulty in this respect at initial inteviews, although it may come up later as a feature of an unsatisfactory sexual relationship. About 10 per cent of women who attend a psychosexual clinic do so because of *dyspareunia*, pain during intercourse.

Physical factors such as diabetes and multiple sclerosis, or deficiency of testosterone may occasionally be responsible for impotence or lack of ejaculation. Impotence and loss of libido are common secondary features of affective illness. And they are not uncommon side effects of drugs, particularly antidepressants and antihypertensives. But most cases of impotence and premature ejaculation have a psychological cause.

This follows similarly with women, although scarring following a clumsy episiotomy, vaginal infection, atrophy, or pelvic pathology is sometimes the cause.

Anxiety, anger or guilt are frequently present in these patients.

> A young couple had a mutually satisfying sexual relationship for three years before marrying. On the honeymoon the man became impotent and lost desire for his wife. She responded by becoming increasingly angry, and then withdrawing physically. Husband and wife were seen together six months later. It transpired that the man had not wanted to marry, and had only done so when the woman threatened to leave him. He had felt resentful and uneasy during the marriage ceremony. When, on the wedding night, his wife had talked about having children he had felt intense anger. It became clear that neither partner had much understanding of the other's emotional needs. Their sexual problem was very much a reflection of this.

Some individuals are only able to enjoy sex when it is closely interwoven with love. They feel 'protected' by a loving relationship, and can then allow themselves to lose control and experience orgasm. But there are others – men and women – who cannot enjoy sex with someone they love. Sex with their wife or husband is dull, and only exciting with a comparative stranger, or even someone they actively dislike.

Fear of pregnancy and the responsibilities of parenthood were probably important factors in the past, but effective contraception has largely removed this. Sometimes sexual difficulties are due to a mixture of ignorance and anxiety. Given the number of books, newspaper articles and broadcasts on the subject of sex, as well as school lessons on human biology, it must be rare today for anyone to be ignorant of male and female sexual anatomy. And the availability of the contraceptive pill allows sexual exploration to develop in safety and without fear, and therefore at the individual's own pace. There are plenty of misconceptions about what is 'normal'; good sex does not mean that each partner should necessarily experience orgasm everytime they make love, least of all at the same time. The insecure man or woman who refuses to 'come' until his or her partner reaches orgasm will sooner or later create sexual difficulties. In any case, some women cannot experience orgasm, or satisfying orgasm, through vaginal intercourse alone. Masturbation, or oral or anal intercourse are important for them in this respect.

Treatment of these common problems ranges from simple to complex. A thorough understanding by the therapist of the nature of the difficulty is essential, and it is best to see each partner alone (assuring each of confidentiality) and then together. The expectations and motivations of each must be explored. It is pointless offering treatment if their relationship seems doomed to end. The nature of the treatment which is being offered should be fully explained, and the commitment to it of the couple emphasised. It is essential that both partners recognise and accept that a 'cure' involves changes not only within themselves but, more important, within their relationship and how they view and treat one another.

When the difficulty is of recent onset, discussion, exploration and reassurance may be all that is required. But all too often the condition has become deep seated, through time and the inevitable vicious circle that is created through anxiety and resentment.

We believe that behavioural psychotherapy, based on the work of Masters and Johnson, is the most effective form of treatment. Masters and Johnson's work has had considerable influence on the way therapists think and on the shape of therapy. Its original elements included highly motivated couples, mostly paying sizeable sums for treatment in a holiday atmosphere, and the exploration, with a male and female therapist, of their sexual relationships and values. High success rates were reported by Masters and Johnson. These were claimed to depend on information imparted, as opposed to the correction of misinformation, desensitisation in vivo to the anxiety surrounding sexual intercourse, and increased awareness of sexual pleasure, and diffuse specific techniques, but most of all to the improved communication which developed between each of the partners.

Two important advances since that initial work are discernable. The first concerns the orgasmic training of the dysfunctional woman, and the second focuses not only on the reduction of sexual anxieties but on the heightening of sexual arousal. In orgasmic training, women move from visual and tactile exploration of their genitals to self stimulation, with a vibrator if necessary. In so doing they desensitise themselves to the former anxiety aroused by strong sexual excitement. They are encouraged, in relaxed circumstances, to enact the disinhibited behaviour they fear during loss of control in orgasm. This enactment is at first alone and then with a trusted, understanding partner.

Sexual arousal may be increased by the use of fantasy or by slides, photographs and films. If part of the problem is that one partner is less appealing to the other than the fantasy or visual material, an attempt is made to switch to him or her in the seconds before orgasm. The objective is to pair the orgasmic response to the real life stimulus partner so that a classical conditioning link is established.

Most sexual therapists speak little about the relationship of the couple to the therapist. Yet the momentum of therapy depends to a large extent on how the therapist is seen: his understanding, knowledge and competence, his trustworthiness and attachment, and how much each partner likes him.

Interpretative psychotherapy and psychoanalysis alone are not often helpful we feel in resolving sexual problems. Group therapy may be useful for some couples. The technique here involves setting tasks for each member, whose performance is then discussed and criticised by the group.

Drugs are occasionally helpful, for instance mild anxiolytics, but not on a long term basis. Marihuana has helped some couples, through its disinhibiting effects, but the drug is at not at present legally prescribable.

Homosexuality

Homosexual behaviour 'in private', between consenting adults over 21, became legal in England in 1967. It is important to distinguish between homosexual acts and homosexuality. Surveys, which are notoriously unreliable, place the incidence of exclusive male homosexuality between 1–3 per cent, and around 1 per cent for women. Homosexual experiences at some time after puberty occur to many people of both sexes, but only 3 per cent or so are persistently homosexual. Society is comparatively tolerant of homosexuals today, although to acknowledge openly that one is homosexual is still liable to influence, albeit in subtle ways, the individual's social and working life.

The causes of homosexuality are not known, although a genetic effect, operating *in utero*, may well be important. Monozygotic twins for instance are much more likely each to be homosexual than dizygotic twins, although this can of course be explained on environmental grounds.

Most homosexuals today accept their identity, although some express guilt and dissatisfaction, and a desire for heterosexuality and children. It is a waste of time, and arguably unethical, to attempt to alter someone who is exclusively homosexual by means of behaviour therapy, or to suppress his sexual feelings by means of a drug such as cyproterone acetate. Rather, any treatment should be aimed at helping the homosexual not only to accept his role but to widen his life and social activities.

Many homosexuals live openly together today, although promiscuity on the part of one or both partners is generally higher than among heterosexual partners. Sexual problems similar to those discussed above may arise, and can be treated along similar lines.

Fetishism

Some people are attracted strongly to objects other than human beings. These people are known as *fetishists*, and the object of their sexual desire a *fetish*. Most fetishists are male. Common fetishes are female clothing, especially underwear, shoes, hair, rubber and plastic sheets, silk and fur. The majority of fetishists are heterosexual. In psychoanalytic eyes the fetish symbolises and replaces a woman, and thereby becomes the object of sexual desire and the means by which the fetishist achieves sexual orgasm. A fetishist may be able to have intercourse with a woman and reach a climax, provided he can fantasise his fetish. Thus a *transvestite* wearing his wife's underpants and stockings was able to make love to his wife without difficulty. When she objected and refused to let him dress in her clothing he became impotent.

Fetishists tend not to enjoy intercourse to the full unless they can associate their female partner in some way with their fetish. *Exhibitionists* are only capable of erection and satisfying orgasm when they expose themselves to an unknown woman. Peeping toms or voyeurs who masturbate while watching an unknown woman undress, and the obscene telephone caller who has no knowledge of his female listener, thus achieve their most satisfying orgasms.

Sadism and *masochism* occur normally in both sexes in a minor degree. Extreme sadomasochistic behaviour is probably more common in the male. The sadist is aroused to orgasm by tying up his partner and subjecting her to 'discipline', i.e. by reprimanding and then beating her. The masochist can only obtain satisfaction through being ill treated and beaten. Some degree of sadomasochism is common in the fore play to lovemaking of many couples, biting, hair pulling, and so on, but it is then of secondary, not primary importance. For the masochist and the sadist, sexual pleasure is impossible without bondage and punishment. Occasionally the sadist's sense of reality is totally lost. He becomes carried away by his sadistic needs and seriously harms and even kills his partner.

Transvestism is a condition affecting for the most part men, to whom clothing of the opposite sex is a fetish. Single articles, usually underwear or stockings, may be worn, or the transvestite may dress himself as a female, complete with wig, makeup and high heels. The smell and feel of the clothing causes intense sexual excitement and orgasm. Many transvestites are ashamed of their behaviour and keep it secret and under control. Others involve their wives or women friends, in the hope of having intercourse dressed in female clothing. Some gradually lose control of their fetishistic behaviour, which then comes to dominate their lives. They spend as much time as possible dressed as women, visiting public places, sometimes with a willing accomplice.

Transvestites are mostly heterosexual and are often married with children. They are capable of leading normal sexual lives, although the pleasure they derive from this is a pale shadow of what they attain from the fetish. They have no wish to change their sex, i.e. their gender is firmly male, unlike transexuals.

Like other fetishes, transvestites are often aware of the pleasure and attraction of their fetish from an early age, although its sexual nature only becomes apparent at puberty. Cross dressing usually begins during adolescence, although it can appear later, perhaps under the influence of depression or early dementia.

Treatment Treatment is difficult, perhaps because the fetishist's motivation is poor. Many transvestites only come for treatment under pressure from wives who have inadvertently learnt of their husband's behaviour, or have become increasingly repelled by it. Psychotherapy, behavioural techniques, and most of all the co-operation of the partner, are necessary for success.

Transexualism

Transexualism differs fundamentally from transvestism in that the transexual wishes to change his or her sex. The transexual, who can be male or female, feels from an early age that he or she belongs to the wrong sex, wishes to change physically to the opposite sex, and be accepted as such by society. There are many examples of sex changes on record. One of the best accounts of changing from male to female is by Jan Morris. In her case the change seems to have been effective on all levels and resulted in a happier and more satisfying life. But this is not always the case. Above all, the personality of the transexual must be a sound stable one for him to be able to encompass such a total change.

13
Drug Addiction and Dependence

Ann Dally

No subject in psychiatry produces more disagreement than drug dependence, particularly when the drug is heroin or methadone. Most authorities, if pinned down, will admit that no one knows how to treat it and that the overall results are bad. The usual figures quoted are that no more than 10–15 per cent of patients become and remain drug-free. Nevertheless feelings run high and sometimes absurd claims are made, particularly about whether or not addicts should be prescribed drugs as part of treatment and in what form, or whether help should be limited to counselling and social support, leaving addicts to find their drugs on the black market. Since the argument is not based on scientific evidence it has become a political and moral, rather than a psychiatric issue. This unfortunate situation often prevents addicts from receiving help, which is particularly regrettable because drug dependence has become increasingly important in recent years. Heroin and other drugs have spread across the world in ever-increasing quantities, bringing with them a huge crime wave and a new 'Mafia'.

Human beings have always been liable to take in substances that are neither food nor water but which have calming or excitant effects. This is part of the search to make life more pleasurable or bearable. Spices, tea, coffee, tobacco, alcohol and opium are just a few that go back several centuries or more. More recently we have had heroin, glue and manufactured drugs. Some of these are derived directly or indirectly from natural substances, e.g. morphine and heroin from opium and cocaine from coca. Others are totally synthetic, such as methadone, barbiturates, amphetamines and benzodiazepines. During the last century increasing ease of transport and other economic factors have spread round the world what had hitherto been more localised natural substances, e.g. cocaine and marihuana. The twentieth century pharmaceutical industry has also produced powerful manufactured drugs, and this has contributed to a climate of opinion which tends towards the view that there must be 'a pill for every ill'. Drug dependence is by no means confined to illegal drugs. Many more people are dependent on drugs prescribed by doctors than on drugs obtained illegally. Recently there has been concern about the amount of 'hidden' drug dependency among people whose drugs are prescribed legitimately by doctors. The benzodiazepines in particular have come under attack. These have been prescribed on a wide scale ever since they were introduced in the 1960s and even more so since the medical profession has been warned about the dangers of amphetamines and barbiturates.

Terminology

The words 'addiction' and 'dependence' tend to be used interchangeably. Because of the difficulty of defining the word 'addiction' the World Health Organisation (WHO) has recommended the term 'drug dependence', defined as the persistent periodic excessive consumption of a drug for non-medical purposes (although initially the drug may have been prescribed for medical reasons and sometimes both doctor and patient have the illusion that it still is). In recent years moral judgments have crept into the terminology including phrases such as 'drug abuse', 'drug misuser', and 'problem drug taker'. Such terms are confusing for a number of reasons. First, there is a confusion of legal, social and medical situations in that smoking a 'joint' of cannabis (which is illegal) would be described as 'drug misuse', whereas smoking the same cigarette containing only tobacco probably would not. This is illogical. Second, it confuses moral with physiological situations. Even if one accepts that the addict 'misused' drugs to become addicted in the first place, it is difficult to say whether, having become addicted, he is 'misusing' when he takes the drug to be normal or when he abstains and therefore makes himself ill. It is probably wiser to avoid these moral issues.

Dependence should be distinguished from *habituation*.The majority of people who take nightly sedatives, daily laxatives or vitamin pills are *habituated* to these dugs. Physical dependence and tolerance do not develop and the dose remains constant.

Increasingly since the early 1960s young people have experimented with drugs, especially cannabis, lysergic acid (LSD) amphetamines and heroin. Cannabis and LSD are not strongly addictive but recently, especially when supplies of cannabis are short, they have tried *heroin*, which is strongly addictive. When heroin is short they often take whatever they can get, perhaps amphetamines, barbiturates, or even cleaning fluids and other chemicals.

Some drugs are more addictive then others. People vary in the ease with which they become addicted and the ease with which they give it up. This can be seen by observing a 'respectable' addiction such as cigarette smoking.

Any substance which alters mood or has a calming or excitant effect is an addictive drug. Addiction occurs after a period of regular or frequent use. This period may be only a few days or it may be years. Addiction involves certain changes, physical, psychological or both. These changes are:

1. The addict, until he has overcome his addiction, does not feel normal, and often cannot behave normally, unless he has a regular supply of the drug. The idea of 'drug-crazed' addicts performing evils deeds is likely to describe either those who have taken amphetamines or other stimulants or else addicts who are unable to get their supplies. This is important in view of the current confusion in terminology and the public hysteria about heroin.

2. The addict deprived of his drug develops unpleasant symptoms known as 'withdrawal symptoms'. Prolonged use of some drugs brings about changes in the central nervous system which cause physical symptoms and signs when the drug is suddenly stopped. The drugs most likely to cause this are opioid drugs (including morphine, heroin, pethidine and methadone), barbiturates, benzodiazepines and alcohol.

3. The addict craves for his drug and becomes increasingly upset if deprived of it. One has only to see the restlessness of the heavy smoker in a no-smoking situation to appreciate this. With the most addictive drugs, e.g. heroin, addicts will resort to any means – even violent crime – to obtain the drug. Thus a highly addictive drug that is forbidden is inevitably associated with a high crime rate, either to obtain the drug directly or to obtain money with which to buy it on the black market.

4. The addict becomes increasingly tolerant to the drug. A 'hardened' addict may be able to take a dose that is 10 times or even 200 times more than what would be a lethal dose for a non-addict and show little or no signs of it. In fact, addicts of stable personality can control their intake and remain normal on the same dose for many years, provided they have access to the drug. In this they resemble people who are dependent on alcohol or tobacco but nevertheless are able to control their intake to conform with socially acceptable behaviour.

Types of addiction

Opioids

This is the current word to cover not only opium and all its derivatives both natural (such as morphine) and semi-synthetics (such as heroin) and also synthetic drugs of similar chemical structure such as methadone, pethidine and dipipanone. All opioids have similar chemical structures and pharmacological effects and are to some extent interchangeable. They are all powerful killers of pain, both physical and mental and this quality and also their euphoric effects which make the user feel on top of the world, are intimately bound with their addictive qualities. Many addicts feel able to face the world and to lead normal lives with opioids but not without. Some of these are underlying alcoholics and resort to alcohol as soon as their dose of opioid is reduced. But many addicts dislike alcohol and have never been able to find the relief that many people find in it.

Symptoms of withdrawal begin about 6–8 hours after an opioid addict's last dose of heroin and 12–24 hours after a dose of methadone. These symptoms are anxiety, restlessness, yawning, sweating, running eyes and nose, nausea and vomiting, pain in the limbs, abdominal cramps and diarrhoea. Although it is often said that the withdrawal symptoms are no worse than a bad attack of 'flu, addicts will do almost anything to avoid them and this is when they are most dangerous to society and liable to commit crime as a means to obtain drugs.

Heroin, or diacetyl morphine, is the commonest opioid of addiction at present. A small amount of heroin is made legally in Britain and is sold for doctors to prescribe for the dying, for intractable pain and (by doctors holding special licences) to those few addicts who still receive it legally. But nearly all the heroin sold and used in Britain today has been smuggled into the country and sold illegally.

By no means everyone who tries heroin becomes addicted. Indeed it may be only a small, though significant, proportion. Many of those who experiment with it lose interest but an increasing number persist until they are addicted. This may happen quickly or only after years of intermittent use, often at weekends only. The idea that heroin is only addictive if injected and not if taken orally or sniffed or smoked is false. Many addicts are created by this myth. Smoking heroin is the current fashion. This is called 'chasing the dragon' and is done by sucking the smoke from heroin which has been placed on silver foil and then heated. Many people who have a horror of injecting themselves become addicted by this method and many of these go on to injecting because this is the way of making the most of what is there. Heroin is expensive. At present a heavy heroin habit costs between £50 and £100 per day. When an addict begins to inject, this is usually initially in order not to waste any. But many addicts then become as dependent on the sensation of injecting (i.e. 'needle fixation'), commonly known as a 'buzz', as on the drug itself.

Heroin addicts have a reputation derived from the worst of them, as criminal types who hang about the streets dirty, unkempt and malnourished. Yet many heroin addicts are respectable citizens with normal jobs and family lives. They keep their addiction hidden from others and have a regular source of supply that does not necessitate overt criminal activity.

Methadone ('Physeptone') is a synthetic opioid widely used in the treatment of heroin addiction, though its advantage over heroin is increasingly questioned. It was introduced as a 'non-addictive' alternative to heroin but its addictive qualities have now become apparent and some say that they are worse than those of heroin itself. As a result of its use there are now a number of methadone addicts. Methadone is similar in action to heroin but the effects last longer so that doses do not have to be so frequent and many addicts find it is more difficult to become 'high' on this drug. But withdrawal symptoms similarly last longer and many addicts and doctors believe that it is harder to overcome an addiction to methadone than an addiction to heroin. Thus the current standard treatment may actually militate against the cure.

The complications of opioid dependence are different from popular ideas about it. In itself the drug produces few side effects and, as far as is known, does not shorten life unless an overdose is taken, which may kill. Most of the long term complications are the result of illegality and of injecting. Injecting usually starts because of illegality. The constant search for drugs, the need to find huge amounts of money and the inevitable criminality lead to self neglect, malnutrition and chronic anxiety. Injecting, particularly with dirty needles and syringes, tends to introduce infection. Abscesses, septicaemia, pneumonia, hepatitis and acute bacterial endocarditis are all common in heroin addicts and kill many of them. Recently the disease AIDS has been spreading among them.

Cocaine is often said to be non-addictive but this is untrue. It is probably less addictive than heroin, but often leads to a strong psychological, though not physical, dependence. It produces increased energy and sexual drive and a sense of well-being, followed by depression, which leads to another dose being taken. It is usually taken either by injection or as snuff, often combined with heroin. If sniffed it causes ulceration of the nasal mucosa. If it is taken for long there may be toxic symptoms, such as paranoid and psychotic states, and a sensation of insects crawling beneath the skin (formication).

Amphetamines and stimulant drugs (phenmetrazine, methylphenidate, diethylpropion). In recent years the medical profession has been discouraged from prescribing amphetamines. Since this group of drugs is relatively easily manufactured by someone with a little training in chemistry, there is now a big black market of illegally made amphetamines, known popularly as 'sulphate'. These drugs create a sense of euphoria and increase activity. They may induce a strong psychological dependence, though physical dependence does not occur. They impair insight and often lead to antisocial acts, particularly of an aggressive nature. Excessive amounts (more than 50 mg per day) may lead to toxic psychosis resembling acute schizophrenia. Withdrawal leads to depression, fatigue and irritability.

Barbiturates. In recent years the medical profession has been discouraged from prescribing barbiturates. The advent of tranquillisers, particularly diazepines, has made this unnecessary in most cases. However dependence on barbiturates is still common. Smallish doses of 200–400 mg at night probably do little harm, although the electro-encephelogram pattern of sleep is altered. Daily doses of 800 mg or more, taken for several weeks, create physical dependence and result in tremor, ataxia, slurred speech and confusion. Sudden withdrawal of the drug can be dangerous, causing epileptic fits and sometimes delirium not unlike that occurring in alcoholism. Barbiturates are often combined with amphetamines.

Hallucinogenic drugs. The commonest used in western society are cannabis and lysergic acid (L S D). Psychological dependence is not uncommon. Physical dependence does not occur. The psychic experience caused by the drug is frequently over-valued. With L S D 'bad trips' occur, especially in vulnerable personalities: acute anxiety, depersonalisation and psychotic episodes may persist for months or years. A 'bad trip' may occur after many experiences of 'good trips' so no one is safe from the experience, which may lead to jumping out of a window or similar acts.

Cannabis does not create physical dependence or tolerance. But frequent use is liable to lead to withdrawal from social activities, apathy and inertia. Depersonalisation and psychotic episodes sometimes occur. There is no convincing evidence that the use of cannabis leads a person to take other drugs, except through social links. A common cause of heroin addiction is a sudden lack of availability of cannabis, leading to substituting heroin.

Treatment

Treatment ideally aims at complete and permanent abstinence from drugs. There is controversy over what help should be offered to those who feel unwilling or unable to achieve this in the near future.

Withdrawal of drugs in a patient who is unwilling is doomed to failure. If the patient is serious in intent, drugs can be withdrawn slowly on an out-patient basis or rapidly in hospital. Social and psychological support and rehabilitation are essential to both.

Heroin is traditionally treated by substituting methadone, though many now doubt the wisdom of this since increasing evidence suggests that the new addiction is more difficult to overcome than the old. It used to be thought that an alternative was a regular 'maintenance' dose of methadone or heroin. This treatment is now unpopular in official circles in Britain and drug clinics are trying to wean their addicts off all opioid drugs. It used to be thought that methadone prevented the effects of heroin but this is true only for short periods. Many addicts take methadone in the morning and heroin later in the day.

Heroin addicts who attend casualty departments with signs of withdrawal should be given 20 mg methadone orally, repeated an hour later if necessary.

Once a patient has been withdrawn he will need support and separation from his drug dependent friends. Specialised hostels, supervision, encouragement and suitable work, individual and group psychotherapy are important in his rehabilitation, which will take at least two years. Ultimately the prognosis depends on the patient's personality and motivation to remain off drugs. Ex-drug addicts have formed communities such as Phoenix House to help the rehabilitation of patients with promising results for some addicts. *Barbiturates* must always be withdrawn slowly and antidepressant drugs may be useful later, but care must be taken not to substitute one drug dependence by another.

Withdrawal from drugs is usually achieved without great difficulty in motivated addicts but relapse is common. Like the alcoholic, once addicted there is always danger of relapse, particularly during crises or even the normal stresses and strains of life. Addicts need to be helped in achieving understanding of this so that they can build up their own protective and preventive mechanisms. Finding a substitute in the form of work, an interest or in social and family relationships can make all the difference. When these are absent, unsatisfactory or geared to drugs, the prognosis is hopeless.

Barbiturates are the most dangerous drugs of addiction and withdrawal as outpatients should only be attempted with great care.

Amphetamines and *cocaine* can be stopped abruptly.

Nursing care

The nurse must seek to form a friendly relationship with her patient, aimed at restoring his self-confidence and respect. She should let him know the ward rules and routines and be positive and firm in her attitude. She must be able to recognise genuine symptoms from false ones. Particularly in the first stages of treatment drug dependent patients produce all kind of reasons why drugs should not be withheld, and they may resort to self-injury as a means to this. But they may also become depressed and suicidal. Vigilant observation is always necessary.

Needless to say patients should be searched for drugs on admission, and care taken that they do not obtain drugs from other patients or visitors. It is a sobering thought that lines of communication for future supplies of illegal drugs are often formed through new contacts and friendships made with other patients in hospital drug units.

14
Alcoholism

Definition

Addiction to alcohol is analogous to other drug dependencies. But its high, and increasing incidence, and the seriousness and width of its effects – not only on the individual, but on his family and society as a whole – make alcohol a far more serious problem. Taking alcohol in reasonable amounts is a beneficial and socially accepted custom in our culture. It is, therefore, not easy to define alcoholism. The World Health Organisation defines alcoholics as 'those excessive drinkers whose dependence on alcohol has attained such a degree that it shows a noticeable mental disturbance or an interference with their bodily or mental health, their interpersonal relations and their smooth social and economic functioning; or who show the prodromal signs of such development'. It is important to recognise that considerable differences exist in the amount of alcohol which is excessive for any one drinker and that leads eventually to his losing control over his drinking. Many of us have a degree of psychological dependence on alcohol. The alcoholic's dependence is extreme. Physical dependence occurs late in alcoholism and is always an ominous sign. Many doctors are still reluctant to make a diagnosis of alcoholism because of the stigma attached to the term.

Alcoholism is a complex problem, involving not only the medical profession but magistrates, police, lawyers, clergy, welfare workers and educational authorities among others.

Incidence

The World Health Organisation estimated in 1955 that there were about 350 000 alcoholics in England and Wales (11 per 1000), of whom 86 000 had mental and physical complications. And there is evidence that it is increasing, especially among young people. In the last 20 years the consumption of spirits has more than doubled, and of wine quadrupled. A recent survey concluded that at least half a million people had a serious drinking problem. Alcoholism occurs at all levels of society and intelligence. The incidence is six times higher in men than women but the difference is steadily diminishing.

Types of alcoholics

'Problem drinkers' is a term preferred by some authorities, as more suggestive of the width of the problem. Jellineck, who should be remembered for his pioneering work on alcoholism, constructed a classification which, although clumsy, is still useful: the *alpha* type, who drinks to relieve pain or emotional distress; the *beta* type, whose drinking has produced physical effects, such as cirrhosis, gastritis; the *epsilon* type, whose drinking is periodic, at first only at weekends or on holiday perhaps (sometimes called *dipsomania*); the *gamma* type, who has lost control and cannot stop drinking; the *delta* type who is unable to stop because of severe withdrawal effects. These types are overlapping, and a drinker may move steadily towards the two final types.

Diagnosis

Alcoholism frequently goes unrecognised for all too long. Doctors, nurses, clergymen, even those closest to the alcoholic fail, or refuse to see the problem until serious consequences make it impossible to ignore any longer. The alcoholic deceives himself, as well as others, about the amount of alcohol he regularly consumes, either openly or in secret. It is always necessary to ask how much he depends on drink, at what times of the day he drinks, especially when he starts, whether alone or in company, if he becomes drunk, suffers from loss of memory, hangovers and physical symptoms of withdrawal and how much his work and family life are affected. The young alcoholic has a strong head for alcohol and is rarely troubled by hangovers. He enjoys drinking with others and is usually one of the last to leave a party. At this stage his dependence is largely psychological.

Tolerance for alcohol progressively develops, and the alcoholic needs increasing amounts to create the same effects. He drinks in secret before parties or meetings and keeps supplies hidden in his home and workplace. His life becomes organised around his need to drink. Family finances suffer and marital problems arise. He may attempt to control himself, and to abstain altogether for days or even weeks. But sooner or later he again takes a drink, and increasingly he finds he cannot control the amount drunk. One drink leads to another and he only stops when supplies or money are exhausted. Physical changes and dependence appear. Tolerance suddenly begins to drop, so that he now becomes drunk after only a few drinks. Tremor develops. He wakes up early feeling ghastly, nauseated, shaky, unable to remember the events of the night before. He needs an immediate drink to control withdrawal symptoms, and drinking now extends through most of the day. Personal relationships suffer, he loses his job, family life is disrupted and there is a steady social decline.

Signs of physical change now appear. His manners and habits deteriorate. Judgement, insight and memory are affected. Self-control is lost. Unless he has treatment serious mental and physical complications will supervene. The more important of these are the following:

1. *Delirium tremens.* Usually, although not invariably, this follows two or three days of abstinence, the result perhaps of infection or a stomach upset. It is ushered in by tremulousness and sometimes hallucinosis. The patient is confused and frightened. Illusions, hallucinations, which are usually visual, and delusions are prominent. He is restless, sweating, pyrexial, anorexic and sleepless. Dehydration and electrolyte disturbances may be profound. Pneumonia is a common complication. Delirium tremens lasts for between 1–2 weeks, but death can occur, usually in the first week. In the recent past, the mortality rate was around 10 per cent; it is still not insignificant even with good treatment.

2. *Alcoholic hallucinosis.* The occurrence of auditory hallucinations in the setting of clear consciousness, sometimes but by no means always following withdrawal of alcohol, is not uncommon. Most cases resolve spontaneously in a week or so, but occasionally hallucinations persist for months. Sometimes hallucinosis is followed by delirium tremens, rarely by a schizophrenic illness.

3. *Paranoid states* are common in chronic alcoholics, particularly pathological jealousy for a spouse.

4. *Korsakov syndrome.* This syndrome which often develops after an episode of delirium tremens, consists of a marked loss of memory for recent events, disorientation and confabulation. The patient sometimes cannot remember what was said or done a few seconds beforehand. To fill in memory defects he makes up stories (*confabulation*) which are often convincing. There are usually, but not invariably, signs of peripheral neuritis. The outlook for full recovery is poor.

5. *Wernicke's encephalopathy.* In this condition there is disorientation, associated with paralysis of ocular muscles, nystagmus, ataxia. Like the Korsakov syndrome, which may succeed it, it is believed to be due to acute deficiency of vitamin B1, superimposed on a chronic vitamin B complex deficiency. It is rapidly abolished by injection of a high dose of vitamin B_1.

6. Other complications of alcoholism are *cirrhosis of the liver, peripheral neuritis, cardiomyopathy, acute pancreatitis, and impotence.*

7. *Damage to fetus.* Heavy drinking by a pregnant woman may result in the *fetal alcohol syndrome.* This includes abnormal facial features and retarded growth and development.

The causes of alcoholism

These are multiple, and invariably several interacting factors are present in every case.

1. *Familial.* Alcoholism runs in families. Forty-five per cent of alcoholics have parents who are or have been alcoholics. But this does not necessarily mean that alcoholism is an inherited condition. Alcoholism can be learnt by children imitating their parents' drinking habits. However, there is increasing evidence that genetic factors play some part. For instance, studies have consistently shown that men with an alcoholic parent, adopted in early life, are four times as likely to be alcoholic as sons of non-alcoholic parents. A genetic predisposition to alcoholism must act through as yet unknown enzymatic pathways involved in the body's breakdown of alcohol.

2. *Sex.* Men outnumber women by six to one, but this is probably related to environmental factors rather than to constitutional differences. However, women alcoholics have a worse prognosis than men; they are, as a group, more demoralised and depressed, and it is more difficult for them to regain their self-esteem and abandon their prop.

3. *Racial.* Family and social attitudes to alcohol exert significant effects. Alcoholism is prevalent among the Irish and rare among Jews.

4. *Social.* Although both Italy and France are wine-producing countries, alcoholism is much more prevalent in France. This is believed to be due to the fact that Italians drink mainly at mealtimes. However, the more easily and cheaply alcohol is obtainable the greater the incidence of alcoholism. This was certainly so in Hogarth's England, when a man could be drunk for one penny, dead drunk for twopence. Certain types of work, for instance brewerymen, and activities involving business entertainment, are likely to hold more than their fair share of alcoholics.

5. *Psychiatric.* Anxiety in youth, depression in middle age, and loneliness in old age are conducive to alcoholism. The incidence of depression in alcoholics, especially women, is high, and the risk of suicide much increased compared to non-alcoholics.

Detection of the Alcoholic.

It is claimed that most alcoholics can be recognised by their answers to the following questions:

a) Have you ever felt you ought to cut down on your drinking?
b) Have people annoyed you by criticising your drinking?
c) Have you ever felt bad or guilty about your drinking?
d) Have you ever had a drink first thing in the morning to steady your nerves or to get rid of a hangover?

Treatment

The type of treatment given depends on what has led the alcoholic to his doctor. The alcoholic with physical complications, such as cirrhosis, or who is on the verge of delirium tremens, invariably needs to be investigated and treated in hospital, and withdrawn from alcohol. Less severe cases can be withdrawn and treated on an outpatient basis. Delirium and agitation require sedation and skilled nursing. We prefer large doses of Lorazepam 2.5–5 mg q.d.s., but other diazepines can be used, or chlormethiazole, 1–2 g or more four times a day, up to 20 g a day. If need be the two drugs can be combined for a time. If a patient is delirious and uncooperative, drugs must be given parenterally. Fits are a withdrawal phenomenon and often complicate delirium tremens. Phenytoin is then required for a fortnight or so. Large doses of B vitamins are always given daily for a week, usually intravenously, on the supposition that the alcoholic is depleted of these. (Vitamin B1 has a specific reversing effect on Wernicke's encephalopathy.)

In the past, and still sometimes today, on the dubious grounds that this may lessen the risk of delirium tremens, alcohol is withdrawn gradually, decreasing amounts being given over the course of a week. However, with modern drugs, there seems little advantage in this.

Delirium tremens lasts between one to two weeks. However, it is sometimes four weeks or longer before a patient regains his full mental acumen. The mortality used to be around 10 per cent and is still high in the absence of good medical care.

Long term treatment. Little can be achieved for the alcoholic unless he is prepared to give up alcohol completely. Some patients cannot accept the idea of never drinking again, and with them it may be advisable to agree to a six month period of abstinence, and then to review progress. It is a vital general rule to assume that an alcoholic can never drink again, that he is always likely to be one drink from damnation, however long dry. It is claimed that some alcoholics, 10 per cent or so, can drink socially again, without losing control. This is a dangerous concept, applicable we believe, only to exceptional cases, and where close rapport exists between doctor and patient.

Inpatient treatment rarely needs to continue longer than a month. It provides a framework for the alcoholic to begin to rehabilitate himself, a springboard for the treatment which must follow.

Psychotherapy is necessary from the start. The patient's confidence must be gained, the reasons for his drinking elucidated, and ways of avoiding relapse discussed; the alcoholic may well need to change his daily habits, his acquaintances, even contemplate different work, if he is to stay dry. Steady encouragement and support are essential in the case of every alcoholic. *Group therapy* is helpful for many alcoholics in understanding themselves and their need to drink, and in the support and sense of approval provided by their peers. Meetings once or twice a week, preferably after work, may usefully continue for a year or more. Many patients derive benefit from joining a self help organisation, such as Alcoholics Anonymous, a voluntary organisation run by ex-alcoholics for alcoholics. Other voluntary bodies such as the Church of England Temperance Society and the Salvation Army also cater for the needs of alcoholics.

Drugs may be usefully given, especially at the start of an alcoholic's rehabilitation, to lessen anxiety or depression, although caution is needed in case of dependency. Depression is commonly met in alcoholics and the suicide rate is high. Lithium may be considered when cyclothymia is linked to periodic drinking.

Disulfiram and citrated calcium carbide – drugs which interfere with the breakdown of alcohol and cause unpleasant reactions if a patient drinks with them – gives a patient additional protection at the start of his treatment, or at recognisable times of vulnerability. The drawback to such drugs is that they must be taken by mouth every day. If a patient wakes up and decides to drink that day, he merely omits the drug. Ideally, the patient should agree to allow a spouse or relative or friend to oversee that he takes the drug. Subcutaneous implants of disulfiram are available, which are claimed to be effective for six months, but their effect is probably as much psychological as therapeutic, for the release of disulfiram into the bloodstream is erratic, and often too low to interfere with the metabolism of alcohol. *Aversion* therapy was widely used in the past, but rarely today.

The patient's family – often disrupted by the time he accepts the need for treatment – must never be forgotten. The wife or husband should understand why the partner drinks, how he or she needs to behave to lessen the risk of relapse, and what to do if this happens. He or she may need treatment in their own right, or attend a group with the spouse; Alcoholics Anonymous organise meetings for relatives, known as Al-Anon. Marital, including sexual difficulties, may need to be tackled and husband and wife seen together over a period of time.

For the patient who insists on 'controlled drinking', advice and encouragement and the setting of limits is essential; for instance, he should not drink outside certain hours, or only at meal times or at weekends, never on his own, and so on. Failure to follow the agreed rules must be recorded by the patient and the reasons discussed and recognised, and a lesson learnt. The more a patient willingly accepts responsibility for his behaviour, and recognises the danger and signs, the more hopeful the long term outlook. Biofeedback techniques may be helpful. The patient learns to control his intake – using a breathalyser or similar instrument – so that the level of alcohol in his blood never rises above say 50 mg %.

Treatment of the Chronic Drunken Offender. Each day, on an average, the Courts deal with some 200 drunken offences. In the past these drunks, usually homeless, jobless and friendless, revolved through Court, prison, drunkenness, Court, ad infinitum, a degrading, expensive, recurring, futile procedure. Now rehabilitation, instead of repeated prison sentences, is being attempted by means of detoxication centres, and 'skid row' hostels.

Prognosis

Prognosis depends on the patient's motivation, good support from his family, and from outside sources, whether it be individual treatment, group therapy, or attending Alcoholics Anonymous meetings. The longer a patient attends for 'help', the better the outlook, ideally five years. An alcoholic must never be abandoned. Relapse is always a possibility. The alcoholic must never be, or feel, rejected by his helpers; rather, each relapse contains a lesson to be elucidated and learnt.

John is 47 and works in advertising. He is married with 3 children. Ambitious and hard working he found himself relying increasingly on alcohol to get through his day successfully. At business lunches he averaged several gins before the meal, a bottle of wine with food, and brandy and liqueurs afterwards.

His consumption in the evening grew until his wife began to complain. He then took to drinking secretly. Eventually his performance at work declined, and he was warned by his boss. Persuaded by his wife he reluctantly sought medical help.

He refused to give up alcohol altogether, but agreed to a trial of controlled drinking. Limits were set; at a business lunch he was allowed a glass of wine, at home one whisky in the evening and 1 glass of wine shared with his wife. He was never to drink alone. His wife was interviewed with him and agreed to the programme. He himself was seen fortnightly. After two months he confessed that he was cheating and that he could not carry on without alcohol. He was now depressed in mood and anxious about his future. At this vital point he was persuaded to give up alcohol totally and to take disulfiram each morning for the next six months. His wife was closely involved and both agreed that she should give him the tablet each day to ensure compliance. Husband and wife were now seen together regularly and dissatisfactions with each other and their lives discussed, and ways in which these might be overcome.

Six years later both are more content and John still does not drink alcohol.

John Davis

The care plan for John Davis involves the initial nursing care necessary while he suffers the physiological effects of alcohol withdrawal. The emphasis of his care will have to be changed to embrace his psychological and social needs once physiological effects are minimised.

Despite the care stressing his physical needs psychological support from nursing staff is important from the beginning of his admission. His wife is involved in building John's self esteem in the care headed 'expressing sexuality'.

Once John's physical state is satisfactory a new nursing plan should be devised. It is vital that such a plan fits with the medical philosophy used on the ward to treat alcoholism. For example if a behavioural approach using antabuse is to be used, the nursing care should reflect this. It is not helpful to patients if the multi-disciplinary team's approach is not consistent. Thus discrepancies in approach by members of the multi-disciplinary team should be sorted out amongst themselves, not by demonstrating their differences to patients.

Nursing Information Sheet

Hospital No: **Wards:** / / / **Date of Admission:** 20/9/84

Surname DAVIS Forename John
Address 6, Southport Road, London
Likes to be known as: John
Date of birth: 19/7/1932 Age: 52 Sex M
Marital status: Married
Religion: R/C Nationality: English

Relevant Psychiatric and General Medical History

John first began drinking heavily two years ago after his father's death. He is now physically dependent on alcohol and has attended out-patients where he asked to be admitted for withdrawal. His raised B.P. is felt to be due to anxiety as no physical abnormality has been found by the medics.

Is patient formal or informal?

Informal

Section

Occupation and past work history

Off License Manager - Self-employed

Source of finance:

Wife still running the shop

Next of kin: Wife, Joan Davis
Address: As above
Tel. no.: 761 0091
Person to contact in case of emergency: (if different from above)
Address:
Tel. no.:

Home conditions

John lives in a large maisonette above and behind his off license shop. The premises are well maintained and there are no problems with rent.

Significant persons in life

Wife. Two teenage sons, Cliff and James

Community resources (CPNS voluntary agencies)

Has been in contact with Alcoholics Anonymous but not attended. Wife attends Al-Anon

---

Patient's profile

Height 5 ft 10
Weight 70 kgs
Build Medium
Complexion Ruddy
Hair–Colour Sandy
Eyes–Colour Blue
Marks and Scars Burn scar on left leg

Special nursing observation

Four hourly T.P.R. and B.P. during withdrawal. Ensure that no one brings John any alcohol

---

T.P.R. T 38°C P 96 R 16
B.P. 180/100
Urine Nothing abnormal detected

Reason for admission:

Withdrawal of alcohol

Referred by: Waiting List Admission
Accepted By:

G.P. Tel No.:

Dr Peter Jones 761 9991
17 High Street
Stretton
London

Present Situation	Actual and Potential Problems (Level of independence/ dependence)
1. Maintaining a safe environment Smokes about 20 cigarettes a day and at present has difficulty in lighting matches due to his hands shaking	John has difficulty lighting his cigarettes. He could burn himself
2. Personal hygiene John is sweating considerably due to alcohol withdrawal. He is able to wash and shave, although his hands shake.	He might cut himself shaving or become uncomfortable due to excess sweating
3. Special factors B.P. 180/100 on admission. T 38°C. No other physical symptoms related to withdrawal at present	Side effects of alcohol withdrawal re. raised TPR and B.P.
4. Care of clothing John was neatly dressed on admission and his wife is happy to take any washing home if necessary	
5. Co-operation in ward life John has made friends with an elderly patient and reads the paper to him. He seems to be willing to join in with activities appropriately	Potential problem that other patients may become dependent on John which may cause increased anxiety during withdrawal
6. Attitude toward medication He understands the need to take medication at the moment to prevent withdrawal symptoms	That withdrawal symptoms will occur if medication is not given 6-hourly
7. Working and playing – social mixing John still has his job but his social life involves mixing with othersin the licensing trade, he believes this could be a problem in the future	That John will drink again with his friends on discharge

Aim of Nursing Intervention	Plan of Care
To ensure that John does not burn himself or set light to anything	Assist John unobtrusively to light his cigarettes. Explain that he must not smoke in bed and why.
Prevent John cutting himself shaving. To keep John clean and comfortable	Ask John to use an electrical razor and explain why. Allow him to wash/bath frequently. Change bedclothes if necessary
Minimisation of alcohol withdrawal symptoms especially anxiety	Observe B.P. P.R.T 4-hourly. Inform medical staff if B.P. exceeds diastolic 110. Talk to John to reduce anxiety
To ensure that John has adequate clean clothing	When his wife visits remind John to ask her to take clothes that need washing
Prevent other patients depending on John. To reduce John's anxiety level if necessary	Spend time with John on each nursing shift and listen to him; pointing out he is here to help himself as well as others
Prevention of withdrawal symptoms	John should have his medication at 6 a.m., 12 mid-day, 6 p.m. and 12 midnight. Additional P.R.N. if John feels very anxious and sweats profusely
To prevent John returning to alcohol	Wait to discuss this with John until his physical withdrawal is complete unless he specifically brings the subject up

Present Situation	Actual and Potential Problems (Level of independence/ dependence)
8. Communicating John describes himself as gregarious and outgoing. He has made contact with others quickly on the ward but says he talks a lot to take his mind of wanting a drink	He is anxious and wants a drink
9. Perception John perceives his condition as a problem and is well motivated to give up alcohol. At present no delirium tremens but he says he feels anxious.	John feels anxious
10. Finance and budgeting As yet John's drink problem has not seriously affected the family budget although he says if he continues to drink it may	If John continues to drink financial problems are likely
11. Mobility John is fully mobile	Leaving the ward for alcoho
12. Eating and drinking He has lost weight recently and has been ignoring his mealtimes due to excessive alcohol consuming. He feels a bit 'sick' and doesn't want much to eat	Dehydration Vomiting Weight loss
13. Eliminating John says that he has never been incontinent even when very drunk. He normally opens his bowels every two days but has had frequent bouts of diarrhoea recently after heavy drinking	Diarrhoea
14. Expressing sexuality John says that he has lost his libido and hopes that when he is dry this will return. He expressed concern about how much he loves his wife and how unreasonable he has been to her recently	John might alienate his wif if he continues drinking
15. Sleeping John has been waking early in the morning (4 a.m.) and drinking alcohol at home	Early waking and alcohol craving

Aim of Nursing Intervention	Plan of Care
Reduction of anxiety	Respond to John whenever he seeks attention. Encourage his wife and sons to talk to him when they visit. Explain that his anxiety will reduce with time
Reduction of anxiety	Talk to John as frequently as possible at least twice a shift. Explain that anxiety is common during physical withdrawal and will reduce. Encourage him to relax using deep breathing exercises
To prevent John returning to alcohol	Discuss John's family responsibilities with him. Point out that financial matters are in his control and that his drinking is too
To prevent John leaving the ward for alcohol	One nurse a shift will be named as responsible for observing his whereabouts - John will be told who this is and why and encouraged to talk to the nurse if he feels like this
Prevent vomiting and dehydration	Weigh John weekly - report to medical staff if loss greater than 3 kg . Encourage fluids - 2000 ml/24 hr fluid input chart. Do not force John to eat if he feels nauseated but give him light, small helpings when he can manage. Review daily.
Observe for diarrhoea. Ask John to inform nurses if he has diarrhoea and give prescribed medication if necessary	Ask John to inform nurses if he has diarrhoea and give prescribed medication if necessary
To strengthen John and his wife's relationship	Ask John's wife to express her respect for John in admitting his problem and coming to hospital for help. Leave them alone during visiting
Prevention of alcohol craving	If John wakes early sit with him and give a warm drink. Reassure him that the craving will pass in time. Review daily

15
Psychosomatic Medicine

The study of psychosomatic disease – or psychophysiologic disorders – is little more than half a century old. Disorders such as asthma, neurodermatitis, peptic ulcer, ulcerative colitis, hypertension, coronary artery disease, and rheumatoid arthritis were at one time said to be typical examples of psychosomatic disease, in which emotions played a decisive role, acting through the autonomic nervous system. Deutsch put forward the idea of 'organ neurosis', part of the body sensitised from early years to react to emotional conflicts. Dunbar suggested that there were specific personality types associated with different psychosomatic diseases. Alexander postulated that specific psychodynamic conflicts resulted in certain diseases. The peptic ulcer patient, for example, was seen as having a 'dependency conflict', a powerful but ambivalent desire for love, equated with food, the conflict arising from early dissatisfactions at the breast. An anxiety-provoking situation later in life re-evoked the specific conflict over dependency and (in high pepsinogen secretors) an ulcer was formed; but while many peptic ulcer patients do show such passive dependent conflicts, many others do not. Theories of specificity failed to find confirmation from later research work, and perhaps even more important, no therapeutic benefit accrued for patients. Interest moved away from psychoanalytic ideas to epidemiology, behavioural psychology, psychosocial studies and psychophysiology. No longer is the view held that psychosomatic disorders have a specific single cause. Current beliefs are that a multiplicity of causes are present in most diseases, and that the various factors summate at the final common pathway.

Exactly what disease develops depends on (1) the presence of a pathogen, and/or (2) an organ system vulnerability, innate or acquired. Organ vulnerability may be some analogue of autonomic specificity. It is well known that when anxious, some people develop tachycardia, others get headaches, diarrhoea, or frequency of micturition, yet others outwardly unperturbed have anxiety 'come out of their arm pits'.

The proposition that liability to illness follows inability to counter stress effectively has links with Selye's work on the general adaptation syndrome, with its successive phases of alarm, adjustment and exhaustion (see p. 77). The cluster syndrome of Hinckle and Wolff, that half of all illness occurs in a third of all people, and that illness of all sorts follows 'unsatisfactory years', is another facet of the same notion. It has received support from 'life events' research; much of which is, admittedly, retrospective and open to bias of patient and researcher. The common finding is of a crescendo of life events – bereavement, job loss, marital separation, illness in the family – in the period leading up to the illness under investigation: myocardial infarction, depression, schizophrenia, subarachnoid haemorrhage, accidents and so on. Prospective studies have been few and difficult to do, but have mostly shown modest, positive correlations between event-reporting and subsequent illness.

Experimental work with animals subjected to psychosocial stress has demonstrated the emergence of physical disease. Rats raised in unusual crowded circumstances not only fight more but also develop hypertension and arteriolar changes. Whether sustained essential hypertension in man can be similarly produced is to date unknown.

Sifneos has described 'alexithymia', and suggested that this personality characteristic is often present in psychosomatic patients. They have difficulty in expressing or describing their feelings, and may indeed be totally lost for words in this respect. There is little or no elaboration of fantasy in their emotional lives. It is alleged that an intolerable affect results, and that this in turn leads to physiological dysfunction. However, in practice there is likely to be found a graded dimension of personality, between those who have few words and those who have many for their emotions. Quantitation of this personality dimension is at present under way.

No matter what future research findings are in the physical, psychological and social areas, they are unlikely to alter radically the way in which practising clinicians investigate and set about treating their patients. Adverse life happenings, including illness itself, are likely to have occurred. The patient's defensive and coping strategies have been sorely challenged. Support from kin and friends may have failed, or been inadequate in the patient's eyes. The patient's state of mind is as much a feature of his illness as are the physical aspects. In the threat-dominated mental state, anxiety and apprehension are likely to be all pervasive. When a sense of loss dominates the patient's thoughts, depression, anger, and hostility are more apparent, but depression and anxiety frequently co-exist, and it is rare to find 'pure' states. How a patient presents is therefore often complex and far from straightforward. Some patients see their problems as primarily psychological, but more often than not physical symptoms dominate the clinical picture and the patient's thinking.

A common presentation is with unrecognised somatic features of anxiety and/or depression; palpitations, muscle discomfort, tremor, sweating and the hyper-ventilation syndrome. Gastrointestinal symptoms, with loss of appetite, weight and energy, due to depression, may masquerade as neoplastic disease. At the same time it is essential for the clinician to remain on his toes and remember that neoplasia and depression can co-exist. He must always reassure himself that he has not overlooked some serious organic disease. Only when he has done this is he in a position to set about reassuring his patient and allay the hypochondriacal concern that is frequently present.

The distress of established physical illness is frequently heightened by the patient's dysphoric state. Twenty-five per cent of seriously ill patients on general wards, for instance, were found in one study to be measurably depressed. This often goes unnoticed in a busy ward, and declares itself circuitously in non-compliance with prescribed regimes, ill-advised self-discharge, or simply failure to improve as expected.

Recurring illness like asthma, neurodermatitis, or ulcerative colitis may be complicated by anxiety and depression. It is never easy to be sure which is chicken and which is egg, but in practice both physical disease and emotional upset need to be treated. The patient needs to be reassured, and his fears about the future discussed realistically but sensibly. Since this inevitably concerns close relatives, it is wise to involve them in the patient's treatment from an early stage. Psychotherapy is often ineffective until anxiety has been reduced to a reasonable level by anxiolytics, or the patient's despair has been relieved to some extent by an antidepressant.

The practice of psychosomatic medicine always involves the delineation, along physical, psychological and sociological dimensions of the causes, features and management of a patient's symptoms and distress. The issue is no longer whether or not there are such dimensions for any problem, but how great the contribution of each is to the disorder, how much one or other can be modified to help the patient. The dimensions of course are for convenience of conceptualisation and study. The whole person is affected more or less simultaneously along all three.

Myocardial infarction, sometimes followed by angina of effort, can be used to exemplify the model and to show the place of physical treatment in its total management.

Physical contributions to its causation like smoking and hypertension are too well known to need recapitulation. Their predictive power is low, and there has been an intensive search for contributory psychosocial factors. Suspected sociological influences have included urbanisation, geographical and social mobility, and status incongruity. This last is a measure not of social class (whose association with ischaemic heart disease is obscure) but of incongruity between parameters of a person's standing in society. These were, in an American study, education, occupation, income, housing, neighbourhood, religion and membership of voluntary societies. Good education with a low income, plus a deteriorating house in a well-to-do neighbourhood, would indicate high status incongruity. It is the incongruity, rather than any one parameter, that appears to correlate with ischaemic heart diseases. Job dissatisfaction, with either too much or too little *perceived* responsibility at work, also appears to heighten risk.

Personality studies have particularly highlighted the ambitious, aggressive, competitive, time-pressured Type A behaviour pattern, which is associated with a high risk of coronary artery disease in contrast to Type B behaviour. Life changes requiring adjustment were found to double above base-line rates in the 6 months before myocardial infarction in Swedish and Finnish studies, and to quadruple if the myocardial infarction was a fatal one. Life events of predesignated magnitude that were societally imposed on the individual, or 'acts of God', clustered significantly in the three weeks before the attack in men aged 30 to 65 who survived a myocardial infarction. Bereavement in widowers over 55 carries a 40 per cent increased mortality risk from cardiovascular disease in the ensuing six months.

Preventive efforts may be in the physical sphere, by reducing smoking, blood pressure, beta-lipoproteins, and perhaps by jogging. Social measures include such steps as improving support after bereavement, and psychologically by modifying Type A behaviour, persuading the patient to change to a Type B way of life (Type A – ambitious people who drive themselves to succeed, in contrast to the more relaxed Type B way of life).

Myocardial infarction not only has well known physical features, pain, arrhythmias, hypotension, and so on, but important psychosocial ones. Possible loss of earnings and the relinquishing of social roles while the patient is ill inevitably increase the patient's difficulties in coming to terms with and adapting to his illness. The decision to hospitalise or not after myocardial infarction should be weighed on social as well as medical grounds. For many patients there is little or no survival advantage in admission to a coronary care unit.

Management of the infarction and its sequelae must be along physical, social and psychological lines. Rehabilitation from the illness depends on a number of factors. Lower paid men, especially with previously poor work records, overestimate the disability due to angina or heart failure, and return to work only after prolonged absence. It is all too easy for them to assume the 'sick role' and use this to compensate for their various inadequacies. The self-employed, by contrast, return early to work and underestimate the disability compared with their physician's judgement.

Medication to combat arrhythmias, angina and heart failure may need supplementation by anxiolytics and/or antidepressants. The closer the psychiatric state is to the 'endogenous' depressive profile the more likely it is to respond to a tricyclic antidepressant, but care is required in this respect, due to the side effects of these drugs. Occasionally depression may be so severe that ECT is required. An agitated seriously suicidal patient cannot be left too long without ECT, although an interval of at least six weeks after the infarct is desirable, but the decision to go ahead with ECT at any time must always depend on the balance of risks, between the possibility of causing a fatal arrhythmia and that the dangers of the patient harming himself, either deliberately or through adverse neuroendocrine effects on the heart itself. Reactive depression, often with phobic features associated with left submammary chest pain and cardiac neurosis, is not uncommon sequelae of infarction, and may respond well to one of the MAOI.

Anxiety-heightening times that need special help are the move from the coronary care unit to a general ward, and the period shortly after the hospital is left behind. Patients who are given a firm outpatient appointment are much less likely to become disturbed and anxious than those sent home without a definite one. Many patients, and their spouses, fear that coitus may be harmful, even fatal, and virtually abandon sexual activities. Advice on its resumption, and indeed its advisability, is often important and welcomed. Death in coitus is rare, and when it does occur it usually takes place in unfamiliar surroundings, with an unfamiliar partner. However, if sexual adjustment was previously poor, one or other partner may well use the infarction as an excuse for steadfastly refusing to resume intercourse.

Return to former employment, or some modification of it, is

the usual aim unless recovery is very incomplete. Most patients are able to return to work reasonably soon, and anyone unable to do so, say, within six months of a myocardial infarction, is more likely to be disabled for psychological rather than cardiac reasons. Adjustment to enforced retirement usually needs considerable psychological assistance, particularly for a patient for whom work has been the most important element in his life.

Pain

Pain may arise unassociated with a demonstrable organic cause, or be of far greater intensity than can be explained by the physical lesion present. Such pains include headache, facial pains, left submammary pain, abdominal pain, with or without the irritable bowel syndrome, musculoskeletal pain, especially in the back, and stump and/or phantom pain after limp amputation. More than 50 per cent of patients attending gastroenterological clinics for the investigation of abdominal pain have no structural lesion found to account for their complaints.

A detailed history from the patient, and preferably from at least one close relative or friend, allows the mental state to be evaluated, and the contributory factors, recent and remote, to be assessed. The characteristics, timing, antecedents, and consequences of the pain, not only to the patient but also to those around him, are established; a 'pain diary' may be of help during the early stages of investigation. The absence of an adequate physical cause must be confirmed, if necessary after appropriate investigations, and in consultation with colleagues. Many patients are taking large amounts of analgesics, including alcohol, when first seen. Quantities are determined, for not only may these drugs paradoxically be contributing to the patient's discomfort and dysphoria, but success in subsequent treatment can in part be measured by reduction in their consumption.

Thoroughness in this appraisal contributes to an informed treatment strategy and engages the patient in the therapeutic task ahead. Particularly when pain has been present for some time an antidepressant drug may effect a 'miracle', rapidly diminishing or even removing the pain. It is unreasonable to expect a patient who has had pain in the face say, for several years, and who has already probably seen numerous practitioners without any relief, to accept that pain is psychological, an expression of depression and resentment, however apparent this may be to the psychiatrist. Once some relief has been achieved, however, (and we recognise that some degree of placebo effect is often present) the patient is ready to respond to a psychotherapeutic approach, to accept that his pain may reflect his feelings and relationships. Now family and friends may also need to be involved.

16
Anorexia Nervosa and Bulimia Nervosa

Anorexia nervosa

Anorexia nervosa is a syndrome which occurs chiefly in adolescent females, but can develop in males, and at virtually any age, although rarely before 11 years. It is characterised by (1) loss of weight, often extreme, due to the patient's *active* refusal to eat an adequate amount of food, or preventing food from being absorbed by vomiting and/or purging with laxatives, (2) amenorrhoea (unless on a contraceptive pill) and (3) preoccupation with her weight and the constant terror of fatness.

Anorexia nervosa has increased enormously in the last 30 years or so. Intelligent girls of the upper social classes are most likely to be affected, and the majority are physically attractive. The instance among schoolgirls of 16 or older in England is 1 in 250. It is as high as 1 in 100 among those attending private schools. The peak age of onset is 16 to 17.

It is convenient to divide anorexia nervosa into a *primary* or *typical* type – the majority of adolescent patients – where fear of fatness represents fear of growing up and accepting responsibility for one's own actions; and *secondary* anorexia nervosa which is mostly seen in older patients – the peak age of onset is around 23 – and is an attempt to bypass conflicts and difficulties. Vomiting and the use of laxatives are particularly likely to occur in the latter.

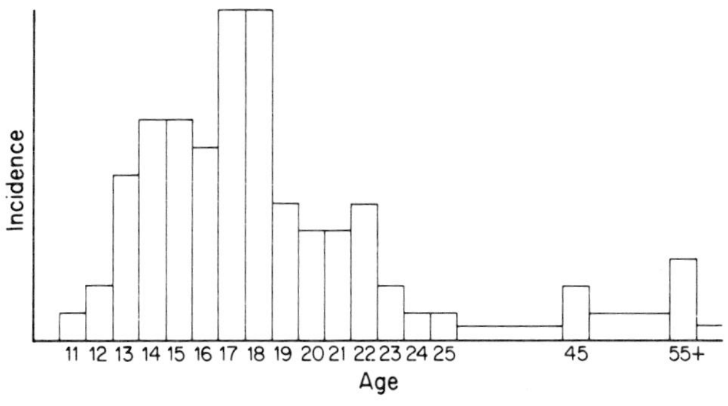

Fig. 16.1 The age of onset of anorexia nervosa

Symptoms

The girl fears that she is too fat – usually around the hips, thighs and abdomen, occasionally breasts and face – and starts to diet. At first it may be in conjunction with her school friends, part of a group activity. Or she may have been overweight and dieted with family approval. Increasingly she omits carbohydrate and fatty foods and eventually she is existing on bran, yoghurt, skimmed milk, fruit and green vegetables, and perhaps cheese. Meat may be eaten, but sometimes she has become a vegetarian even before beginning her diet. Weight can be lost slowly and progressively, or precipitously.

Alison's weight dropped from 59 kg to 36 kg in 5 months. Joanne took nearly a year to go from 54 kg to 39 kg.

Hunger is intense at first, and resisted with difficulty. But with continuing starvation this declines, and in some cases virtually disappears. The patient weighs herself frequently, even several times a day, and is elated when she finds she has lost more weight. She exercises at every available moment to increase the loss, rises from bed an hour or more earlier than usual to 'take the dog for a walk' or go for a bicycle ride. She cannot keep still for long. She looks at her emaciated figure in the mirror with satisfaction, and yet after a time this satisfaction is tinged with horror. At this stage she feels energetic and well, triumphant at her success. She is still able to concentrate on her work, although her mind is concerned with the next meal and weight. Sooner or later her family, or the staff at school if she is a boarder, become concerned. She is urged to eat more. Scenes occur at mealtimes as parents and siblings insist, ineffectually, that she must eat more. She resorts to various subterfuges, often so successfully that relatives – and nurses in hospital – are convinced that her diet is adequate and that an organic disease is responsible for the weight loss. She may insist on cooking her own meals, or eating her meals separately from the family.

After a time, although she continues to insist that she has no problem, and is still physically active, she begins to feel tired and has to push herself to keep going. Concentration is impoverished and her work deteriorates. She can think of nothing but the next meal and how to avoid eating too much. She often spends much time cooking for the family, eating nothing of what she prepares. Inwardly she is miserable. Part of her now realises that she is ridiculously, even dangerously, thin, yet another stronger part tells her that she is still too fat and distorts her perception of her body image, of how she sees herself. She withdraws from her friends, feeling that she is unlikeable and unwanted, explaining that she finds them 'boring'. She feels safer with older people. Her behaviour at home becomes more childlike. She clings to her mother, is jealous of her siblings, critical of her father. An increasing sense of ineffectualness grips her. She feels useless and incapable of almost any positive action.

Symptoms and signs of starvation add to the girl's discomfort and alarm of those around her. Downy hair grows on her back, face and limbs. The extremities become become blueish red and the skin cold and rough. Carotenaemia causes her palms and the nasal area of her face to become orange coloured. The face otherwise has a pallor which creates an illusion of anaemia. She feels desperately cold. The pulse slows, and blood pressure drops. When emaciation is extreme dependent oedema appears.

Severe weight loss itself can bring about mental disturbance, and occasionally a transient schizophrenic-like state. Certainly emotional reactions from conceptual thinking are invariably impaired. The patient by now is helplessly trapped, unable to help herself. Her image of herself is grossly distorted, and she can no longer distinguish between satiety and hunger; a morsel of cheese, a spoonful of spinach, produce a sense of uncomfortable distension and a terror of fatness.

Causes

Anorexia nervosa never, or rarely, has a single cause. In most cases a number of factors interact to produce the condition. There are at least six factors to be considered:

1. *Social and cultural.* Our culture encourages thinness in women, looks down on fatness. The thin model or actress glamorised in the mass media, provides many young women with their ideal. Anorexia nervosa is especially common among fashion students and ballet dancers, where thinness is important for success. Much more is now expected of women scholastically than in the past, and academic success looms large in their mind, particularly among those attending private schools where there are often considerable pressures to succeed. An important exam, O or A levels, frequently seems to precipitate anorexia nervosa by exaggerating the patient's unrealistic fear of failure. In a childlike way, these patients need to succeed in order to please their parents and other adults close to them, rather than themselves. They equate failure with lapse from grace.

2. *Struggle for Adult Identity*. This is an exaggeration of the normal adolescent conflicts and the ways in which they assert themselves and express their emerging sexual needs. There is often a strong conflict between desire for academic success and developing sexuality (for they tend to be both intelligent and physically attractive). Most patients are, in fact, sexually timid and immature. A scandal, involving a member of her family or a school friend, may become incorporated with her fantasies, and arouse considerable anxiety about her own self control. Strict control of her appetite through dieting reassures her that she is still in charge of herself, although of course she has virtually given up freedom to develop any real identity and autonomy.

3. *Psychobiological regression.* In addition to reassuring the patient that she is in control of herself, much loss of weight has the effect of reducing libido and sexual conflicts and allowing her to regress from emerging adulthood to childhood. So long as she starves she will not 'grow up'.

4. *Primary hypothalamic disturbance.* The hypothalamus contains the 'centres' which control feeding. Disturbances in the hypothalamus certainly exist in anorexia nervosa, especially along the hypothalamic-anterior pituitary-gonadal axis. However, it is generally believed that these changes are due to weight loss, rather than being responsible for it.

5. *Family pathology* (see p. 30 on Systems Theory). Patients with anorexia nervosa come from all types of family. Yet it is now widely accepted that anorexia nervosa is not due simply in intrapsychic conflicts. It can only be fully understood and treated if the family and the patient's role within the family are taken into account.

Many anorectics' families preserve an outward air of family harmony. Even when considerable tensions exist within a family they are not openly faced by its members. Sooner or later, often in response to a change of circumstances which upsets the earlier equilibrium, one of its members takes on a 'sick role'. Worry and concern are now directed on to him or her, and the family tensions are ignored, if not forgotten. The victim may 'punish' the parents through her demanding behaviour, but the gain to the parents is often considerable. Such parents have therefore a vested, if subconscious, interest in maintaining the child's illness.

> Mary was 16, the younger of 2 girls. Father was an obsessional man, dissatisfied with his job, continually declaring at home that

he continued his work only to provide comforts for his family. Mother was an attractive woman who always gave into her husband's demands because she disliked rows. As a result she was treated as though she were a child, and indeed behaved like one in her husband's presence. Mary was close to and sided with her mother, while her sister Alice took her father's side. Three years before Mary developed anorexia nervosa, mother began an external university degree course. She began to speak up more for herself. Tensions grew, although open rows did not occur. Mary began to diet and lose weight. Both mother and father and Alice became increasingly preoccupied and united over Mary's condition. Battles developed between Mary and the rest of the family over her eating. She always won.

She was admitted weighing 38 kg. When she regained weight family therapy sessions were held. Family relationships were explored, and Mary's fears that her parents would separate if she recovered were discussed.

In this instance both parents responded positively to treatment, the atmosphere at home improved, mother obtained a degree and started work, Mary maintained a normal weight and went on to take A levels and acquired a boy friend.

6. *Masked Depression*. The incidence of depressive illness and alcoholism in the families of patients with anorexia nervosa is raised. This increase is particularly so in secondary anorexia nervosa and in bulimia nervosa. Depression of mood is common among these patients, particularly when the illness is chronic. Suicide gestures are not unusual and the suicide rate is around 5 per cent. While depression in a parent, particularly the mother, often has an important influence on anorexia nervosa in a young adolescent patient, it seems unlikely that depression per se presents in disguised form as anorexia nervosa. Certainly antidepressant treatment has little or no lasting beneficial effect on the condition.

Precipitating factors are very varied and do not differ greatly from those found in other psychiatric illness.

1. *Loss* which upsets the patient's sense of security and equilibrium:
   (a) Fear of failure in an important exam.
   (b) Death of a family member or close friend.
   (c) Family misfortune – father's redundancy, moving from a much loved home, family loss of status.
   (d) Separation, such as going to boarding school, parents moving abroad.

(e) Children leaving home, which affects particularly older post-menopausal patients.

2. *Illness*, such as glandular fever.
3. *A family scandal*, which is usually of a sexual nature, and which arouses the patient's fears of her own self control.

Differential diagnosis

Loss of weight from refusal to eat or vomiting can occur in a number of psychiatric conditions. Severe depression can cause anorexia and amenorrhoea. A schizophrenic may refuse to eat because of delusional ideas about being poisoned. Anorexia, loss of weight and menstrual irregularities commonly result from anxiety, particularly psychosexual, in immature women. Organic conditions must be excluded, such as thyrotoxicosis, Crohn's disease and pituitary or hypothalamic lesions. It is usually not difficult to exclude these. Any signs of anaemia or vitamin deficiency should immediately raise doubts about a diagnosis of anorexia nervosa, except in much older patients and secondary anorexia nervosa.

Treatment

Before discussing the details of treatment it may helpful to list certain axioms:

1. It is essential to gain the patient's trust and co-operation from the start. Without this, a lasting recovery is unlikely. You will only gain her trust when she recognises that you understand her agonising dilemma; that part of her wants desperately to be of normal weight, but another aspect is literally terrified of putting on any weight at all.
2. Except for some patients with chronic anorexia nervosa who have been ill for years, the patient does not want to kill herself. The last thing she wants, in fact, is to die.
3. The natural history of many psychiatric disorders is towards recovery. This applies to anorexia nervosa, but emaciation blocks recovery. It is therefore vital to restore weight as quickly as possible. Psychotherapy and family therapy are, by and large, unhelpful when a patient is emaciated.
4. Anorexia nervosa invariably involves the family (or a spouse if married). Unless their problems, vis-à-vis the patient, are dealt with the hope of lasting improvement is reduced.

(A) The initial interview is of enormous importance, not only for recognising the problem and glimpsing its causes, but for therapy. The patient should be seen on her own, and then with her family. Subsequently it may be helpful to see parents or a spouse without the patient being present, but it is vital to respect the patient's confidence and always to obtain her agreement for such an interview. On occasions, particularly when weight loss is not extreme and the illness has lasted less than 18 months, and family conflicts are not excessive, the patient begins almost immediately to recover. A vicious circle has been broken due to everyone seeing the problem anew, in a different light. But more often it is apparent that the patient cannot regain weight at home and needs to come into hospital. It is useless to threaten her or to force her unwilling admission. The therapist must strike a bargain with her, after having explained why it is so vital to regain weight. Either she proves that she can increase her diet at home by gaining 1 lb a week over the next 3 weeks or if she cannot she comes into hospital. Such a bargain is nearly always accepted and adhered to. If she does begin to gain weight satisfactorily, then it is reasonable to continue to treat her on an outpatient basis, provided weight continues to move towards a mutually agreed target. If not, she is admitted.

Only in a life saving situation is it justifiable to admit a girl to hospital for refeeding against her will, usually on a Section 2 or 3 Order.

(B) In hospital most emaciated patients are at first confined strictly to bed and allowed no visitors. A final weight is agreed upon and the patient is reassured that she will not exceed this. A bland milky diet is given at first, of about 1500 calories a day – to avoid such complications as gastric dilatation or paralytic ileus – and slowly increased over about 10 days to 4 or 5000 calories a day. On this regime a patient will gain at least a kilogramme a week. Water retention often occurs at first and is later lost, which can give a distorted picture of weight gain.

Charts

It is helpful for the patient to have a weight chart kept by her bed. Targets are set on this chart which, when attained, are rewarded. Rewards include getting up for toilet, being allowed to use a telephone, to have visitors, to be up all day, choose her own diet, go home for weekends, and finally, go home for good.

Many of the younger patients are tearful and miserable, feeling abandoned and alone. It is at this point that a nurse can do so much good, taking over the role of mother to the patient, reducing her fear of putting on weight, and making her feel that she is in safe hands. It is best for an experienced nurse to bring the patient her first small meal and to remain with her. Until she has gained sufficient weight to be allowed up a nurse has to sit with the patient during each meal. As far as possible this should be the same nurse, who will then get to know the patient and develop a mutual understanding and liking.

If a patient reacts aggressively by throwing food away or regurgitating, the nurse picks up the remains and asks the patient to eat them, or if this is impracticable obtains fresh supplies. The strain imposed on the nursing staff is considerable, and it is essential that they are given adequate support. No doctor can manage any but the mildest cases of anorexia nervosa without devoted co-operation from the whole of his team.

Many patients begin to eat surprisingly quickly, and need little pressure. The initial fear and resistance give way, with friendly encouragement from the bedside nurse. The nurse must insist that she eats everything, however long she takes. In addition to supervising her eating, the nurse chats with the patient, gets to know her interests, the outline of her life, and how she sees her friends and family. Later on she can tentatively explore the fears that underlie the anorexia nervosa. When visitors are allowed there may be important observations to make, particularly the effect of one or both parents (or husband), or a sibling, on the patient's mood and her subsequent eating.

> Ellen lost a kilogramme over the week her parents began to visit. This was discussed with her, and led to Ellen confessing that she was frightened that her parents might separate. These fears were later aired during the family therapy session.

A few patients remain recalcitrant in spite of every encouragement. After 10 days or so of this, chlorpromazine should be given, the dosage ranging from 75 to 300 mg or more a day. This reduces a patient's anxiety and encourages eating, far more effectively than a benzodiazepine. Once the patient is eating readily the drug can be stopped. Older patients in particular may show signs of depression, and here a tricyclic antidepressant drug is useful. ECT is only needed today as a life saving measure. It is given on successive days. Two or three treatments only are needed before the patient begins to take nourishment. ECT is preferable to tube feeding in our view.

Once the patient has reached a reasonable weight and is out of bed, individual and group psychotherapy are started; the nature of her relationships, her fears and doubts of herself, the limits she sets for herself, are explored. Doctor and nurse, or occupational therapist or social worker, often become for a time, in the patient's eyes, parent substitutes or extensions.

The patient is now responsible for what she eats and her weight. She reaches a weight at which she can spend weekends at home. The reasons for her losing weight after a visit home are discussed, for this suggests that she is still vulnerable to family tensions. The weight chart of many patients, before they finally leave for good, become erratic, reflecting their self-doubts and uncertainties about their ability to cope. But eventually they reach and maintain their weight target.

(C) The last stage, in which the patient comes to accept her adult role and feel sufficiently confident to move away from home, to find work and make friends of both sexes, is often the most difficult. Relapse must be guarded against. It is essential therefore to see the patient regularly after she leaves hospital, to offer her support, advice and understanding. If a fall in weight persists she may need to return to hospital for a short spell, not so much for 'fattening' as to give her a rest from the tensions which are building up at home.

The majority of patients recover, but sometimes the patient is unable to free herself from her fears. After 7 years or more the condition must be regarded as chronic, although recovery is always possible if circumstances change.

> Joan developed anorexia nervosa at 17, in the year leading up to her A levels. She went on to university and subsequently trained as a teacher. Until the age of 29 her weight never rose about 40 kg and several times fell to 34 kg. Her father died suddenly and unexpectedly. She spent 8 weeks in hospital and went home to her mother weighing 40 kg. Five months later mother met and married a man not much older than Joan. Joan left home and within 4 months was living with a man almost as old as her father had been. Her weight rose to 52 kg, and menstruation resumed a year later.

Depression is common in chronic anorexia nervosa. Antidepressant drugs, or even ECT, may be indicated.

Prognosis

The vast majority of young women with primary anorexia nervosa never need to see a psychiatrist, and improve with little or no specific treatment within a year. Those who require specialised treatment are likely to take several years; 75 per cent are of normal steady weight four years after the onset, although a proportion are still preoccupied with thoughts of food.

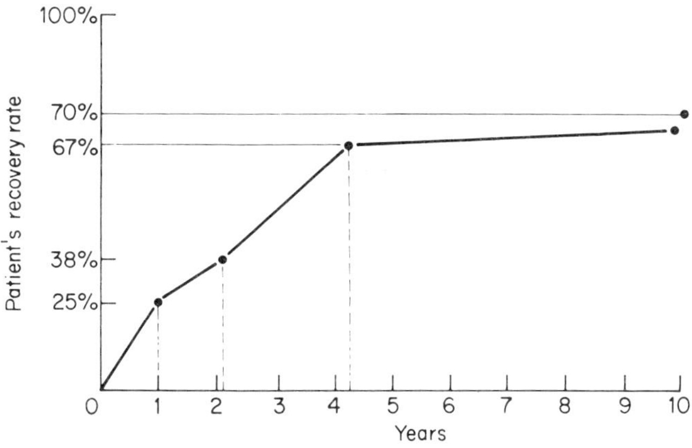

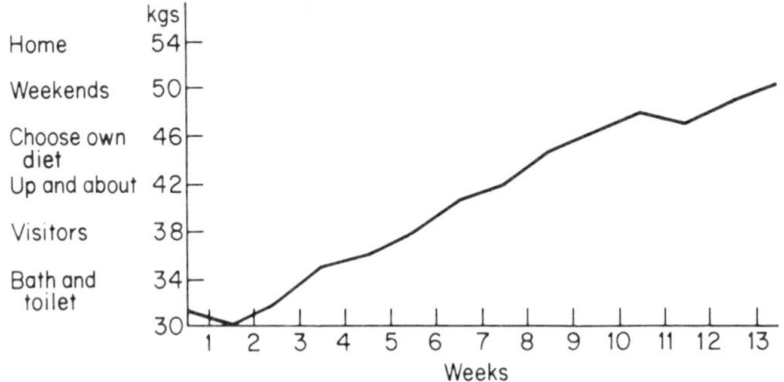

Fig. 16.2 Charts of recovery from anorexia nervosa

Those who fail to recover a normal steady weight either go on to chronic anorexia nervosa, remaining emaciated; or bouts of bingeing develop, and anorexia nervosa alternates with bingeing; or the condition evolves into pure bulimia nervosa.

Menstruation follows return of normal weight in most patients, although there may be a delay of up to a year or more. We prefer to wait for at least a year before giving clomiphene; 50–100 mg are given daily for 7 days. This is usually followed within a week by bleeding. The cycle may not immediately become regular. Although it is possible to induce menstruation in underweight patients there is no therapeutic value in doing so.

Fertility in anorexia nervosa is not later reduced. Patients who recover are able to become pregnant without difficulty, and the birth weights of their babies are normal. Indeed some patients have become pregnant before menstruation has even resumed.

Binge eating and Bulimia Nervosa

Bingeing – solitary, secretive stuffing of food excess – occurs in the obese and is not uncommon in the non-obese, especially among women. American researchers claim to find very high rates among students, as high as three-quarters of the females and nearly half of the male students. In the U K figures are more conservative. Fairburn reported 7.5 per cent of women attending a family planning clinic binged at least weekly.

Obviously, if bingeing occurs frequently, the individual must become obese unless she takes steps to prevent absorption of the food. Some bingers therefore resort to vomiting, or the use of large amounts of laxatives, separately or together, a pattern of behaviour which has been increasingly recognised in the past 10 years, and which has been named *bulimia nervosa* here and *bulimia* in the States.

Bulimia nervosa is characterised by:

1. Powerful and intractable urges to overeat.
2. Avoidance of the fattening effect of food by vomiting and/or the abuse of laxatives.
3. A morbid fear of becoming fat.

Bulimia nervosa clearly has features in common with anorexia nervosa. In fact about one-third of patients recovering from anorexia nervosa go through a transient bingeing phase. Some of those who remain ill develop pure bulimia nervosa. Others develop a mixture, or alternating phases of bulimia nervosa and anorexia nervosa. This may follow on immediately from strict dieting, or may appear some time after apparent recovery of weight.

Anorexia nervosa	Alternating anorexia nervosa and bulimia nervosa	Bulimia nervosa

Fig. 16.3 Relationship between anorexia nervosa and bulimia nervosa

Like anorexia nervosa, bulimia nervosa is far and away more common in women. The usual age of onset is the early twenties, but it can develop earlier or later.

Symptoms

The patients are gripped by an overwhelming urge to binge, which can arise suddenly 'from out of the blue', or at the end of a build up of desire which culminates in 'loss of control'. The woman may have been preoccupied all day long by thoughts of food, and may have planned a binge and bought sweets, cakes and biscuits earlier in the day. Arriving home a patient described herself as 'like an animal. If anyone interrupted me I'd go mad'. The food binged is one of the kind she normally avoids; quickly absorbed, sweet, starchy foods. But if these are not available she clears whatever is in the larder. The amount eaten is sometimes gargantuan.

> Jean ate 6 Mars bars, 2 packets of sweet biscuits, a large loaf of bread, a pot of jam, 2 lbs. cheese, 2 tins of rice pudding, a packet of fish fingers, and a large iced cake. She scarcely tasted the food, swallowed rapidly, barely chewing, and only stopped when her stomach was painfully uncomfortable. She felt heavy and depressed, but nonetheless relaxed, for she knew that she was about to get rid of the food. She drank a pint of water and vomited into the lavatory. Afterwards, cleaning her teeth she experienced a mixture of disgust and despair.
>
> Diane had been concerned about her weight since her teens. At 18 she had begun to binge and her weight rose to 81 kg. She dieted, sometimes going without food for several days at a time, but sooner or later gave in and binged. Eventually she heard about vomiting through a radio talk and began practising this after every meal. Her weight fell dramatically, but eventually she stabilised it around 52 kg. Occasionally now, if bingeing has been extreme and her weight has increased in spite of vomiting, she takes laxatives, usually 2 packets of Exlax, and very rarely a diuretic. She recognises that the habit is ridiculous, potentially harmful, and expensive, but she cannot break the habit. She is

deeply ashamed and keeps her behaviour a secret, even from her husband.

Bulimic behaviour may be continuous, the woman's life revolving round thoughts of food and weight, or episodic, occurring in response to disturbing events. The continuum kind, when extreme, brings normal working and social life to a halt. Binges occur several times a day. The woman may not be able to afford an adequate supply of foods, and resorts to shoplifting. One woman even took up prostitution to obtain enough of the 'right' food. But the majority of continuous bulimics can keep their behaviour within containable limits unless their lives become stressful. Being alone is especially dangerous for the bulimic patient. Boredom and restlessness build up and end in a binge. The housewife, alone at home, preparing the family's meal, is particularly vulnerable. She gives in gradually, picking at the food until eventually she has a full scale binge. Episodic bingers tend to have a low self esteem, and the slightest upset to their precarious equilibrium is liable to set off a bout of compulsive eating. Depression follows, and it may take weeks to regain her equilibrium. During this time she is particularly prone to further binges, and it is all too easy for a vicious circle to develop. Menstruation is usually unaffected, but bingeing often increases during the premenstrual period.

Depression of mood is common, and suicide gestures may occur which occasionally result in death. Alcohol and tranquillisers are abused, particularly by those who feel completely out of control. Smoking tends to be excessive. Compared to patients with anorexia nervosa, those with bulimia nervosa are impulsive, with little control of their appetites. Sexual activity, except after a binge, is unimpaired.

Complications

A huge binge can cause acute dilatation and paralysis of the stomach, but this is rare. Hypokalaemia and alkalosis result in cardiac arrhythmias, renal damage, tetany, paraesthesiae and fits. A painless swelling of the parotid is sometimes quite prominent. Most common is erosion of the enamel of teeth, recession of gums, and inflammation of the gastro-oesophageal junction.

Possible causes

1. Many patients were fat as children and ashamed of their state.
2. Cultural attitudes, as in anorexia nervosa, are clearly important.

3. Depression may play an uncertain role, for affective disorders and alcoholism are common in the families of bulimics.

Treatment

It is essential to gain the confidence of these patients from the start. Many of them have had bulimia nervosa for years, and have eschewed seeking medical help through shame. A patient needs to feel accepted by the therapist, and that he understands her powerlessness, and is prepared to help. A detailed account of the patient's pattern of eating must be obtained, and it is useful for her to keep a diary in which she records where, when and what she eats, and what circumstances may have triggered off a binge.

Most patients are treated on an outpatient basis, on a combined psychotherapeutic and behavioural approach. A contract is established from the start. The patient must eat three regular small meals a day, irrespective of whether she binges, make herself chew food slowly and methodically, and avoid situations which she knows from past experience are liable to provoke bingeing. If she feels she is about to be overwhelmed she must immediately describe in writing, taking at least 3 minutes, her feelings, before allowing herself to eat. (This in itself can sometimes avoid a binge.) Vomiting must be gradually reduced. When she has been regularly vomiting, three to four times a day, she must begin to reduce this progressively until after three to four weeks she has stopped vomiting, irrespective of whether she continues to binge. If she fails in this she must explain the reasons at her next interview.

The patient's ideal weight has been agreed upon by therapist and patient from the outset, and weighing must be restricted to times when she visits the therapist. The reasons for unusual weight gains or losses, and their emotional effects on the patient, must be considered.

Drugs are occasionally useful, particularly at times of crisis, or if a patient seems to have come to a serious halt. A small dose of a tricyclic antidepressant at night will relieve tension. A short-acting hypnotic – chloral hydrate is especially useful – can get a patient to sleep quickly and reduce the risk of a binge. Very occasionally an anorectic drug such as diethylpropion can interrupt a spell of increased bingeing, but more often than not it does more harm than good.

At first the patient needs to be seen weekly for 6–8 weeks. Once a normal pattern of eating has been established the intervals between interviews can be steadily lengthened over the next 6 months. Relapse is common, but is often transient, and the therapist need not despair provided the patient remain motivated. For treatment to stand a chance of lasting success, a patient's emotional problems must be explored. Frequently there is a distorted relationship with a key figure. Many patients with bulimia nervosa are living with a husband or partner, a high proportion of whom know nothing about the behaviour. This invariably reflects unexpressed conflicts and a lack of close communication. From the start of treatment the partner must be told by the patient. Ideally he should be seen by the therapist and brought into treatment.

Such treatment is time consuming. Group treatment is more economic, but not all patients respond. Lacey has devised a treatment programme over 10 consecutive weeks, which can be conducted by non-medical staff. The patient is seen for half an hour weekly to discuss her specific problems, followed by 1½ hours of group therapy. Lacey's success rate is high, because he chooses individuals who are highly motivated, and excludes anyone with a history of alcohol abuse, or of earlier anorexia nervosa.

None of the above methods is successful with patients who have totally lost control of their eating, are bingeing and vomiting repeatedly and taking large quantities of laxatives and diuretics. Such patients need to be treated in hospital, where a framework is provided wherein they can regain self control. The patient must contract not to binge or vomit, and to ask for immediate help from the nearest staff member if she feels the urge to do so. Her eating pattern improves rapidly in these protected circumstances. However, she is bound to relapse on returning home unless emotional problems are effectively tackled.

17
Affective Disorders

Depressive illness

Definition

A feeling of sadness, despair or inexplicable disinterest, is experienced by most people at some time. Characteristically it follows the loss or abandonment of some much wanted ambition or object. When personal loss is severe sadness deepens and becomes grief. The mourner for a time becomes preoccupied by painful memories and thoughts. Gradually these fade and life resumes its former course.

But sometimes sadness and grief are prolonged and exaggerated beyond what seems reasonable. Depression ceases to be merely a symptom and becomes an illness, involving widespread depression of mental and physical functions. The patient appears slow and indecisive, increasingly unable to cope with his everyday problems. Physical symptoms are often prominent, not only because bodily functions are upset but because depression lowers the tolerance for discomfort and pain.

The incidence of depression increases with age and reaches a peak in late middle age. It is rather more frequent in women than men. Depression seems to be rising in the United Kingdom, to judge by first admission rates to psychiatric hospitals and units. About one in ten of the population is liable to develop a depressive illness at some stage of his life. Recent studies have shown that adolescents and young adults quite frequently experience depression – and a number of them treat themselves with illicit drugs. The rising suicide rate in young people, when suicide as a whole has been diminishing for the past twenty years, emphasises the seriousness of depression in youth.

Classification of depression

It is still far from satisfactory. Most psychiatrists use a simple, practical classification, dividing depression into two groups, reactive and endogenous. *Reactive* depression implies that there is a strong precipitating factor, which the patient can recognise, often concerned with the loss of something or someone. Clinically, depression of mood is not deep, and may even be denied, masked by somatic symptoms and anxiety. *Endogenous* depression, on the other hand, is seen as caused mainly by a biological imbalance, arising from genetic influences, external factors being of secondary importance. Depression of mood is more severe and liable to reach suicidal depths, and instinctive activities such as sleep, appetite and libido are greatly affected.

Reactive depression is most likely to appear in middle age, although it can develop at any age, given a strong precipitant. Endogenous depression is a recurring condition of depression alone, or interspersed with mania; first attacks may develop in late adolescence or early adulthood, but can delay appearing until old age. A family history of depressive illness is more likely to be present in patients with endogenous depression.

Although psychiatrists still disagree over whether reactive and endogenous depression are separate entities, or form a continuum, stretching uniformly from reactive to endogenous, they all recognise the complexity of depression, how impossible it is to ignore environmental stresses, sociocultural factors, a patient's personality and temperament, and his psychobiological vulnerability. Nonetheless, it is clinically and therapeutically useful to make the distinction.

A classification along almost the same lines divides depression into *neurotic* and *psychotic*. *Neurotic* depression implies a highly vulnerable personality, liable from an early age to overreact to minor upsets and 'losses' with affective symptoms. *Psychotic* is similar to *endogenous* depression, genetic factors being of paramount importance.

More recently, as a result of interest in and work with lithium, endogenous depression itself has been categorised into unipolar and bipolar depressions (see below).

Symptoms

Symptoms of depression are protean. A sense of misery and sadness is usually, although not invariably present, accompanied by some degree of withdrawal from the world into oneself, loss of interest in other people, and self-preoccupation. Normal behaviour may break down; a depressed mother, for instance, reacts irritably, even violently, to the demands of her children. Fatigue is almost always present, whatever the type of depression, and is often the main complaint. Severe depression is usually unmistakable. The patient looks miserable and pessimism colours his view of himself and his future. He is indecisive, hopeless, and continually blaming himself for past peccadillos or imaginary failures. He sees only ruin and disgrace ahead; sooner or later self-punitive thoughts appear. He may show marked retardation with little spontaneous movement or talk. He may be extremely *agitated,* continually pacing the floor, wringing his hands and clasping his head. Very often there is a curious mixture of *retardation* and *agitation.* His sleep is nearly always disturbed and typically he wakes in the early hours, when depression is likely to be at its worst. In the beginning depression may lighten as the day lengthens, but later there is no lift whatever. There is usually profound anorexia and loss of weight. Constipation is a common complaint and there may be delusional ideas of being blocked or rotting internally, with hypochondriacal preoccupation. Sexual interest is lost and menstruation may cease. There may be depersonalisation and unreality feelings.

Milder depressions are less obvious and present in a variety of ways. Occasionally the patient smiles and jokes about his symptoms, although underneath he may be suicidal. Often he complains merely of fatigue and irritability, of waking tired and unrefreshed, or of no longer being able to cope with his work.

Many patients deny feeling depressed and complain only of physical symptoms for which no organic cause can be found; this is sometimes called a *masked depression.* Abdominal pain and nausea are common symptoms, and may lead to prolonged investigations. Careful questioning reveals, after negative investigation, that the patient is depressed, that the pain is really an unpleasant churning sensation in the epigastrium, at its worst on wakening. Headaches are severe and persistent and take the form of a tight band, or heavy pressure, often associated with a feeling that the head is packed with cotton wool. Pain in the back is common, and many a 'slipped disc' hides depression. Pain from muscle tension may be felt in the limbs, and is often interpreted as 'arthritis'. Any part of the body may give rise to persistent discomfort. Cardiovascular symptoms are sometimes attributed to 'blood pressure' and treatment with antihypertensive drugs makes matters worse. Palpitations, dizziness, shortness of breath, chest pain, and flushings lead to increasing anxiety; in women all this may be attributed to 'the change'. Loss of sexual potency and interest are less likely to be regarded as organic, but are sometimes dismissed as due to middle age. They can sometimes lead to marital troubles, for instance, when a wife attributes her husband's failures to infidelity.

Some depressions present as anxiety states and the underlying depression may easily be overlooked. Phobias connected with travelling, harming people, of madness or of some fatal disease are common. When these occur suddenly in middle life without apparent cause, they should always bring depression to mind. Many of the differences in depressive symptoms are the result of individual differences in personality. For instance, when very obsessional people become depressed they often develop obsessional ruminations or compulsions. One woman who has had recurring bouts of depression since her husband died is compelled during an attack always to rent an expensive flat, far beyond her means, although she has a comfortable home of her own. Another patient is impelled to steal goods from display counters. Such behaviour is distressing to the patient and she is unable to resist when depressed. In other depressed patients psychopathic behaviour is released. A faithful spouse suddenly goes off the rails, becomes promiscuous and leaves his family, or starts to drink or gamble excessively. Unless it is realised that a medical rather than a moral opinion is needed, a previously happy home is broken.

There is invariably some loss of insight in depression and a patient's explanation of his illness should often be doubted until confirmed by others. He may blame an unsatisfactory job, home or marriage for his depression, whereas the reverse may be the case. It is essential to prevent the patient from taking any action which he may later regret. Any suggestion that he should change his job or leave his wife should be firmly opposed until he has fully recovered. Only then is he capable of making responsible decisions.

Depression may occur at any age. Some authorities deny that it occurs in children, but this seems to be a quibble rather than a fact, and a condition resembling depression is clearly seen in some children. Moodiness in adolescence is normal, but full-blown depression is by no means uncommon, although this may herald a schizophrenic illness. The incidence of depressive illness increases steadily with age until the senium. Recent work has shown how frequently recoverable depressions occur in old age and how important it is to distinguish them from senile dementia whose prognosis is hopeless.

Clinical categories of depression

These are briefly described.

1. *Reactive or neurotic depression.* Symptoms of *anxiety* colour and often mask those of depression. Depression of mood is not generally deep rooted and may be temporarily lifted by pleasant

company or a change of surroundings. Symptoms tend to be at their worst at the end of the day when the patient is alone. Symptoms of anxiety and tension have often been present for many months, even years, before the onset of depression. Suicidal feelings are common but suicide itself is rare, although self-poisoning gestures may occur. These patients are more likely to attribute their troubles to other people than to blame themselves.

2. *Endogenous depression*

(a) *Bipolar or manic depression.* Kraepelin (1896) was the first to link mania and depression. He pointed out the good prognosis for spontaneous recovery, but also the tendency for recurrence. Manic depression can start at any age, but the first attack is usually in early adult life, and depressive in nature. Many patients never have an attack of mania. In others mania alternates with depression or occurs intermittently. A few patients have attacks of mania only.

Patients with manic depression tend to be of an endomorphic/mesomorphic type of body build, and to have cyclothymic extroverted personalities. Many are successful in their work, and the onset of depression with loss of drive and zest, unreasonable anxiety and pessimism creates considerable problems. Retardation is often prominent. Delusions of guilt and unworthiness may develop into delusions of persecution. Anorexia, weight loss and insomnia are marked. Physical changes are sometimes striking, the skin becomes pale, bouts of sweating occur, hair lacks lustre, boils and skin infections develop, eyelids droop and muscle tone diminishes. Depressive attacks last from a few days or weeks to years. The average time is between six to 18 months, but each patient tends to follow his own characteristic pattern. Attacks often develop suddenly with little or no prodromal warning signs, and may lift as dramatically. Attacks may occur at the same time each year, particularly spring and autumn, several times a year, intermittently at long intervals, or once only.

Recovery from depression is usually followed by an upsurge of energy and enhanced sense of enjoyment. This can be looked upon as normal, and gradually disappears. But in some patients mania or hypomania (a mild form of mania) develop.

(b) *Unipolar depression.* This describes recurrent attacks of depression without mania. There is some genetic evidence that unipolar differs from bipolar affective illness, but it is usually impossible to rule out the possibility of a manic episode in the future.

(c) *Involuntional melancholia.* This type of depression, beginning in middle age, is characterised by agitation rather than retardation (although in practice a mixture of both is usually present), hypochondriasis and paranoid delusions. If untreated, it has a poor prognosis. In fact there is considerable doubt as to whether involutional depression is a separate entity. In any case the prognostic significance of the diagnosis is lost since patients respond well to ECT and antidepressant drugs.

(d) *Depression in childhood* (see p. 201).

Aetiology

1. Genetic factors are probably important. In manic depression a dominant gene with incomplete penetrance (meaning that the condition may skip a generation) has been postulated. The concordance rates for identical and non-identical twins is 68 per cent and 23 per cent respectively, which suggests a strong genetic influence. The risk of first-degree relatives of a patient developing manic depression is considerably greater than in the general population, approaching 15 per cent. Men and women are equally affected.

A clear relationship exists between age of onset at first attack and genetic factors. Patients who develop depression for the first time after 50, and even more after the age of 65, are much less likely to possess a positive family history of affective disorder than young patients. In older patients therefore physical illness and external stresses are perhaps of greater causal importance.

2. Biochemical changes are known to be associated with depression and mania, although these may be the result rather than the cause of the attack.

The monoamine theory of depression is based on findings that dopamine, noradrenaline and 5-hydroxytryptamine (5HT), which are neurotransmitters in the brain (see p. 73), are depleted in depression and increased in mania. The evidence for this comes from (a) animal studies, (b) changes in the concentration of these substances in the CSF during affective disorders, (c) depleted amounts of monoamines in the brains of people who have committed suicide, and (d) evidence from the use of drugs in man, which either increase or deplete brain amines. Work has also been done on cyclic adenosine 3-, 5-, monophosphate formation (cAMP) and phosphodiesterase activity in the brain. It is possible that noradrenaline acts as a neurotransmitter through forming cAMP in the neuron.

Output from the adrenal glands is increased in both depression and mania, probably a stress effect secondary to the disorder itself.

3. Early childhood experiences, both psychological and physical, are important and may, by a conditioning process, invest the factor precipitating the illness with its emotional significance. Thus the loss of a parent in early childhood predisposes that person to depression in later life following a 'loss' (see p. 43).

4. Cultural influences affect both the incidence and the symptomatology of depressive illness. It is claimed that affective disorders are most common among 'people who have a high degree of social cohesion and are group centred'. Depression is inversely related to the open expression of aggression. Depressive illness and suicide rates invariably drop during times of war and during riots (see under Suicide, p. 224). Depression rises during times of unemployment.

Depression seems to be comparatively uncommon in primitive societies, and when it does occur tends to be characterised by hypochondriacal and paranoid symptoms. Self-blame and a sense of guilt, which occur so frequently in our culture, are almost never seen and suicide is rare. In our socity depression is thought to be increasing, particularly in older patients and young adults, although whether the increase is real or only apparent is hard to say.

A sense of isolation often results in depression. Old people living on their own, hampered perhaps by deafness or bad eyesight, are prone to become depressed. Lonely single people are more likely to kill themselves than those living with their families. But even families are not immune from isolation and depression. A survey of a new estate has shown that the incidence of neurotic illness is about 50 per cent higher than the average for the whole country, 'neurotic reactive depression in women' predominating. The conclusion from this survey was that each family 'kept itself to itself' producing loneliness and social isolation that led to psychiatric symptoms. Brown has shown that working class mothers who have to stay at home with young children, and who have no close communication with a partner, are particularly at risk with depression.

The menopause, between the ages of 45 and 55, is a time when women are particularly vulnerable to depression. Life suddenly appears empty, the last child has left home, a husband appears disinterested, it seems too late to take up new activities or work. The more depressed the woman feels, the more difficult it is for her to adapt and assume new roles.

5. Depression frequently causes and mimics organic disease, but especially in middle age, depression may be secondary to physical

disease, especially malignancy, where it is sometimes the first symptom.

Depression often occurs after a virus infection such as influenza, infective hepatitis, glandular fever, after operations, particularly hysterectomy, the puerperium and with endocrine disorders. Drugs such as cortisone or L-dopa may also cause severe depression. It has been estimated that about 10 per cent of patients treated for hypertension with reserpine developed depression. Weight loss can also be a precipitating factor and too-enthusiastic slimmers are sometimes seen in psychiatric clinics. Psychological factors have already been discussed and it is apparent that no single factor alone is sufficient to explain the occurrence of depression.

Differential diagnosis

Depression sometimes ushers in schizophrenia; inexplicable depression in an adolescent should always raise this possibility. Depression may be secondary to drugs, legally obtained or otherwise. The possibility of organic diseases, particularly malignancy, has already been mentioned.

Dexamethasone Suppression Test (DST)

Dexamethasone suppresses the activity of the hypothalamic–pituitary–adrenal axis. In normal people 1 mg dexamethasone given at night will inhibit corticotrophin secretion, which in turn stops cortisol production, for 24 hours. In many depressive illnesses this inhibitory action of dexamethasone does not occur. This is the basis of the DST. At bedtime 1 mg dexamethasone is given. The level of cortisol in the blood is determined next morning by a blood sample. While the test is statistically significant for depression, false positive and negative results do occur and it is an unreliable biological marker for individual patients.

Treatment

1. When discussing the value of treatment in affective disorders it is necessary to remember that spontaneous recovery, sooner or later, is virtually the rule. It may well be that time, as much as specific therapy has resulted in recovery.
2. The vast majority of patients can be effectively treated as outpatients. Inpatient treatment is indicated if the patient is a suicide risk—if a patient with endogenous depression cannot promise his doctor that he will not kill himself in the near future, he

should be admittted at once; depressed patients rarely lie, and do not 'play games'. Patients who have had numerous treatments over a year or more, without improvement, those with a particularly stressful environment, and patients who are vey much underweight may also benefit from admission. Day Hospital attendance may be advantageous for some. In many areas today, community psychiatric nurses are available to visit the families of patients treated at home.

3. Psychotherapy is particularly important in reactive depression, where emotional problems are likely to be prominent. It is important to establish a strong rapport with the patient, on which trust and mutual understanding can grow. The more neurotic the type of depression, the longer psychotherapy is likely to be needed. Psychotherapy is important even in endogenous depression, for however psychotic a patient is he still needs and is able to respond to a therapist to whom he can confess and whom he trusts. It is best to avoid comments and interpretations, or even advice, to a psychotic patient for fear of increasing his sense of guilt and, at the start, precipitating a suicidal attempt.

Group therapy, or marital therapy may be considered later.

4. Chemotherapy. Antidepressant drugs are thought to exert their therapeutic effects by raising the level of catecholamines and indolamines in the central nervous sytem. But in addition, they often improve sleep, and in small doses they are effective anxiolytics.

Tricyclic antidepressants are particularly useful in endogenous forms of depression. There are now at least twelve different kinds to choose from, and it is essential to gain experience of say three. Amitriptyline was one of the earliest tricyclics, and remains one of the most effective. It has strong sedative properties (although these often disappear after the first week), as well as being an antidepressant. Clomipramine has less marked sedative effects. It is particularly indicated when obsessional symptoms are present, and in bipolar disorders. Biochemically, its action is almost entirely confined to blocking the reuptake of 5HT, and therefore raising the concentration of that substance.

Doxepin is especially useful in old people, because anticholinergic side effects are less. It is also less likely to cause cardiac complications, and is the tricyclic of choice for a depressed patient with coronary disease.

A different group of antidepressant drugs are the monoamine oxidase inhibitors (MAOI). They are of specific value in reactive depression, and in chronic anxiety and in phobic anxiety states.

Tranylcypromine, which resembles amphetamine in its molecular configuration and in some of its effects, is very useful in reactive depression. Its antidepressant activity can be enhanced by combining it with trimipramine (see p. 360). MAOIs such as phenelzine and isocarboxazid are best used in anxiety and phobic anxiety states.

Recently, new groups of drugs have been introduced as antidepressants. The clinical indications for their use are still far from certain. *Quadricyclic* antidepressants, with four benzene rings in their central structure, include maprotiline and mianserin. Maprotiline, which biochemically blocks the reuptake of noradrenaline, seems to be useful in reactive depression; it reduces anxiety and helps sleep. Mianserin, which increases dopamine in the CNS, also seems to be most effective in reactive depression, particularly with older patients.

Although a patient with endogenous depression should be given a tricyclic antidepressant as the first choice, and one with reactive depression a MAOI, or possibly maprotiline, it is impossible to be too didactic over such choices; even today it is often a matter of trial and error. In most cases it is best to begin treatment with a tricyclic antidepressant since this is safer than a MAOI, and it is easier to change quickly to a MAOI than vice versa if the patient fails to respond. With most antidepressants there is a delay of up to a fortnight, usually five to ten days, before therapeutic effects begin to show, while side effects appear almost immediately. It is important to tell the patient about this. The antidepressant drugs are not curative. They suppress symptoms and allow a patient to cope and if necessary sort out his life problems until spontaneous remission occurs. They must be continued therefore for years if necessary. Stopping the drug too soon brings on relapse. (For details of dosage, side and toxic effects etc., see p. 356).

Lithium. Lithium has antidepressant properties, although its main action is to prevent recurring attacks of depression and/or mania. Long term lithium treatment should not be started indiscriminately. Three episodes of manic depression within two years, or an attack of depression each year for four years, unresponsive to maintenance treatment with antidepressants, are good reasons for giving lithium. Once begun and found to be effective, it may have to be given indefinitely.

Amphetamines are now rarely used. Their euphoric effects tend to be transitory and are sometimes followed by an increased sense of depression. There is also a danger that the patient may become dependent on the drug.

Tranquillisers, either diazepine derivatives or small doses of a phenothiazine such as trifluoperazine or perphenazine, are often combined with an antidepressant if anxiety or agitation are severe. The tranquillisers have no specific antidepressant action but many anxious patients undoubtedly feel more cheerful when their anxiety is relieved. Older patients in particular, with symptoms of mild anxiety and depression often respond to a tranquilliser alone.

L-tryptophan, which is the precursor of 5HT, is claimed to relieve depression and to have few side effects. It may potentiate the action of the MAOI group, but alone or with the tricyclic antidepressants its effectiveness is still uncertain.

Electro-convulsive therapy (ECT) is still the most effective treatment for depression and should be given at once if there is a serious risk of suicide. It should never be withheld for too long when a patient fails to respond fully to antidepressant drug therapy. ECT and drugs can be combined with safety. ECT is still occasionally used for the treatment of mania. It must then be given much more frequently, once or twice a day, until there is improvement, usually within a few days.

Prefrontal leucotomy may rarely be considered for chronic agitated depression which has responded well but transiently to ECT in the past (see p. 380).

Nursing care

Nursing care involves attention to all the physical symptoms which may accompany a depressive illness. Psychological care is aimed at increasing a patient's feeling of worth and self confidence, but it is not easy to convince a depressed patient that life is still worth living. The nurse should encourage the patient to participate in ward activities and entertainments, but should not force him before he is ready. He should not, on the other hand, be allowed to isolate himself completely.

If the patient expresses suicidal ideas the nurse must be especially vigilant.

Jane Miles

Jane is a 29-year-old girl who shares a flat with her boyfriend Jock. She has recently been made redundant and has become increasingly withdrawn since this occurred. She has been admitted informally with a medical diagnosis of depression.

In order that Jane's self esteem is preserved the successes of her life are promoted in her care plan. Friends are encouraged to visit and her boyfriend is asked to tell her when she looks good.

The care plan outlined may need frequent review but if she responds to the approach described her admission could be brief. It is not desirable to hospitalise anyone in her position for long as this can cause stigma (both from within the patient and society) and labelling as a psychiatric patient. Jane has been treated for depression as an Out-patient in the past and discharge to similar status may be possible soon after admission.

Jane evidently has had difficulty in adapting to her unemployed state and the nursing staff could discuss this with her. The alternatives open to Jane include getting a new job (which may be difficult) or coming to terms with her situation; free discussion about these may help Jane.

It is to be hoped that her fears of being talked about by others will reduce with her social contact on the ward. It would be important to ensure that she was not discharged to sit alone at home where such fears may return. Therefore, Day Hospital placement may be considered if she had not found new employment.

Nursing Information Sheet

Hospital No: 1234567 Wards: 1/ / / Date of Admission: 27/10/1984

Surname MILES Forename
Jane Elizabeth
Address 7A Rye Lane
Horchester, Kent

Likes to be known as: Jane
Date of birth:
7/3/1950 Age: 29 Sex: F
Marital status: Single
Religion: C of E Nationality: British

Relevant Psychiatric and General Medical History

Jane was depressed while at University in 1975. This was treated with medication by her General Practitioner over a period of six months.

Is patient formal or informal?
Informal

Section

Next of kin: Mother, Mrs A Miles
Address: 26, Church Street,
Horchester, Kent

Tel. no.: Horchester 76942
Person to contact in case of emergency: Mother A/A
Address:

Tel. no.:

Occupation and past work history

Degree in Biological Sciences. Has been working as a fashion store manageress. Recently made redundant.

Source of finance:
Unemployment Benefit

Home conditions
Jane lives in a two bedroomed flat with her boyfriend Jock. He owns the flat.

Community resources (CPNS voluntary agencies)

Significant persons in life
Boyfriend - Jock Cristy

Patient's profile

Height 5ft 7in
Weight 7 stone 12lbs

Build Medium
Complexion Sallow pale
Hair–Colour Brown
Eyes–Colour Hazel
Marks and Scars None

T.P.R. T 36.50°C 75 15
B.P. 120/80
Urine
Ward Urinalysis - nothing abnormal detected. Sample sent for drug screening, 27/10/84

Special nursing observation
Suicide risk

Reason for admission:
Jane has become increasingly withdrawn since being made redundant. In the last week she has been expressing fears about the neighbours talking behind her back. Her boyfriend eventually persuaded Jane to go to her G.P. who referred her for assessment.
? Psychotic
? Depression - Drug Abuse

Referred by: Accepted by:
Registrar to Dr Watson
G.P. Tel No.:
Dr John Walters
The Surgery
Manor Road
Horchester
Kent

Present Situation	Actual and Potential Problems (Level of independence/ dependence)
1. Maintaining a safe environment Jane is mobile and in touch with reality - she is considered to be potentially suicidal	Jane is a potential suicidal risk
2. Personal hygiene Jane said she normally bathes every morning and washes her hair twice a week. At present she has not bathed for a week because she says 'I'm a filthy person and no amount of washing will cleanse me'	Personal hygiene poor, Jane may be avoided by other people unless she washes regularly
3. Special factors Jane is considered to be a suicidal risk by the medical staff	Potential suicidal risk. Request for close observation by medical staff
4. Care of clothing Jane says she doesn't care what she wears any more. On admission she was dressed in ill matching clothes and had ladders in her tights. Her boyfriend says her appearance is upsetting him as Jane is usually immaculate and dressed well	Jane's dress is upsetting her boyfriend and contributing to her own sense of being worthless
5. Co-operation in ward life Jane responded politely when introduced to other ward members but expressed a desire to be left alone for a while in order to 'settle in'	Jane may become increasingly isolated if left alone too long to settle in to the ward
6. Attitude toward medication Jane is not on any medication at present	
7. Working and playing – social mixing Prior to being made redundant, Jane efficiently managed a dress shop - she said that she lost her job because the shop was sold, not for any other reason. She has not made any attempt to get another job. Jane enjoys shopping in markets and her social life tends to be orientated towards doing this with Jock. She has begun to isolate herself - does not go out without Jock at all	Jane's friends may stop visitin[g] if she does not respond to them The longer Jane has no job the less likely she is to get one.

Aim of Nursing Intervention	Plan of Care
To prevent suicidal attempts	See 3. Establish that Jane has no dangerous objects that she could hurt herself with re. scissors, tablets
To encourage Jane to re-establish her normal pattern of personal hygiene	Jane should have a bath and wash her hair at least twice a week. If she wishes to bathe more often, this should be encouraged. Ensure she has wash things, towel, etc. Do not allow her to lock herself in the bathroom at present
	Observation of Jane at all times. At the beginning of each shift nurses should be allocated for 1-2 hours at a time to do this
To improve Jane's self-esteem and improve Jock's feelings of distress when seeing Jane so untidy	Encourage Jane to wash and iron her clothes. Ask her to select clothes to wear that she normally wears together
To give Jane a period to settle in to the ward prior to encouraging her to join in activities	Jane should be allowed time to herself. Review this in 3 days. Encourage her to mix with other patients at mealtimes
1 To establish Jane's social life 2 That Jane applies for jobs	Welcome Jane's friends and see that they know the visiting periods. Jock can take her for a walk when he visits if he wants to. Review in 1 week. Talk to Jane about the kind of work she would like in the future. Review in 1 week with regard to job applications

Present Situation	Actual and Potential Problems (Level of independence/ dependence)
8. Communicating	
Jane speaks clearly and quietly when spoken to. She does not initiate conversation. She looks away when eye contact is established and when sitting alone stares into space and hugs her arms to her body	Jane is isolated and is giving non-verbal messages that she wishes to be alone
9. Perception	
Jane says that she feels a failure, that she has let everyone down. She also says that Jock can't love her anymore and he has given her up by bringing her into hospital. In addition she believes 'she is dirty' - See 2	Jane's self-esteem is very low. She feels that admission is a rejection by others
10. Finance and budgeting	
Jane is entitled to earnings related employment benefit. She contributes to the flat finances but has saved money both while in employment and during unemployment	Jane manages her finances well
11. Mobility	
Jane is physically mobile and there is no evidence of any problems. She does sit alone for long periods but moves appropriately. NORTON SCALE 4	Jane is fully mobile (refer to 1)
12. Eating and drinking	
In the last six weeks Jane has lost over a stone in weight. She says that she is not interested in food, can't be bothered to prepare it and often feels physically sick when presented with a meal	Jane has lost weight and feels sick when presented with food
13. Eliminating	
Jane reports no problems with eliminating. Urine - nothing abnormal detected	Potential problem of constipation if Jane does not eat or take any exercise
14. Expressing sexuality	
Jane looks unattractive at the moment. Her boyfriend says that they usually have a 'normal' sex life but that Jane's libido has reduced since she has been at home all day	Jane looks ill-kept and unattractive. Her libido is reduced
15. Sleeping	
Jane has never required medication to help her sleep. At the moment she reports having difficulty in going to sleep and this causes her anxiety. She sleeps well once she is asleep. Sometimes a warm drink helps at home	Jane has difficulty in going off to sleep

Aim of Nursing Intervention	Plan of Care
1 To listen and talk with Jane 2 That Jane initiates conversation	Jane's nurse should initiate conversation with her for at least ½ hour in each shift. Observe Jane's self-esteem and willingness to communicate. Review 1 week
To improve Jane's self-esteem and reduce her feelings of rejection	Point out to Jane how successful she has been and encourage her visitors to do same. Assure her that she is <u>not</u> dirty and try to divert this type of conversation into positive areas (i.e. washing, the future)
To establish that Jane continues to claim her benefits while in hospital	Refer Jane to the social worker to ensure she gets benefits while in hospital
	Ensure that Jane does not leave the ward unaccompanied. This is the responsibility of the nurse observing Jane
That Jane is well hydrated and begins to put on some of the weight she has lost	Weigh weekly. 1500 ml fluids/day on a fluid chart. Jane likes hot chocolate made with milk - she can be given this in place of a meal if she feels sick. Review 1 week
Prevention of constipation	Encourage light exercise i.e. walking around the grounds. Fresh fruit if Jane will eat it. Ask Jane to tell us if she is constipated
To improve Jane's appearance and raise her self-esteem	Encourage Jane to use make-up as she does normally. See 2 and 4. Ask Jock to tell Jane when she looks nice
Observe Jane's sleep pattern. Reduce Jane's anxiety if she cannot get off to sleep. Try to help her to go to sleep before midnight	Observe Jane's sleep pattern. Give her a warm drink to aid sleep as appropriate. Try not allowing her to sleep during the day as this may prevent her getting off to sleep at night

Mania and hypomania

Definition

Mania is the opposite of depression. The patient is elated, optimistic and extremely quick, both mentally and physically. In his conversation he shows *flight of ideas,* and the topic is likely to change continually. But the changes are always understandable and connected to one another, unlike the disconnected talk of a schizophrenic. The manic patient is lacking in tact, disinhibited and often very amusing. He is always on the go, is distractible and easily irritated; at times he can become paranoid and deluded. Grandiose schemes are started only to be dropped for something even greater. There is generally little time for food or sleep, but sometimes he is promiscuous and spends money recklessly. Judgement is faulty and he may run foul of the law.

Extreme states of mania result in patients becoming unmanageable outside hospital. Delusions, hallucinations, both visual and auditory, and aggressive overactivity may develop. The milder forms, known as *hypomania,* merge imperceptibly with normal states of elation.

Treatment

Mania requires treatment in hospital. Up to 1000 mg or more of chlorpromazine, combined with up to 80 mg of haloperidol may be needed every 24 hours for the first week or so. If a patient is uncooperative, intramuscular injections are necessary (100 mg chlorpromazine, 30 mg haloperidol, every four hours). If previous attacks of mania and/or depression have occurred, it may be as well to begin lithium at the same time, starting with 1600 mg a day. When, as occasionally happens, it is still difficult to control the patient and persuade him to eat and drink adequate amounts, intramuscular flupenthixol decanoate 40 mg, or fluphenazine decanoate 25 mg, is helpful, although 48–72 hours elapse before the effects of these drugs begin to be apparent. In the event of the patient remaining overactive and uncooperative (a dangerous situation) ECT can be given if he is not taking fluids; this can be a life-saving measure. One or two treatments are given each day for two or three days; this rapidly calms the patient.

Differential diagnosis

Mania needs to be distinguished from acute catatonic schizophrenia and schizoaffective states, confusional states, and conditions induced by drugs such as amphetamines.

Nursing care

Manic patients should be nursed in quiet, non-stimulating surroundings; ideally in a single room, under sedation. Full nursing care is necessary, with special attention given to an adequate fluid intake, diet and personal cleanliness.

The nurse should be tactful in her dealings with the manic patient, who may laugh with her at one moment but become angry the next. These patients are meddlesome and interfering and can cause havoc in a peaceful ward. When the patient is up and about, it is best to provide him with some occupation. It is useless, however, to expect him to continue with one activity for any length of time.

Rebecca Stanley

On admission to the ward, Becky is clearly out of touch with reality suffering from a hypomanic phase of a manic depressive illness. She is a formal patient held under Section Two of the 1983 Mental Health Act.

Owing to Becky's state, her initial care plan has been designed with her safety in mind and does restrict her actions to some degree. However, in order to prevent unnecessary irritation, her opinions are sought and met when appropriate. An example of this is given in the Plan of Care for Elimination – where it is suggested that she show any diarrhoea to the nurses but, that if she refuses to so, this issue should not be forced.

At the beginning of each shift a 'nursing rota' is organised to ensure that Becky is closely observed. A rota is considered to be preferable to one nurse being responsible for a whole shift. The reasons for this are that it can be very stressful for the nurse involved to observe a hypomanic patient for long periods and that by changing over this may be reduced.

Becky's care plan will require frequent evaluation while she is in the acute stage of her illness and should be changed appropriately. It is suggested that her care should be reviewed every twenty-four hours for the first few days.

Nursing Information Sheet

Hospital No: 72099792 Wards: / / / Date of Admission: 7/6/1984

Surname STANLEY
Forename Rebecca Edith
Address 11, St James' Road,
Donchester,
Hants

Likes to be known as: Becky
Date of birth: 12/7/1948 Age: 36 Sex: F
Marital status: Married
Religion: R/C Nationality: English

Relevant Psychiatric and General Medical History

Admitted to psychiatric hospital first in 1962 - frequent recurrent admissions with hypo-mania. Depressed twice in 1973 and 1976 after birth of children.

Is patient formal or informal?

Formal

Section Two 1983 MHA

Occupation and past work history

Trained shorthand-typist. Has not worked since Jane, her eldest daughter, was born.

Source of finance:

Husband's income

Next of kin: Mr Stephen Stanley
Address: As above
Tel. no.: Donchester 69174
Person to contact in case of emergency: (if different from above) A/A
Address: Police Station, Real Row, Donchester
Tel. no.: (Work) Donchester 44241

Home conditions

Three bedroomed house in good repair

Community resources (CPNS voluntary agencies)

C P N generally visits monthly. Has been going daily during the last week.

Significant persons in life

Husband, two children Jane, 11
Isobel, 8

Special nursing observation

Reason for admission:

Hypomanic phase in patient with a previously diagnosed manic-depressive illness.

Mr Timothy James Snr Reg.

Referred by: C P N Accepted by:

Dr P. Smith

G.P. Tel No.:

Dr Roger Bradley
The Surgery
Chotley Street
Donchester

Patient's profile
Height 5ft 3in
Weight 52 Kg
Build Small
Complexion Fair
Hair–Colour Red-bright
Eyes–Colour Blue
Marks and Scars

T.P.R. T 36°C P 96 R 20
B.P. 120/85
Urine Nothing abnormal detected

Present Situation	Actual and Potential Problems (Level of independence/ dependence)
1. Maintaining a safe environment Becky is not to leave the hospital as she is considered to be a danger to herself due to elevated mood. She has been walking in tights with no slippers and she offered to change a light bulb in the dormitory because it was not working	Potential danger to herself due to elevated mood. May hurt herself slipping over or doing a job to be helpful
2. Personal hygiene Cleans teeth slowly for about 5 seconds because her mouth is dry. Says that she has not got time for a bath but will wash when requested to. No deodorant, which is necessary because of excessive perspiration	Poor personal hygiene due to excited/hurried state. No deodorant
3. Special factors When 'irritated' by a request or someone's behaviour she becomes verbally aggressive, swearing at anyone. Apparently she never swears under normal circumstances	Verbally aggressive outbursts due to irritation
4. Care of clothing Clothes look rather untidy - she has given up ironing as it is a waste of time. Reluctant to wash items separately and some of the dye in a red shirt has coloured most of her underwear. Dresses appropriately for the weather. Normally immaculate	Damage to clothes due to inappropriate cleaning. Clothes untidy
5. Co-operation in ward life Very cheerful towards both patients and nurses. Talks loudly and rapidly which some of the other patients find irritating. Volunteers to lay the table because she is 'quick' at it	Iritates other patients at times but tries to be helpful
6. Attitude toward medication Becky says she feels on 'top of the world' and does not see why she should take any medication. When asked to take it when it is presented, she swallows it 'to keep the peace'	Without medication regularly her irritation/excitable state may increase
7. Working and playing – social mixing Becky has been unable to manage the house over the last ten days. Very inappropriate with her children - dancing with them in the playground rather than making them go into school	Inappropriate social mixing causes her family embarrassment

Aim of Nursing Intervention	Plan of Care
Prevention of harm to herself	At the beginning of each shift a timetable of nurses who will 'special' Becky will be organised by the nurse in charge. The special nurse will be responsible for knowing where Becky is and ensuring that she is not in any danger (i.e. proper shoes, etc.)
To promote personal hygiene	Daily bath, either morning or evening. Encourage Becky to clean her teeth at least twice a day properly, and to wash her hair when necessary. When husband visits ask him if he could bring in some deodorant
Prevention of verbal aggression	When Becky is obviously becoming irritated try to move her away from the source by diverting her attention elsewhere, e.g. if she is in the Day Room take her into the quiet room
Ensure clothes washed and ironed so that Becky looks better	Explain to Becky that it is important that her clothes are clean and properly washed. Stay with her while she washes them herself and only intervene if necessary (i.e. if she becomes irritated)
To prevent others being irritated by Becky without hampering her desire to help	Encourage Becky's enthusiasm to help but stay with her while she does so i.e. lays the table. Explain that there is plenty of time and that everything does not have to be done quickly. Thank her when she has done the task. Point out the fact that she is irritating others when appropriate
Ensure that medication is given regularly to prevent escalation of her mood	Ask her to take her medication quietly but firmly at the appropriate times - see drug chart
Prevention of inappropriate behaviour	When Becky is behaving in an excited manner i.e. dancing, explain 'quietly and firmly' that this is inappropriate. Do <u>not</u> join in with excited behaviour

Present Situation	Actual and Potential Problems (Level of independence/dependence)
8. Communicating Wishes to be called 'Becky'. She talks very quickly and loudly for long periods without waiting for an answer i.e. She said, 'What do you want me to do for you?'	Talks loudly/quickly, rarely listens for others to speak. Irritates some patients
9. Perception Feels that she is very well. Does not accept the need to be in hospital, but is willing to stay 'for an easy life'. Says she is worried that people think she is 'mad' when she is 'sane'	Does not accept that she is ill
10. Finance and budgeting Husband took control of the housekeeping when Becky first became ill. He says that she normally manages well, but when excited is prone to spend money on luxuries and forget necessities	Unable to manage family budget but husband coping with this
11. Mobility Overactive - dashing around the ward. She knocked a flower vase over this morning and this upset her. Did not stay off the corridor floor when it was being polished despite a request to do so. Likes badminton	Overactive and potential problem of falling due to this
12. Eating and drinking Weight 52 kg. Will drink very quickly when given something even if it is very hot - nearly burning her mouth. She says she has not much time to eat and tries to eat so quickly that she chokes; has not finished a complete meal for 4-5 days	Potential dehydration. Poor fluid and diet intake
13. Eliminating Passing urine satisfactorily. She says that she is having 'diarrhoea', but when asked to call a nurse to see it prior to flushing chain she simply laughs	? Diarrhoea
14. Expressing sexuality Stephen her husband, has complained that Becky has been demanding sexual intercourse several times over the last week, which he finds exhausting. She leaves her buttons undone and exposes her breasts but will do them up when requested to do so	Exposing breasts on the ward. Sexually demanding of husband
15. Sleeping Sleep pattern at home has been very irregular : when she is exhausted she sleeps for several hours at any time, and is wide awake at night and restless	Irregular sleep pattern resulting in nocturnal restlessness

Aim of Nursing Intervention	Plan of Care
To prevent Becky irritating others and to encourage her to listen to others	Spend short periods of time (i.e. not more than 15 minutes) talking with Becky. Ask her to speak more quietly and slowly if necessary and to give time for you to speak. Encourage her to listen to other patients, explaining that their opinions are valuable too
To orientate Becky to 'reality' as far as possible	Explain to Becky that she does not have to be 'mad to be' in hospital but that she is very excitable and that this has been interfering with her everyday life and needs to be treated. Point out that it has happened before and she got over it.
	Husband coping well. Review situation in 1/52
Prevention of falling or hurting herself due to mobility	See 1. Try to divert Becky's attention into calmer activity i.e. reading or washing up; but be aware her attention span is short. In the afternoon take her to the gym to play badminton and see if this chance to be active helps her. Report any escalation in activity
Prevent dehydration, ensure adequate diet	Weigh weekly. Fluid chart - encourage her to drink at least 2000 ml/24 hours. If she cannot sit still long enough to eat an entire meal give her toast and milky drinks at three-hourly intervals or when she asks for them
Observe for diarrhoea	Observe how often she is using the toilet. She has been asked to 'sho the nurses' any diarrhoea. She may have, but do not force this issue
To ensure Becky is modestly dressed. Prevent overt sexual demands on the ward	Ask Becky to do up her shirt buttons if they are undone. If she initiates discussion about 'sex', listen to her and respond appropriately, but do not encourage fantasy. If she makes overt demands of others - intervene and report this
Promote sleeping at night to regularise pattern	Try to keep Becky awake during the day so that she will be tired at night. If she does fall asleep in a chair, wake her within an hour. Observe and chart pattern

Suicide

The official suicide rate in England and Wales has declined over the last ten years from 120 to 80 per million but has now started to increase. Men still outnumber women by two to one but the female proportion is increasing, particularly in elderly women; suicide is also increasing in adolescents. There is disagreement about how reliable these official figures are. The majority of people who kill themselves, probably over 90 per cent, are psychiatrically disturbed; most of them are depressed. Many, just before their death, have gone to their GP but failed to obtain help. Many have made one or more abortive attempts before the final act. In other words, suicide rarely comes out of the blue but is preceded by warning signs. Late middle age is when suicide is most likely. Alcoholism increases the risk. So also does the presence of physical illness.

Many factors contribute to suicide. It was Durkheim who pointed out the relationship between suicide and the way in which a person is integrated in his society and controlled by its norms and values, especially those concerning death and suicide. Those who are and feel socially isolated are more prone to suicide. Marriage and children, active religious faith, a settled home, all lessen the risk of suicide. The suicide rate is highest among the single, divorced and separated, among those who emigrate or move to an unfamiliar area, and is greater in urban than in rurual areas. Sudden stress, particularly bereavement, financial worry, and legal disputes may prove the last straw for the middle-aged depressive already near breaking point. Drugs are the common method of suicide, usually obtained from a doctor. In the past gassing was frequently used, but natural North Sea gas has removed that possibility. Depressives sometimes employ particularly unpleasant methods; throat cutting, swallowing corrosive liquids, hanging, drowning, jumping in front of a train. Suicide nearly always arouses considerable guilt among members of the suicide's family and in his medical attendants.

Greater medical awareness of depression and suicide, the introduction of antidepressant drugs and in particular of natural gas, may all have contributed to the falling suicide rate. The Samaritans, a voluntary organisation available at any time to help people in despair, may also have had some influence. Paradoxically, as the suicide rate has fallen, the number of cases of attempted suicide or self-poisoning has risen alarmingly. In 1970, one in five of all emergencies and one in ten of all admissions to medical wards was due to self-poisoning. Unlike suicide, women outnumber men by at least two to one and the majority are aged between 15 and 40. Barbiturates, tranquillisers and aspirin are the drugs most frequently employed. The act of self-poisoning is often an impulsive one, not intended to be fatal, expressing a variety of feelings, anger and aggression, threats and appeals, and often represents a way of escaping from an unpleasant situation.

Since 1961, when the Suicide Act became law, attempted suicide has ceased to be a criminal offence. It is now looked upon as a medical and social problem. But the problem, involving between 80 000 or more cases a year, is a huge one, and the area of responsibility is ill defined. Only about 20 per cent of patients seen after self-poisoning can be considered psychiatrically ill in the strict sense, although many of them are 'disturbed personalities', with considerable social problems. Adolescent female self-poisoners are likely to be promiscuous and to have had an abortion. A number of self-poisoners repeat their actions in the future, and not a few in fact do kill themselves eventually. There is an inverse relationship between on the one hand depressive illness and suicide, and on the other, open aggressive behaviour. During both world wars there was a sharp drop in suicides. And in Belfast during 1969–70, the suicide rate fell by almost 50 per cent; there was a corresponding increase in homicide and crimes of violence.

18
Pregnancy and the Puerperium

Pregnancy

Pregnancy results universally in psychological and physiological changes, the one interacting with the other. Some women feel marvellous almost as soon as they conceive, but the majority experience varying degrees of emotional and physical distress. The first three months tend to be the worst. The primiparous woman must face and prepare herself for new and changing roles. She is soon to become a mother, responsible for her child's safety and upbringing. If she already has children she must face the likelihood that the new addition will alter family dynamics. Her husband will see her in a new light, not always to her advantage. Her own dissatisfactions with her marriage, if these are present, may be highlighted and demand redress. She may have to curtail her much liked job or career. Ideally this question should be resolved by husband and wife together before conception. When the pregnancy is unexpected, husband and wife should reach mutual agreement as soon as possible. The ambitious woman who wishes to continue her career must, for her peace of mind, feel that she has the full support of her husband in this matter.

She has also to cope with nausea and sickness, and often to struggle against exhaustion and depression. Nausea usually stops by the fourth month, but rarely vomiting (hyperemesis) increases and continues through most of pregnancy. It is sometimes said that this reflects an underlying wish to reject the child. Occasionally this explanation may be tenable, but usually the emotional disturbances on which such a view is based seem more likely to result from the vomiting than to be the cause.

Mood changes are common, especially during the first half of pregnancy. The extent of these depends on the personality and emotional maturity of the woman, the quality of her marriage, and how much she and her husband want the baby. Depression and emotional lability are most common in the first trimester and lessen progressively with time.

When depression continues and perhaps deepens, it is likely that the woman harbours resentments towards her husband, feels rejected and unwanted, and wishes she were not pregnant. These feelings need to be brought into the open and discussed, ideally with the nurse or doctor supervising the pregnancy, and including her husband. Rarely, depression may deepen to psychotic depths or pose a risk of suicide. (It is rare for functional psychoses to manifest themselves in pregnancy, even when there have been earlier episodes.) In such an event termination may have to be considered (see below), and possibly treatment with psychotropic drugs or ECT. But for emphasis we repeat that this is very unusual. The vast majority of depressed pregnant women only need to talk about their problems. Rarely do they require drugs.

Anxieties are liable to develop at any time. Fears that the fetus may die or be deformed are not uncommon, particularly among women who have had an abortion. So also are fears of the woman dying in childbirth, or of her husband abandoning her. These anxieties, which reflect neurotic conflicts arising out of the woman's need to adapt to her changing life, are relatively easily assuaged by a sympathetic understanding attendant.

Appetites, like mood, fluctuate, particularly during the second trimester. At least 60 per cent of pregnant women experience sudden cravings for unusual foods and those they formerly avoided, or become averse to foods they enjoyed. An intermix of physiological and psychological influences are probably responsible. *Pica,* the eating of non-nutritive material like dirt or paint, is a rare occurrence suggestive of psychosis or mental impairment. Compulsive eating throughout pregnancy, with undesirable weight gain, is most likely to occur when a woman is depressed, or has bulimia nervosa. The depressed woman cannot be bothered to control her appetite, for depression saps motivation and self control. Many women with bulimia nervosa can only reduce their excessive intake for a time, although out of fear of harming the fetus they can usually stop vomiting or abusing laxatives. The result is that they may be much overweight after nine months.

Libido declines, especially in the early weeks and in the last trimester, but in between not a few women experience heightened desire for intercourse, from both a real increase of sexual appetite and a need to feel wanted by and close to their husbands. Sometimes a woman refuses to have intercourse throughout pregnancy for fear that this may bring on a miscarriage. This may be reasonable if she has previously miscarried. But more often than not it is a sign of deeper marital conflicts. Such behaviour is liable to arouse the husband's resentment and exacerbate their problems.

Few primiparous women are able to visualise the fetus or even accept fully that they are pregnant until movements can be felt. (Where there is much anxiety an immature woman may occasionally refuse to accept that she is pregnant, almost up to delivery. Such denial is not simply lying, but seems to involve a mixture of hysterical dissociation and suppression.) The child then begins to take form in the mind's eye of the mother, he comes to life in her thoughts, and emotional attachments develop.

Pregnancy invariably makes demands on the husband. He must understand that his wife's emotional lability or irritability is not unusual, and not a sign of moral weakness or ambivalence to their child, and requires him to provide her with extra support and proof of his affection. Many husbands are now present with their wives throughout labour. Not everyone is psychologically capable of benefiting from sharing thus, but among many of those who do, trust and love are strengthened, and the man's ability to relate to and fully accept his child is made easier.

Delivery

Childbirth may be perceived as a frightening event. Antenatal classes, talks, relaxation, and exercises have not entirely dispelled this fear, although it is much less now than it was 20 or 30 years ago.

Today women are encouraged to have their first babies in hospital. Medically it is safer, although psychologically it may be more satisfying to have the baby at home. Sometimes conditions in the labour ward are far from satisfactory. Women may be left alone in labour for several hours, frightened and in pain. Labour can be prolonged by the woman's own anxiety. Overworked midwives become impatient and tell the woman to hurry up, to stop behaving like a baby. Resentment and guilt build up. An exhausted, demoralised woman may have little emotional feeling left for her child when at last he arrives.

As soon as the child is born he is usually handed to his mother. Maternal feelings need to be reinforced by the child's presence, and if for any reason mother and child are separated for the first few days these are inevitably impaired to some extent. Most women experience a surge of pleasure and satisfaction at this moment. This experience is lessened if the mother has been bullied or treated unsympathetically during her labour, or if she has been heavily sedated or anaesthetised. Apart from the value of this in stimulating maternal feelings, many women become anxious if they do not see the child, fearing that he is dead or deformed.

Breastfeeding is usually encouraged in hospital, although there is disagreement as to how far women should be persuaded. Some women feel disgusted and embarrassed by breastfeeding and are upset if they are forced to conform. Modern artificial foods are probably as good nutritionally as breast milk, and an infant probably cannot distinguish a bottle from a breast in his first weeks of life. But there is little doubt that many mothers experience increased maternal feelings when they breastfeed, and this may result in the breastfed infant being fondled more than the bottlefed one. Recent work has suggested that it is the amount of handling a child receives rather than the way he is fed that influences his early development. And certainly intimate contact between mother and child in the early days after birth is enormously important for their future relationship, and especially for the mother's depth of attachment.

A woman may actively dislike her child at first, in spite of her sense of guilt and strong efforts to reverse the feeling, perhaps upset that he or she is not the sex she envisaged. Such reactions have complex causes and usually include earlier conflicts between the woman and her own mother. Something about the child or the nature of the birth reactivates suppressed childlike aggression in the mother, which then becomes displaced on to the child. Sympathy and encouragement can usually help mothers and their husbands over this sometimes difficult phase.

Some mothers like their children to be totally dependent on them and these women are often model mothers with young babies. Sometimes a woman loses interest as her children become independent. Women of strongly obsessive personality may have difficulty in coping with their children when they start to assert themselves, unable to accept that they cannot completely control the child and what he does. Another woman may dislike the helpless state of a young baby, and only begin to enjoy her children later when she feels that they have their own separate existence.

Puerperium

About 70 per cent of women experience short-lived emotional upsets three or four days after delivery, burst into tears for no obvious reason, feel depressed and fuss about their competence to care for the baby. This state probably results from a number of factors, the most important being the hormonal changes that follow birth. For the most part '*maternity blues*' disappear spontaneously and they are of no lasting significance. But sometimes the 'blues' are deeper and more prolonged than usual and may presage a breakdown. However, the relationship is far from certain and for the most part severe 'blues' should not be cause for alarm, but rather ensure that signs of a postnatal psychosis are not overlooked – not difficult if the woman is in a busy hospital ward.

Puerperal psychosis

Approximately 1 woman out of every 600 deliveries develops a psychotic illness, mostly within 2–3 weeks of delivery, but never within the first 3 days. There is disagreement as to what constitutes the actual period of the puerperium, but we take 12 weeks to be the outside limit for the onset of this condition. Some authorities, and these include the WHO's International Classification of Diseases, do not recognise puerperal psychosis as a separate clinical entity. Others regard the relationship between the psychosis and childbirth as clear cut.

The early symptoms include depression, irritability, insomnia, anxiety and restlessness, generalised worrying and lack of zest and concentration, not differing markedly from the 'blues'. Symptoms are often mild at first and only deepen after the woman returns home. But they can deepen quickly and psychotic symptoms appear after 5 or 6 days. Depression may predominate, and suicide and infanticide become a serious risk. There may be clouding of consciousness, with hallucinations and excitement. Schizophrenic features may appear. Although the illness may present as predominately schizophrenic or affective, it is this mixture of depressive, schizophrenic and confusional signs and symptoms that is so characteristic of acute puerperal psychosis.

> Mary returned home from hospital with her first child, a boy, after one week. The pregnancy and delivery had been uneventful and she had looked forward to the birth. She started breastfeeding without difficulty. On the second and third day she repeatedly burst into tears and worried unreasonably about the baby receiving sufficient milk. She calmed down after reassurance from nurses, and returned home in what seemed to be good spirits. She had a flat she liked, and a husband she loved, who gave her plenty of support. And for the first fortnight her mother came to stay to help with the baby. All seemed well for the first five days at home, but then she began to behave strangely. Her sleep became broken and she kept getting up to look at the child, repeatedly saying that he was starving, that she could see his bones protruding through his skin. Reassurance from her husband and mother was at first effective, but

subsequently began to make her agitated and at times violent. She refused to eat, saying that the food was poisoned and was killing the child through her milk. A doctor was called who prescribed diazepam. That night, while attempting to breast-feed, she suddenly rushed from the room into the garden. Her husband pursued her, she tried to scramble over a fence, dropped the baby and attacked her husband. When admitted to hospital (with the baby) she appeared confused, and incapable of giving a coherent account of herself.

Causes

Puerperal psychosis can occur after any child, although the risk is greatest with the first. A breakdown after the first child may be succeeded by one or more uneventful deliveries, or the illness may only appear with the second or third child. Nonetheless the danger of recurrence is high. Once a woman has had a postnatal psychosis, the risk of further illness rises enormously from the statistical norm of 1 in 600 to less than 1 in 10.

Women who have had earlier episodes of manic depression, unconnected with pregnancy, are also at similar risk after childbirth. Indeed, a strong family history of manic depression should always alert doctors and nurses to the possibility of trouble in the postnatal period. There seems to be no such clear relationship between schizophrenia and puerperal psychosis. A past schizophrenic illness is not usually reactivated, nor is current schizophrenia necessarily exacerbated. Nonetheless some puerperal psychoses are essentially of a schizophrenic nature.

There are virtually no known aetiological factors. Social class, age, housing, marital harmony or otherwise play no obvious part. Biological mechanisms – still unknown – together with genetic vulnerability, are likely to be responsible. It is significant that termination of pregnancy is not associated with the risks of full term delivery. Post-abortion psychosis is almost never encountered, presumably because biological changes have not proceeded far enough to render the woman liable to breakdown.

Treatment and Prognosis

Every woman who develops a puerperal psychosis should be admitted to hospital, together with her child. Ideally she should go to a mother and baby unit, but these are few and far between, and often a long distance away from the patient's home. Most are looked after in a single-bedded side room in a psychiatric hospital unit. Mother and child should remain together, unless there is a risk of infanticide, or she is too confused and disorganised. The infant must then be kept apart from her, but frequently shown to his mother in order to further mother/child 'bonding'.

Physical treatment is usually necessary, dependent on the patient's clinical condition, and follows the same lines as for non-puerperal psychotic states. Drugs vary in the degree to which they enter breast milk; antidepressants are present in small amounts, neuroleptics and tranquillisers rather more, and lithium builds up to a comparatively high concentration (see p. 362). In general it is advisable for the woman not to breastfeed, but to suppress lactation and bottlefeed the child. In any case, markedly psychotic behaviour makes breastfeeding hazardous, if not impossible.

The role of the nurse is a changing one. Initially she has to care for the patient's physical as well as mental state. Many women have not eaten or drunk adequately for days, and may be dehydrated and generally debilitated. They require encouragement and reassurance in addition to medication, and help in returning to reality. The infant has to be cared for, and frequently shown to the mother. As the mother improves she is encouraged to take increasing responsibility for the child. Her self confidence and feelings towards the child are boosted. Her husband is made to feel a welcome and necessary visitor, and helped with the anxieties and doubts that the catastrophe must inevitably have aroused in him. Future problems, real and possible, need to be discussed, including the advisability of further pregnancies, of contraception, and even sterilisation.

The average stay in hospital is around 6 weeks, but most patients need to be followed up, at decreasing intervals, for at least 6 months and preferably a year. Maintenance therapy with an antidepressant or neuroleptic drug, or lithium, depending on the clinical condition, may be necessary for a time. Home visits from the Community Psychiatric Nurse may be advisable if there are doubts about the woman's ability to cope at home on her own. It is vital to remember that neurotic problems may succeed or complicate a psychiatric breakdown, and interfere with full recovery. Overall the outlook for full recovery is good. In the long term however, about one-third are liable to develop an affective illness, unconnected with pregnancy.

Postnatal Neurotic Illness

The incidence of depression is increased over the next nine months, but particularly in the three months following childbirth; about 1 in 10 women are affected. The woman becomes irritable, miserable, complains of lack of energy and inability to cope, and is often in tears. She feels that she is an inadequate mother, a poor wife, generally useless. In some cases phobic anxiety and obsessional symptoms are prominent. A vicious circle arises when her child responds by becoming difficult and demanding, the more so when her husband is unsympathetic. The picture is quite different from that of puerperal psychosis, and is largely understandable in terms of the woman's personality and her environment. Women who are strongly obsessional (requiring for their peace of mind to ensure that they are firmly in control of their lives) exhaust themselves, especially with their first child by struggling for perfection in the child's management. The child reacts, and what may seem to the woman a life and death struggle develops. A sense of failure, inadequacy and depression follows. Social factors such as poor housing, loss of company and isolation through having to give up a job, and marital difficulties may be contributory factors. A woman whose pregnancy was unwanted may still harbour ambivalent feelings towards the child. Her hostility leads to guilt and anxiety which may increasingly turn into depression, especially when she cannot turn to her husband for support. Unresolved conflicts within an immature woman's personality, stemming back to childhood and her relationship with parents, especially mother, are sometimes important. A woman's anger towards her mother is now turned against herself. To oversimplify, she now becomes the 'bad' mother against whom she fought and struggled to free herself when younger; depression is the consequence.

Treatment and Outcome

The majority of these women recover spontaneously within six months or sooner, often without any help, as the condition commonly goes unrecognised. In a few, symptoms persist for a year or more, and occasionally continue a fluctuating course for many years. Exploration, explanation and reassurance are especially helpful in the early stages and probably shorten the illness. Antidepressants or tranquillisers may be needed, especially if depression is impairing the woman's ability to cope at home, or when it persists for more than a few months.

Stillbirth

A stillbirth may be followed by a psychosis, but the incidence is no more or less than after a normal live delivery. Reactive depression is understandable and may be severe and prolonged. This is the more likely if the stillbirth has been followed by 'a conspiracy of silence'; disinclination by doctors and nurses (often out of a sense of their own guilt and failure) to discuss details of the birth and possible reasons for the baby's death. It is essential that the woman – and her husband – grieve openly for the child (which should be given a name), and express the sense of anger and guilt which, suppressed, so often prolongs depression. See also the case study on p. 219.

Termination of pregnancy

The Abortion Act of 1967 allows pregnancy to be terminated by a gynaecologist, provided that two medical practitioners agree that (a) continuance of the pregnancy involves risk to the life of the pregnant woman, or of injury to the physical or mental health of the woman, or any of her existing children, greater than if the pregnancy were terminated; or (b) there is a risk of the child suffering from such serious physical or mental abnormalities that it would be seriously handicapped.

Before 1967 a psychiatric opinion was almost invariably sought, as pregnancy could only be terminated if the woman's life or physical or mental health were likely to be endangered by the pregnancy. Today psychiatrists see far fewer patients, and these are mainly referred by gynaecologists prepared to terminate but anxious to know the possible harmful effects of abortion on the patient. Of the women seen by psychiatrists, abortion is recommended in around 70 per cent. Of those refused termination, only about one in four or fewer produces a live baby, and few of these keep the child.

Some psychiatrists didactically state that there are no psychiatric grounds for termination. Even if social factors are ignored, for instance, a 43 year old woman with two young mentally impaired children, or a depressed woman hardly able to cope with her family of four children and habitually drunk husband, both of whom have inadvertently become pregnant again, there are still justifiable psychiatric grounds. A woman who has had a severe prolonged puerperal psychosis, or repeated attacks of manic depression, and therefore has a 1 in 5 chance of developing a psychosis if she proceeds to delivery, must surely be justified in requesting termination.

Termination seems to cause little or no adverse emotional effects in women of previously stable personality (a post-abortion psychosis is almost unknown), although some of them may react with more guilt than is apparent. This may account for the increased incidence of depression and anxiety in pregnancy among those women who have earlier had an abortion (see above). On the other hand, chronically neurotic and unhappy women may displace their depressed mood and sense of failure onto the abortion, and attribute most of their troubles and dissatisfactions to the operation, never ceasing to regret it was done.

Termination can be carried out at any time before the fetus is legally viable, 28 weeks. But unless the delay is not the fault of the patient, doubts must be cast on the wholeheartedness of her wish for termination if she has dithered for so long. If termination in the NHS is refused, young women are likely to seek for a private or even illegal method of abortion, the latter with sometimes disastrous consequences. The risk of suicide is increased. Parasuicide attempts are not uncommon with overdoses or wrist slashing. Depression is certainly common, and adds to the difficulties many of these women have in accepting and loving the child. This may affect the child's development adversely. There is evidence that the children of women refused abortions are more likely than other children to develop psychiatric disabilities.

In all this one has to recognise the problem abortion poses to the nurses and doctors directly concerned. It is a destructive operation, destroying a life of sorts, irrespective of whether one cares to deny a 10 week old fetus a human identity. Staff with strong religious principles may understandably refuse to participate. Neurotic reactions are readily aroused. Those who hold didactic views for or against abortion are lucky. For most of us it is a matter of summing up and weighing the pros against the cons.

Sterilisation

Sterilisation of the woman, or vasectomy in the husband, are carried out frequently today. Psychiatric complications are unusual, provided there are good realistic reasons, and both partners are in agreement. Neurotic men and women may subsequently hide behind the operation and attribute sexual and marital difficulties to it. Gynaecologists sometimes 'pressurise' a woman to be sterilised after abortion, particularly if she has had more than one. Since the woman is not always in a sufficiently detached frame of mind to make a proper decision, it is as well to leave the question until later.

Elizabeth Yatton

Liz was formally admitted to the ward with her daughter who is four days old.

Liz's care plan embraces her physiological needs which are special in that she has so recently given birth. Similarly her daughter will need special attention. A care plan for the daughter should be constructed. For the purpose of Liz and her baby's post-natal care the Community Midwife will visit the ward until the baby is ten days old. The ward staff should seek advice as appropriate from the midwife to ensure all physiological needs are met.

Liz's prime psychological need is that of 'safety' for herself and baby. This is emphasised in her care plan and a 'special nurse' is delegated to co-ordinate the care on each shift. This nurse also has the role of close observation of Liz's physical and mental state. Any changes in Liz's state will be reported to the nursing and medical teams.

Simon, Liz's husband, is involved in her care to a degree. It is important to view the situation from his standpoint and offer him relevant support. It may be that a simple gesture like giving him a cup of coffee and asking how he feels will give him a chance to express his doubts and fears. As far as possible the family unit should be preserved within the nursing plan.

The nursing care plan will need to be reviewed at least every twenty-four hours in the initial few days of admission. As soon as appropriate, Liz should be encouraged to become closely involved in her baby's care and her new role as 'mother' promoted.

Occasionally, nurses find it difficult to give babies up, when they have been closely involved with them. Liz's health is of paramount importance and this should be remembered if such attachment occurs.

Nursing Information Sheet

Hospital No: Wards: Date of Admission:

Surname YATTON
Forename Elizabeth Jane
Address 7, Tintern Avenue
Laucenster

Likes to be known as: Liz
Date of birth:
5/4/1956 Age: 28 Sex: F

Marital status: Married
Religion: C of E Nationality: British

Relevant Psychiatric and General Medical History

Liz had a much wanted baby daughter on 17 November (4 days ago) and has become increasingly withdrawn since she is now mute and has been admitted under Section 2 of the Mental Health Act 1983 for assessment

Is patient formal or informal?
Formal

Section
Section 2 21st November, 1984

Occupation and past work history

Shorthand secretary to a solicitor prior to leaving to have her baby

Source of finance:
Husband's income and maternity benefit

Next of kin: Husband, Simon Yatton
Address: A/Above
Tel. no.: Laucenster 17716
Person to contact in case of emergency:
(if different from above) A/Above
Address: Workplace Smiths Factory
Tel. no.: Laucenster 77426 ext. 234

Home conditions

A two bedroomed modern house which Elizabeth has always kept beautifully according to her husband. No obvious problems at home

Significant persons in life

Husband, New baby daughter - Sarah

Community resources (CPNS voluntary Agencies)

Community midwife visited Liz prior to childbirth and will visit her and the baby here until baby is 10 days old

Patient's profile

Height 5ft 2in
Weight 56 kg
Build Medium
Complexion Pale
Hair-Colour MidBrown
Eyes-Colour Hazel
Marks and Scars

Special nursing observation

Closely observe Elizabeth whenever she is with her baby. At no time is she to be left unaccompanied with the baby

Reason for admission:

Emergency for Assessment, due to character change and 'muteness' after childbirth

T.P.R. T 36 °C P 72 R 16
B.P. 120/80

Urine Nothing abnormal detected on routine examination

Referred by: G.P.

Accepted by: Dr J Jones Register Consultant Psychiatrist after assessment of Liz's mental state at Mile Lane Maternity Unit

Tel No.:

Present Situation	Actual and Potential Problems (Level of independence/ dependence)
1. Maintaining a safe environment Liz doesn't seem interested in her baby daughter but the medical staff fear that her disinterest could result in injury to herself or the baby	Risk of injury to Liz or her baby
2. Personal hygiene Liz washes very slowly but manages to achieve this. She still has a slight vaginal discharge and engorged breasts due to not feeding the baby	Infection of breasts. Forgetting to change sanitary towels
3. Special factors Care of Liz's baby daughter. Engorged breasts and Liz's disinclination to either breastfeed or express her milk	Daughter's needs may not be met. Painful engorged breasts
4. Care of clothing Liz keeps putting the same rather dirty nightdress on after washing. She clasps this to her body when encouraged to change it.	Liz is wearing a dirty night-dress
5. Co-operation in ward life She is completely withdrawn and just lies on her bed - there is no response when asked if she would like to come to the table to meals or into the sitting room to mix with other patients	Liz is very isolated. Potentially cut off from others and withdrawing into fantasy
6. Attitude toward medication At present Liz is not written up for any medication except paracetamol for soreness in her breasts. She has refused to take this when it is offered	Pain in breasts - refused to take paracetamol
7. Working and playing – social mixing Liz is on maternity leave and she hadn't decided whether to return to work as she thought she would do this after the baby was born (information from husband)	Possibility that Liz will have difficulty in making this decision

Aim of Nursing Intervention	Plan of Care
Prevention of injury to Liz and her baby	Each shift a nurse will be delegated to 'special' Liz and her baby. This person will liaise with everyone involved in Liz. Changes in Liz's behaviour should be reported to Dr Jones who is going to work with her
Prevention of infection Promotion of personal hygiene	Discuss with midwife care of breasts and follow advice. Remind her to wash and change ST's as appropriate
That baby is looked after. Liz's breasts - reduction of pain and engorgement	See separate regime for baby. Midwife will try to teach Liz to express her milk and clean her breasts. Ward nurse to be present and report to rest of team about how often this should be done
To get Liz to change her clothes regularly	Try to build up 'trust' with Liz by offering to wash her nightdress with her and giving her a clean one. Do not insist she changes it as yet
To keep Liz in touch with the reality of her surroundings	Talk to Liz when involved with doing things with her - explain what is going on. Talk clearly and concisely
Reduction of breast pain by taking paracetamol	Explain to Liz what the drugs are for - show her the bottle to prove what they are. If she refuses do not pressure
To relieve the anxiety of making a decision at the moment	Together with Simon reassure her that no one expects her to take big decisions at the moment

Present Situation	Actual and Potential Problems (Level of independence/ dependence)
8. Communicating At present Liz is mute and has not spoken for two days. She lies curled up on her bed hugging her knees and has confused looking facial expression	Withdrawn, lack of communication with daughter may inhibit bonding
9. Perception It is difficult to assess if Liz is deluded or hallucinating, or how she is feeling. She does appear to be suspicious of her surroundings in that she looks around and then clasps her chest and rocks	Suspicious about the hospital
10. Finance and budgeting Simon, Liz's husband says that he can manage at the moment but would like to speak to the social worker about maternity benefit at some time	Maternity benefit/grant may not be paid
11. Mobility Liz can walk, and does when actually asked to but she lies for long periods without moving at all	Pressure sores. Deep vein thrombosis - especially post-childbirth
12. Eating and drinking Liz will not join others to eat. If given a tray of food by her bed she gulps it down very fast and looks around suspiciously	Does not want to eat with others
13. Eliminating Liz was incontinent of urine prior to admission but when asked to go to the toilet she does so	Incontinent of urine. Liz could harm herself if left alone in the toilet
14. Expressing sexuality At the moment Liz seems to be denying her new role as a mother and is not looking after her breasts. She turns over and faces the wall when her husband visits	Rejection of mother role sore breasts rejection of husband
15. Sleeping Liz slept well at the maternity unit. She lies on her bed during the day, so might not sleep well at night	May not sleep at night

Aim of Nursing Intervention	Plan of Care
To bring Liz out of herself and establish a relationship with her daughter	Spend time with Liz showing her how to bath the baby etc. Encouraging her to help. Ask Simon to talk to Liz about a name for the baby
To reduce suspicion Observation for any change in Liz's behaviour	Explain to Liz what you are doing when you are with her. Observe for any signs of hallucinations or delusions - encourage Liz to talk about how she is feeling
To introduce Simon to social worker	Arrange for Simon to see the social worker
Prevention of pressure sores and DVT	Encourage Liz to change position and walk around the ward - if she won't get off the bed - passive leg exercises. Explain the reasons for this
To ensure that she eats and drinks adequately	Fluid chart - at least 2000 ml/24 hour intake. Allow Liz to eat and drink alone. Review daily
To prevent urinary incontinence and Liz harming herself	Remind Liz to go to the toilet - go with her but allow her to go into the bathroom alone. Wait outside
Acceptance of role to care for her own breasts. Communicate with her husband in some way	Reinforce Liz's role with her daughter. See 3 re. breasts. Leave Liz alone with her husband for a few minutes at visiting
Accurate assessment of Liz's sleep pattern	Night nurse 'special' to closely observe and record Liz's sleep pattern. If Liz is awake try to communicate with her and establish how she is feeling

19
Schizophrenic Illnesses

Schizophrenia

Definition

Schizophrenia probably embraces a group of diseases, all characterised by disorders of thought, feelings and volition and a tendency to retreat from reality into an inner world of fantasy.

Historical

Throughout the 19th century there were descriptions of what we now recognise as schizophrenic states. But it was Kraepelin in 1896 who first brought them all together under the term *dementia praecox*. (The term means *early dementia*.) He described the various symptoms in detail, but emphasised what he thought to be the crucial feature, the progressive deterioration of personality which ended ultimately in a state of dementia.*

This gloomy prognosis was challenged by the Swiss psychiatrist, Eugene Bleuler, in 1911. He introduced the term *schizophrenia* as descriptive of the splitting or fragmentation of psychic functions which occurs. (This must be distinguished from a 'split personality' which is described under hysteria.) He considered the basic fault in schizophrenia to be a disorder of the associative processes. Ideas split into unrelated parts, and emotions are not linked to appropriate thought content. He thought of schizophrenia as a group of diseases which, although likely to scar the personality in some measure, might remit at any stage without severe deterioration.

Bleuler's concepts are responsible for some of the diagnostic disagreement that exists today, especially between America and European psychiatry. In America any unusual psychiatric state is liable to be labelled schizophrenia. Indeed the term *pseudoneurotic schizophrenia* covers a range of what in England would mostly be considered to be severe personality or borderline personality

* True dementia does not occur in schizophrenia. Formal intelligence remains intact, although the behaviour of a deteriorated schizophrenic may resemble that of a dement. Nor does it necessarily begin at an early age.

disorders. Today attempts are being made to standardise the criteria by which psychiatrists diagnose schizophrenia.

Incidence

Schizophrenia is a widespread disabling disease. Between eight and ten people out of every 1000 born today are likely to develop schizophrenia at some time in their lives. Men and women of all ranges of intelligence are affected. More than half the patients in psychiatric hospitals today have schizophrenia. It occurs in all countries and cultures. Although cultural factors colour symptoms, the basic disorder is common to every patient.

Age of onset

Schizophrenia typically begins in late adolescence or the early twenties. However, it can develop at any age. The later the age of onset, the slower the splitting of psychic function and the more the personality remains intact.

Diagnosis

Since many schizophrenics exhibit protean symptoms, it is vital from the diagnostic point of view to recognise which are primary and which secondary. Bleuler distinguished four fundamental symptoms, present in every patient, and accessory symptoms which might or might not be present. Fundamental symptoms included disruption of the *normal association of thought, ambivalent feelings* (love/hate, joy/sorrow), *autism* (which results in a lack of interest in people and the outside world), and *affective incongruity*; accessory symptoms included hallucinations, delusions, ideas of reference, automatism, among others. Today many psychiatrists rely upon Schneider's 'first-rank symptoms' to distinguish schizophrenia from other functional psychoses. Schneider listed these as:

1. Certain types of auditory hallucinations, particularly the patient hearing his own thoughts being repeated aloud, voices arguing and criticising his actions.
2. Somatic passivity experiences, such as outside influences playing on his body.
3. Thought withdrawal and other interference with thought.
4. Diffusion of thought, so that other people are able to read and experience his thoughts.
5. Delusional perception and feeling.

6. Impulses and acts experienced by the patient as the work or influence of others.

If one or more of these symptoms is present the diagnosis is schizophrenia. But in fact first rank symptoms are absent in at least one-third of schizophrenics, and they are not uncommonly present in mania. Bleuler's concept is still very much in use. The onset of the illness may be acute or insidious. Symptoms fall into six main headings.

1. *Disorders of thought and speech.* The normal association of ideas become disconnected and it may be difficult or even impossible to follow a patient's flow of talk. It is curiously woolly and never quite to the point. Thinking is over-inclusive, the normal framework of conceptual thought is lost and irrelevant ideas are brought in. Sometimes he stops in midsentence and, after a puzzled silence, begins a different topic. One patient described this *thought blocking* as, 'they suddenly start up the vacuum gap'. He believed his thoughts were being sucked from his mind by other people. Some patients complain that their thoughts are shared and experienced by everyone else (*thought broadcasting*). At other times thoughts race through the mind so quickly that the patient has no time to speak (*pressure of thought*), or irrelevant ideas constantly intrude into his thoughts and cause total incoherence. In chronic schizophrenia thinking becomes empty and rather facile, although the patient may attempt to cover this up by reading and talking about philosophy or psychology.

Rational thinking is gradually replaced by *fantasy thinking* (see p. 7) dominated by his emotions. *Condensation*, *displacement* and *symbolisation* occur. *Condensation* is a mixing of ideas which have something in common, regardless of whether this is logical. *Displacement* refers to the use of an associated idea in place of the correct idea. *Symbolisation* is the misuse of symbols, due to abstract being replaced by concrete thought. For instance, a schizophrenic said: 'I've an elephant in my head,' meaning that he had a long memory. *Neologisms*, newly constructed words, are formed: a *word salad* occurs when these are so numerous that speech cannot be understood. The speech of a chronic schizophrenic is often stilted and strange. Writing is similarly affected.

2. *Disorders of emotion.* During the early stages of schizophrenia depression is common. Sudden outbursts of panic, bewilderment or elation understandably occur, but these lessen as the illness progresses. Once the disease is established emotional feeling becomes blunted (*flattening of affect*), and the personality appears insensitive and even callous. Social isolation increases as the

schizophrenic withdraws from his friends. The emotional coldness and withdrawal may be 'felt' at the first interview; lack of emotional rapport, described as 'like having a pane of glass between you and the patient', is a useful diagnostic point.

Affective incongruity, the showing of feelings that are inappropriate to the schizophrenic's thoughts or situation, occurs in many cases. A schizophrenic described with a smile how a poison was being injected into his body during sleep. Another laughed as he described his mother's death. Contradictory or ambivalent emotions, like love and hate, may be felt simultaneously and result in contradictory behaviour.

3. *Loss of will-power and drive*. Together with flattening of affect goes loss of will-power and ambition. Patients complain of this in the early stages of the illness. A young man previously active and energetic takes to lying in bed until midday, gazing into space instead of working. Nothing gets done in spite of urgent demands. His appearance is neglected. Dirt and squalor accumulate. He feels changed, that his thoughts and feelings are not his own any more (*ideas of passivity*), that his identity is being lost (depersonalised).

Sometimes this loss of will-power is carried to extremes, resulting in *automatic obedience*. The schizophrenic does whatever he is told or imitates every word (*echolalia*) and action (*echopraxia*) of his interrogator. At other times he shows *negativism*. He disobeys all requests or does the exact opposite of what he is asked to do.

Catatonic signs vary from stilted odd mannerisms and grimacings to the most extreme and bizarre posturings. A curious change takes place in muscle tone. Limbs can be moulded into unusual positions (*waxy flexibility*) which are sometimes maintained for hours on end. Many of the strange postures assumed have a symbolic meaning for the patient. Immobility may suddenly give way to wild destructive outbursts.

Schizophrenic *writing* may reflect this mental disorganisation. Mannerisms, changes of style, word salads, repetitions of words or phrases, curious punctuations and symbols, make their writings as difficult as their conversation to understand.

4. *Delusions and hallucinations*. It is useful, for diagnostic purposes, to distinguish between *primary* and *secondary* delusions. A primary or *autochthonous delusion* is an idea or belief which appears suddenly from out of the blue for no obvious reason and is immediately accepted as true by the patient, despite its obvious absurdity. One of our patients believed that the Pope was in love with her and was sending her messages. Another one suddenly

knew that he was in contact with certain beings on the planet Venus.

A secondary delusion is equally as absurd to everyone except the patient, but develops 'logically' from the patient's attempts to understand his symptoms. He believes that his next door neighbour is interfering with his thoughts or will-power by 'a vacuum gun', by rays through the television set, or by poisoning his food.

Delusional mood refers to a patient feeling that something is going on which concerns him but is being kept from him. A bank clerk had felt thus for several days and was growing increasingly puzzled and anxious. Suddenly, while having supper with his wife, he knew that she was trying to change him into a woman.

Ideas of reference are common. The patient becomes aware that something said or done refers to him. A ticket inspector said, 'Good morning. Lovely weather for H-bombs,' to a young man developing schizophrenia. He at once understood this to mean that the ticket inspector knew that he was a homosexual and was warning other people.

Hallucinations. Auditory hallucinations may consist of indistinct background voices and noises, or be clearly audible. Certain auditory hallucinations, in the setting of clear consciousness, are indicative of schizophrenia. These are hearing one's own thoughts spoken aloud, or voices criticising and abusing the subject. Generally they are unpleasant and may distress the patient if emotional feeling is still well preserved. They may come from inside or outside the head and increase when the patient is unoccupied. From his behaviour, it may be apparent that a patient is hallucinated. At times he may answer his voices aloud.

Visual hallucinations are much less common but do occur, particularly when paranoid symptoms are marked. Hallucinations of other sensations can also occur. A patient had the experience of being raped, smelt semen, and heard a voice telling her that she would become pregnant.

5. *Disorder of perception.* Perception becomes distorted because it is dominated by one particular emotion or idea. External objects and events are still recognised, but their significance or meaning is grossly distorted. An empty milk bottle lying on the ground was recognised by a patient to mean that he should kill his mother. It becomes difficult for the schizophrenic to separate himself clearly from his environment and other people. Schizophrenics, in the early stages of their illness, may complain that they are changing their sex or are becoming someone else. Strange hypochondriacal beliefs sometimes occur.

6. *Physical symptoms.* Cyanosis of hands and feet, and a greasy spotty skin are common in young schizophrenics. Menstruation may become irregular or stop, as in any severe mental illness. Loss of weight is usual in acute schizophrenia.

Formal intelligence, consciousness, memory and sensation are unaffected (but see also Atypical Schizophrenia).

Clinical forms of schizophrenia

Schizophrenia may appear in many forms. It is still usual to divide schizophrenia into four types: *simple, hebephrenic, catatonic* and *paranoid.* These are briefly described below, although in clinical practice we feel that these subdivisions have little value. It is much more constructive to think of the disease in terms of prognosis and probable response to treatment (see p. 251).

Simple. This develops insidiously in adolescence or the early twenties. Apathy and lack of emotional response and drive are the most marked features. Hallucinations are usually absent. Many are undiagnosed and drift from job to job, and finally into vagrancy. The prognosis is poor.

Hebephrenic. The onset may be equally insidious. The patient often presents with depression, even attempted suicide. Later, emotional incongruity and shallowness become more marked. He indulges in outbursts of fatuous giggling and smiling. Delusions and hallucinations are usually present. The prognosis is poor.

Catatonic. Motor abnormalities characterise this type, either of generalised inhibition or excitement, associated with hallucinations and delusions. After a period of depression and progressive withdrawal, the patient's behaviour becomes increasingly negativistic. He refuses food, becomes mute or shows echolalia. Bizarre mannerisms, posturing and grimacing occur; a curious pouting protrusion of the lips (schnauzkamps) used to be seen in the past more often than today. Stupor develops in extreme cases. The patient is unresponsive to what is happening to and around him, although subsequently after recovery it is apparent that he was fully aware of everything done or said. His body may be stiff and resist all attempts to alter its posture, or it may become curiously malleable (waxy flexibility). At any time catatonic excitement may supervene. This is one of the few psychiatric conditions when a patient can be extremely dangerous.

Paranoid (see p. 255). Paranoid schizophrenia starts later than the other forms, usually after the age of 30. Delusions of persecution are the prominent symptoms and the personality is often well preserved for many years. Sexual delusions are particularly common in women. Paranoid schizophrenia in attenuated form, without much personality deterioration, occurring in late middle and old age, is sometimes called *paraphrenia.*

Atypical forms and other terminology

Acute psychotic disturbances in which both depressive and schizophrenic symptoms occur and the outlook for full recovery is good, are sometimes referred to as *schizo-affective* disorders. They are not easy to separate from manic depression, for first rank symptoms can occur in both conditions.

Schizophreniform psychosis is sometimes used in place of *schizo-affective* to describe acute schizophrenia precipitated by severe stress, accompanied by considerable emotion, where the prognosis is excellent. The term *typical, process* or *nuclear schizophrenia* implies, by contrast, a poor prognosis. Schizophreniform psychoses are characterised by an acute onset, vivid dreamlike hallucinations, and catatonic excitement or stupor, in a setting of clouded consciousness. Similar states have been described under the name *oneiroid psychosis.*

Aetiology

The causes of schizophrenia are still not known. There are two main theories. One maintains that the progressive splitting of the mind is probably a biochemical disorder interfering with central integrative mechanisms. The other holds that the cause is purely psychological, schizophrenia being the result of *regression* to an early infantile level. Although there is no conclusive evidence in support of either view, we believe that an organic cause will sooner or later be found.

Some contributory factors are known.

1. *Genetic.* A predisposition to develop schizophrenia under certain circumstances is inherited. The chance of the child of one schizophrenic parent developing schizophrenia is around 10 per cent, compared to about 1 per cent in the general population. If both parents have schizophrenia the incidence increases to 40 per cent.

Identical twins possess the same genes. The consensus of findings of a number of schizophrenic twin studies is that 60 per cent of monozygotic twins are concordant, that is both twins develop schizophrenia. Corresponding studies of dizygotic twins found that only 12 per cent were concordant, the same as for non-twin siblings. No single gene can fit the evidence; only a multifactorial genetic theory is tenable.

2. *Personality*. Typically, schizophrenia tends to occur in people of *schizoid personality*, shy, withdrawn and over-sensitive. Of course, only a small proportion of schizoid personalities develop schizophrenia. But the incidence of schizoid personalities is considerably raised in families who have a schizophrenic member.

3. *Body build.* When schizophrenia starts in youth the body build is often asthenic or ectomorphic. A pyknic or muscular build seems to act as a 'protection' against the illness. People of this build who develop schizophrenia usually do so later in life, and affective symptoms may be prominent.

4. *Child–parent relationship*. The mothers of schizophrenics have been accused of being cold and rejecting towards their child. This is believed to be an important causative factor by supporters of the psychological regression theory. The evidence for this is weak. R. Laing has put forward the idea that schizophrenia is a form of defence, adopted by the patient to protect himself from being engulfed and destroyed; he retreats into his own world where he is safe and secure from intolerable emotional demands that he cannot face. Few people wholeheartedly accept such a theory.

It is often claimed that communication in the families of schizophrenics is distorted, contradictory and 'illogical'; the implication being that the patient learns his distorted method of communication from his family during childhood. However, the evidence for this claim is by no means clear. Bateson suggested the concept of the 'double-bind' parental relationship. The child is confused by one set of parental reactions conflicting with another. Thus a mother may hold out her arms to her child and say, 'Come and give me a kiss', but at the same time her expression and tone of voice are such as to repel the child. When he hesitates she says, 'Don't you love me?'

5. *Sex and Social class.* The sex ratio is equal in schizophrenia. There is no sustained evidence that birth order or the time of year born has any relationship to the disease.

The incidence of schizophrenia is inversely proportional to social class, being ten times more common in class 5 (the lowest) than class 1. Yet investigation of the families of schizophrenics shows that the socio-economic class of the fathers of schizophrenics is the same as that in the general population. What is more, the type of school attended and the academic achievements, at the age of 11, are similar to non-schizophrenic 11 year olds. In other words, schizophrenics are not overwhelmingly born into social class 5, but drift steadily down the social scale as a result of failure to establish careers or work for themselves.

Schizophrenics are found in greatest numbers in the centres of large towns. One theory holds that it is the impersonal conditions of crowded urban centres which cause schizophrenia. But it seems more likely that this feature is due to schizophrenics drifting there, partly because living is easier and cheaper, but also because they are able to avoid making close personal relationships, and can remain anonymous and free of pressures.

It does not seem that poverty or bad housing per se are responsible for schizophrenia.

Emotional overstimulation and understimulation, while being unlikely to be prime causes of schizophrenia, have been clearly shown to be important factors during the course of schizophrenia, and responsible for relapses (see below). Patients living in homes where they are subjected to strong criticism and emotional pressure (Expressed Emotion, known as EE), or overprotected by parents, are likely to relapse. But equally dangerous is the all too common social isolation of the schizophrenic, where there is no social contact to distract him from his autistic world.

Few schizophrenics marry, compared to the general population; this may partly be due to the early age of onset; many of those who do marry are later separated or divorced. The fertility rate of these patients is low.

6. *Physical factors.* It has long been recognised that persistent deafness is liable to cause the sufferer to become withdrawn, suspicious and irascible. Recently the importance of deafness in the development of schizophrenia for the first time in middle or old age has been shown; deaf people are inevitably cut off and isolated socially to some degree. In old age, sensory deprivation of this type alone may be sufficient for paranoid delusions and hallucinations to develop.

7. *Biochemical and Endocrine abnormalities.* Many schizophrenics show clinical and biochemical evidence of endocrine imbalance and abnormalities of body fluid constituents. Some are remarkably insensitive to huge doses of thyroid or insulin. This reflects the schizophrenic's lack of physiological as well as psychological adaptability.

A small group of schizophrenics, with *periodic or recurrent catatonia*, either retain or excrete nitrogen in excessive quantities as symptoms develop.

Schizophrenic body fluids are toxic to some animals. Much work has been done to try to isolate a self-produced toxin, particularly one which may be related to an abnormality of adrenaline metabolism. There is, in fact, strong evidence to suggest that all effective neuroleptic drugs, whatever their class, are able to block dopamine receptors in the CNS (dopamine released in the CNS acts on post-synaptic receptors). However, this is not proof that dopaminergic mechanisms are overactive or abnormally responsive in the brains of schizophrenics. Another chemical system may be at fault, which only indirectly influences the dopamine system.

8. *Hallucinogenic drugs*. These include lysergic acid diethlyamide (LSD) and marijuana. Small doses can cause schizophrenic-like symptoms. At one time it was hoped that the mechanism of action of these drugs would lead to greater understanding of the biochemical causes of schizophrenia. But the resemblance between these drug-induced states and schizophrenia is not very close. Large doses of amphetamine (50 mg or more) are capable of causing acute schizophrenic-like states, and sometimes bring on relapse in remitted schizophrenia. The behavioural effects of amphetamine are thought to result from the drug's ability to increase the concentration of dopamine in the brain. Neuroleptics block this effect.

Precipitating factors may be of almost any nature. Physical illness, childbirth, surgery, head injury, drugs, emotional conflicts may all act as precipitants. There is evidence that the onset of many schizophrenic illnesses are triggered off by a 'markedly threatening event' occurring only a few weeks before symptoms first appear. But in simple schizophrenia the illness usually develops insidiously, without any obvious cause.

Prognosis

Schizophrenia is a disease of remission and exacerbation, with a poor outlook in spite of improved treatment. Research into outcome is bedevilled by such problems as diagnostic difficulties and patient samples and numbers, and what is meant by 'improvement'. Recent work, using Schneider's first rank symptoms and a computer for diagnosis, and the Present State Examination (PSE), gives hope of clearing away some, if not all, clinical confusion over the course of schizophrenia.

Prognostic signs have recently been disputed. Nonetheless, we believe that the following are good signs:

1. Absence of family history of schizophrenia
2. Plenty of emotional response
3. An acute onset
4. An outgoing extroverted personality
5. An emotionally stable home
6. Acute emotional stress immediately preceding the illness
7. Late age of onset

Different diagnosis

Schizophrenia must be distinguished from depression, obsessional states, organic states, drug intoxications, hysteria and epileptic twilight states. Catatonic excitement may at first be difficult to differentiate from mania.

Treatment

Modern treatments have enormously increased the chances of improvement, if not recovery, and lessened chances of relapse.

Acute schizophrenia almost invariably needs to be treated in hospital. As an extension of this, it is fair to say that every schizophrenic, before treatment is instituted, should be admitted to, and thoroughly investigated in, hospital.

Drug therapy

Chlorpromazine, the first phenothiazine derivative, is still the most effective neuroleptic for an excited or agitated patient; 300 mg or more a day in divided doses is needed. On this dosage patients lose their anxiety, their psychotic symptoms gradually fade, and they can again begin to relate to other people. This in turn allows doctors and nurses to develop friendly constructive relationships with them.

Neuroleptic drugs have completely replaced deep insulin therapy. There are now many different effective drugs, but in general chlorpromazine remains the drug of choice for agitated psychotics. For other patients, for instance, a patient with paranoid schizophrenia, one of the piperazine side chain phenothiazine derivatives, such as trifluoperazine, is indicated; it is less soporific in its side effects, and is particularly effective in reducing paranoid thinking and aggressive behaviour; 15 mg is equivalent to 300 mg chlorpromazine a day.

Psychotic symptoms start to disappear after a fortnight or so of treatment. However, the neuroleptic must be continued, even when symptoms have all gone; if the drug is stopped symptoms are liable quickly to return. Most schizophrenics must continue to take a neuroleptic, perhaps indefinitely, if they are to avoid relapse or deterioration. The introduction of long-acting phenothiazine and thioxanthene preparations; fluthenazine decanoate (Modecate) and flupenthixol decanoate (Depixol) has made such treatment more reliable. Regular two to four weekly injections (see p. 348) obviate drug defaulting, and ensure that the drug is fully absorbed.

Recent studies, comparing the effect of long-acting neuroleptics with placebo in chronic schizophrenic patients, confirm the protection provided by these drugs; in one study 66 per cent of patients given a placebo relapsed over the course of nine months, compared to only eight per cent given a neuroleptic. Nonetheless, there are many reasons why a patient may relapse, and it is as well to be aware of this. About a third of all patients who are receiving long term treatment relapse over the course of a year.

The majority of first admission and relapsing patients spend six to eight weeks in hospital. In the past, most schizophrenics could expect to spend the rest of their days in hospital. Today, with good treatment, very few become chronic inmates. However, although this is ideally a splendid achievement, in practice one doubts whether the schizophrenic is always much better off. The Mental Health Acts of 1959 and 1983 put the onus for providing after care facilities on local authorities; hostels, social clubs, day centres, sheltered workshops, group homes. These are, for the most part, lacking in many areas.

Many schizophrenics return to their families. However willing, the majority of families find looking after a chronic schizophrenic relative a considerable strain. Although neuroleptic drugs have undoubtedly improved the behaviour of the schizophrenic, he is still difficult to live with; he may be dirty, untidy and unpunctual, irritating in his habits, and careless of the feelings of others. All too often the hostility and criticism which is said to exacerbate schizophrenia is the direct result of the schizophrenic's own behaviour. Nonetheless, the presence of a high emotional atmosphere at home increases the likelihood of relapse. If relapse threatens, the dosage of the patient's neuroleptic drug should be increased. This is not invariably effective, and other drugs may need to be given as an alternative, or in combination: haloperidol, pimozide, penfluridol, fluspirilene. Attendance at a day hospital or centre will help to lower EE at home. Or the patient may need to be removed from home and spend two or three weeks in hospital in a calmer atmosphere. In the long run he may be better off in a group home or hostel.

Extrapyramidal side effects result from most neuroleptics. AntiParkinsonian drugs, such as orphenadrine, may then need to be given concomitantly. However, they should not be given routinely, since they can themselves cause side effects, and antagonise the therapeutic action of the neuroleptic.

Occupational therapy and the atmosphere of a therapeutic community are important. But care must be taken not to involve the patient emotionally too much in group therapy, as this may act as a threatening event and retard his progress.

ECT is only indicated in catatonic schizophrenia, when it can be a lifesaving measure, or when there is a strong depressive component. It is given concomitantly with a neuroleptic. Antidepressant drugs may also be helpful in combatting depression. Depression is likely to occur in about 60 per cent of schizophrenics at some time or another, and must be regarded as part and parcel of the schizophrenic illness.

Behaviour therapy is sometimes useful in breaking undesirable habits; for instance the use of token economy. Tokens for cigarettes or privileges are awarded when a patient gets out of bed promptly in the morning, dresses neatly, shaves and bathes, attends meals on time, and so on. Such tokens must be given immediately after the desirable action occurs.

Suitable work is of great importance in maintaining morale and lessening the risk of relapse. If necessary a patient can be registered as disabled, under the Disabled Persons Act.

Prefrontal leucotomy is today rarely considered. Only when there is a well preserved personality, and considerable tension underlies the patient's psychotic behaviour, does this treatment even merit consideration (see p. 380).

Problems occurring outside hospital

Medico-legal. Occasionally schizophrenics become involved in crime, sometimes of a particularly callous nature. But usually they lack the emotional drive necessary for planned crime.

Sudden unprovoked assaults may occur, sometimes in response to hallucinations. An innocent bystander may be struck a violent blow. Murder occasionally occurs, and the rare case of matricide nearly always involves a schizophrenic.

If a discharged schizophrenic inexplicably begins to behave

aggressively he should be admitted to hospital for observation without delay.

Marriage and eugenics. A patient with schizophrenia or with marked schizoid traits is unlikely to marry. But for those who recover, marriage raises problems. A relapse is always a possibility. And the chances for any children being affected must be considered. These problems should be discussed fully with both partners.

Childhood schizophrenia. The same disintegration of mental functions and withdrawal from external reality occur in childhood as in adult schizophrenia. But the symptoms in childhood schizophrenia depend on the stage of intellectual and emotional development the child has reached.

There is always a change of personality and *every* aspect of development is affected. The child becomes emotionally cold and withdraws into herself. Speech is lost or becomes babyish or may never develop. Incontinence, unprovoked screaming outbursts, continuous anxiety and negative behaviour may make the management of these children difficult. Deterioration is sometimes extremely rapid.

Childhood schizophrenia is probably made up of a number of different conditions separate from the adult form. Some of these may be clearly organic. Often it is difficult to distinguish mental impairment from childhood schizophrenia. Physical treatment with drugs or electro-shock is of little value, although phenothiazine drugs may be useful in controlling behaviour.

The prognosis is poor.

Paranoid states

Paranoid thoughts – that one or more people are hostile and intent on causing harm or trouble – come to most of us at some time, particularly when anxious or in new and strange surroundings. We project onto others at such times our own anxiety and hostility. In some people paranoid personality traits predominate. They are touchy, suspicious of others, and usually lacking in humour. They possess an inflated sense of their own importance, imagining that everything about themselves and their actions attracts attention. They are unadaptable and rigid in their relationships with others, and are not easy to live with or befriend for long; sooner or later they are likely to take offence and see friends as enemies. Social isolation increases their paranoid feelings.

The reactions of a man with a paranoid personality are largely understandable when related to his everyday experiences. But paranoid reactions may occur which are not understandable, and which are then considered to be delusional and abnormal. Many of these instances are manifestations of schizophrenia, but the personality may be well preserved for years and other signs of schizophrenia be hard to find. The terms *paraphrenia* and *paranoia* are sometimes still used for this type of paranoid schizophrenia.

Paranoid schizophrenia often develops at a comparatively late age, and perhaps as a consequence of this, the personality does not deteriorate so rapidly and to the same extent as in other types of schizophrenia. Deafness and other modes of sensory deprivation are believed to play an important causal role in patients who first develop paranoid delusions and/or hallucinations late in life. Treatment is along the lines already described for schizophrenia, with particular attention to correcting organic defects and social isolation. Neuroleptics frequently have to be continued indefinitely.

Paranoid delusions may occur during depressive illnesses. These can be understood on the basis of a patient's intense sense of guilt and self-reproach. He feels he is being watched by the police and is about to be arrested for his past wickedness. Paranoid behaviour and delusions can also develop during mania. Paranoid reactions are common in confusional and organic states; they are not systematised as in psychotic disorders, and are transitory.

Often it is difficult to say when 'normality' ends and delusion begins, and the patient may need to be seen over a long time. Paranoid litigants, for instance, who believe themselves to have been wronged, may spend their lives bringing court actions, writing to newspapers, Members of Parliament and so on. There may have been a basis of truth initially, but this has now become distorted and lost. Yet in other respects they may seem to be 'normal' people.

Pathological or morbid jealousy, is a paranoid condition which can arise from a variety of psychiatric conditions. When unaccompanied by signs of schizophrenia or psychotic depression, it may stem from a minor unfaithfulness by a spouse. This then becomes the focal point for the partner's sense of sexual inadequacy, and is elaborated to delusional intensity.

Sometimes a sane individual is 'infected' by the paranoid delusions of a close friend or relative and comes firmly to believe them. This is known as *folie á deux*. When separated, the 'sane' partner usually, but not always, gives up the delusional ideas.

Treatment of paranoid states depends on the underlying cause.

Nursing care

The nursing approach should be open and friendly, and care taken not to reinforce the patient's suspicions. Nurses talking together may immediately be seen as threatening. The hospital bleeps now carried by most doctors and senior nurses are often misconstrued as transmitters of unwelcome messages. Their purpose needs to be explained simply to the patient, although it may not be entirely believed at first. Radios and televisions may also be a cause of alarm for the patient, a means by which 'someone' sends them warnings and threats. Paranoid patients are naturally suspicious of accepting anything from staff; food and medication may at first be thought to be poisoned. Even the friendliness of staff is sometimes seen as a subtle ploy to win the confidence of the patient. This basic mistrust is not easy to dispel, but time and consistency of approach gradually does so.

Ali Khari

It can be seen from Ali's care plan that he has a series of problems which are inhibiting his activities of living. Some are actual problems, for example poor personal hygiene and refusing food. In addition the assessment process has highlighted certain potential problems which include the possibility of burning himself with cigarettes and not taking his medication.

With patients like Ali it is essential for the nurse to objectively define potential problems. This is because the nursing team can then plan interventions to minimise the risk of them actually occurring. In order to identify potential problems it is necessary for nurses to have an understanding of mental illness, in this case schizophrenia, so that assessment is theoretically based.

While all of Ali's problems stem from his illness, three of the nursing objectives require the same intervention. For the purpose of this care plan they have been grouped together so that this provides a clear visual display to the nursing team.

The plan is formulated for Ali's initial care but will need to be revised at regular intervals. It is imperative that he is encouraged to be as independent as possible during his admission in order to prevent institutionalisation (Barton, 1960).

Although Ali is an informal patient it is deemed necessary to ask him to stay in the ward and only to go out if he is accompanied. If he refuses to do this his informal status should be reconsidered by the medical and the nursing teams. Naturally, the nurse's assessment of Ali would be valuable in the consideration of whether Ali should be allowed to leave or be formally constrained under the Mental Health Act 1983.

Nursing Information Sheet

Hospital No: 1999724 **Wards:** / / / **Date of Admission:** 20/11/84

Surname KHARI
Forename Ali
Address 14 Great Smith Road,
Hertfonds,
Sussex

Likes to be known as: Ali
Date of birth: 11.6.1930
Age: 54 Sex: M
Marital status: Single
Religion: Muslim
Nationality: British

Relevant Psychiatric and General Medical History

Schizophrenic illness diagnosed in 1952
In-patient until 1980 when discharged into group home. Has been attending day centre from group home.

Pneumonia 1982

Is patient formal or informal?
Informal

Section

Occupation and past work history
Unemployed

Source of finance: Social Security
Sickness Benefit

Next of kin: Mr Sidi Khari (Brother)
Address: 17 Lord Nelson Road, London,
London, NW1

Tel. no.: 01 924 0000
Person to contact in case of Emergency:
(if different from above) As above
Address:

Tel. no.: (Work) 01 000 4241 ext. 721

Home conditions
Own room in group home. Ali has not been cleaning this, and it is described as in a 'terrible state' by C P N. Other rooms in house cleaned by other residents and are O K.

Community resources (CPNS voluntary agencies)
C P N

Significant persons in life
Brother
Six other residents in 'group home'

Special nursing observation

Patient's Profile
Height 5ft 4in
Weight 72 kg
Build Heavy
Complexion Brown
Hair-Colour Black
Eyes-Colour Brown
Marks and Scars

T.P.R. T 36°C P 74 R 18
B.P. 125/80
Urine Nothing abnormal detected

Reason for admission:
Gradual deterioration over the past three months. For reassessment and stabilisation of medication

Referred by: C P N and G P. Accepted by: Dr N. Jefferies Snr Reg.

G.P. Tel No.:
Dr J. Fletcher,
Manor Health Centre
Hertfonds

Present Situation	Actual and Potential Problems (Level of independence/dependence)
1. Maintaining a safe environment Ali is not to leave the hospital without an escort. He is quiet and withdrawn but likes smoking and has been known in the past to set light to his clothes while nodding off with a cigarette	Potential problem of cigarett burning when Ali falls asleep
2. Personal hygiene Ali has not been washing himself or his clothes for about a week. His hands and nails are dirty, as is his hair. He has not shaved either, although he generally does so daily. This appears to be because he is so withdrawn and lethargic	Personal hygiene poor due to lethargy and being withdrawn
3. Special factors See Perception	
4. Care of clothing Ali has not been washing, changing or mending his clothing. It is in a dilapidated state with cigarette burns and dirty patches	Clothes dirty and have cigarette burns
5. Co-operation in ward life Ali is very withdrawn and turns away when he is approached by others. He appears 'frightened' and moves his chair when others sit by him	Very withdrawn and moves awa when approached by others
6. Attitude toward medication Appears to take medication when it is offered, but looks suspiciously at the tablets, turning them over in his hand before taking them. Refuses to open his mouth to demonstrate that he has swallowed them	Suspicious about medication. Potential problem of not swallowing medication
7. Working and playing – social mixing According to the Community Nurse, Ali normally contributes to the upkeep of the group home and particularly enjoys 'hoovering' and watching television. Recently he has refused to do either because of 'noise'	Disturbed by 'noise' which is causing inactivity
8. Communicating Does not initiate conversation. Replies when asked a direct question. He frequently shakes his head and talks into the air - when questioned he says there's so much going on and everyone keeps bothering me.	Conversing with 'no apparen person'. ? Auditory Hallucinations
9. Perception Ali appears to be suffering from auditory hallucinations in that he complains of noises and voices that no-one else hears. He says that his 'blood has air in it, and keeps popping'. He also thinks 'certain people' want to get at him - he appears frightened about this	Frightened - possibility of auditory and tactile hallucinations

Aim of Nursing Intervention	Plan of Care
Prevention of cigarette burns Not to leave hospital unaccompanied	Explain to Ali that he is not to leave the hospital unaccompanied. At the beginning of each shift a nurse will be made responsible for this. Explain that cigarette smoking is not allowed in dormitory, and ask him to leave the cigarettes in the office at night. Observe closely when he smokes in the day and prevent burning if he falls asleep
Improve personal hygiene	Encourage Ali to wash daily and bathe every two or three days. Ensure that he has adequate soap, flannel, etc. Give him the electric razor to use a.m. Prompt when necessary, calmly but firmly
Clean Ali's clothing	Send Ali's dirty clothes to laundry and see what the sewing room can do about the burns. Temporarily use hospital clothing. If Ali refuses to part with his clothes, respect this wish and reassess situation
Prevention of isolation without causing unnecessary stress	For short periods of time i.e. 5-10 minutes try to engage Ali in conversation. Do not press him if he terminates conversation by moving
Ensure that Ali takes his prescribed medication	Allow Ali time to investigate his medication and give him a large glass of water or squash with which to swallow it. Observe immediately afterwards to see that he is not disposing of it
Divert Ali from his pre-occupation with 'noise in his head'	These three areas all require similar nursing intervention Spend periods of time with Ali for as long as he desires. If he asks to be left alone - do so, but return about half an hour later. Explain that while you appreciate his fear and that he is hearing voices they are not audible to you. Try to divert his attention by discussing the here and now (i.e. time of day, weather, what's for lunch). If possible involve him in an activity i.e. washing up, looking at the newspaper. Do not push him to watch television if he does not want to. Observe his ability to concentrate and note anything that seems to increase his fear
Divert Ali from his ? auditory hallucinations	
Try to reduce 'fear' by diverting into reality	

	Present Situation	Actual and Potential Problems (Level of independence/ dependence)
10.	**Finance and budgeting** Ali is dependent on social security and sickness benefit, but his rent is paid directly from D.H.S.S. so this has been done. He has not cashed this week's giro and wants some cigarettes	Has not cashed Giro and requires cigarettes
11.	**Mobility** Ali is able to move freely, but sits still in a chair for most of the day. He does get up to go to the toilet and moves if others get too close to him	Moves if others get too close to him. Sits still for long periods
12.	**Eating and drinking** Ali likes sweet tea with two sugars and plenty of milk (according to C P N). He has refused to eat since he has been on the ward because he does not like the look of anything. He has drunk tea and milk. Weight 72 kg	Refusing food because he does not like the look of it. ? suspicious of its content
13.	**Eliminating** Passing urine, but when questioned did not know when he had last had his bowels open. Has a slight cold and does not wipe his nose unless asked to	Potential problem of rejection by other patients if he does not wipe his nose ? Constipation
14.	**Expressing sexuality** There is no evidence of Ali having been particularly interested in 'sex' during the last four years (C P N information). He does however usually like to look neat and tidy and has joked that he could get a girl if he wanted one	Very untidy but normally neat and cares about his appearance
15.	**Sleeping** Ali says that he can't sleep at the moment, but likes to lie down anyway to 'get away'	Not sleeping well

Aim of Nursing Intervention	Plan of Care
Ensure that Ali has some cigarettes	Arrange for Ali's giro to be cashed by the social worker and obtain some cigarettes for him
Prevention of isolation	As 7, 8 and 9
Promote adequate diet	If Ali continues to refuse prepared food allow him to prepare his own in the kitchen, e.g. scrambled eggs. See that he has plenty of tea with sugar and anything else that is available which he requests. Review daily and weigh weekly
Prevent rejection by others due to poor hygiene. Prevent constipation	Ensure that Ali has sufficient tissues and prompt him to wipe his nose if necessary. If he will eat it, give him bran, fresh fruit and 2000 ml fluid per day
As 2 and 4	As 2 and 4. Unless Ali initiates conversation concerning his sexuality do not discuss this at present
Observe sleeping pattern for 24 hours	Observe and record Ali's sleeping pattern hourly. Try to establish whether he does sleep or just lies down

20
Organic Mental States

Any condition which interferes with cerebral function will result in some degree of psychiatric disorder, manifested in perceptual and intellectual impairment, clouding of consciousness, and changes in mood and behaviour.

A *toxic confusional state (delirium)* is a diffuse, temporary, reversible impairment of mental function. It can occur in a variety of conditions. Although coloured by a patient's personality, and previous neurotic and psychotic states if these were present, delirium has certain characteristic features.

Most striking is the disturbance or clouding of consciousness. The patient is disorientated for time and place. His attention can be held, if at all, for short periods only. He is perplexed and anxious, unable to understand what is happening to him, or to separate real from imaginary experiences. All aspects of memory are upset. He is restless, his mood may fluctuate rapidly between depression and elation, and terrifying dreams interrupt his sleep. Illusions occur; fluff on the bed changes into little animals; cracks on the wall assume the shape of moving faces. Nurses become enemies to be attacked or avoided. Frightening visual hallucinations cause him to panic and react violently. These symptoms are liable to be at their worst at night, for external stimulation, which helps to combat confusion, is then minimal.

In *subacute delirium* consciousness is less disturbed. The patient realises at times that his perceptions are abnormal and tries to understand what is happening to him. But his thoughts and speech remain confused, and it is usually difficult to follow him for long. His level of consciousness and accessibility fluctuate a good deal, and this helps to distinguish delirium from acute mania and catatonia.

Confusional states last from a few hours to days and weeks, depending on the underlying cause.

Aetiology

1. *Infections.* Any systemic infection with high fever may cause mental confusion. Old people and heavy drinkers are particularly vulnerable. Intracranial infections, encephalitis and meningitis, commonly produce some degree of confusion.

2. *Metabolic illnesses* such as hepatic failure, uraemia, hypoglycaemia, dehydration and electrolyte disturbances may be present. Porphyria should always be remembered, for delirium is a common complication.

3. *Nutritional deficiencies*, particularly those of the vitamin B complex. Vitamin B1 deficiency is rarely seen in western countries today, except in association with alcoholism. It is responsible for Wernicke's encephalopathy and Korsakov's syndrome. Deficiency of vitamin B3 results in pellagra. Deficiency of vitamin B12 and folic acid produce permanent brain changes if untreated for long, but when caught in the early stages, mental symptoms are reversible.

4. *Intoxication or self poisoning* is a frequent cause of confusion; almost any drug taken in big enough dosage will do so. Common ones are hypotensive, antiParkinsonian, antidepressant and tranquillising drugs. The elderly, with their lowered metabolic and excretory functions are especially vulnerable. Alcohol potentiates their effects. Large doses of amphetamines, hallucinogenic drugs and opiates are all capable of causing confusion. Alcohol can of course cause confusion, either from the direct result of large quantities, or from delirium tremens, as a result of withdrawal.

5. *Cardio-respiratory*. Cerebral anoxia from pulmonary disease or congestive heart failure is liable to cause confusion.

6. *Trauma and brain lesions*. Concussion; the post-traumatic confusional state which follows severe head injury may continue for weeks or longer, and fluctuates from day to day; subdural haematoma often results in fluctuating confusion and mental symptoms; subarachnoid haemorrhage; cerebral arteriosclerosis; epilepsy (see below); cerebral tumours, particularly when deep-seated; advanced stages of multiple sclerosis.

7. *Miscellaneous*. Post-operative confusional states are short-lived, except in old people or alcoholics. Open heart surgery is often succeeded by confusion for three or four days. Cancer of the lung may be associated with delirium.

Differential diagnosis

Clouding of consciousness and perplexity must be present for the diagnosis of a confusional state. Acute schizophrenic and manic patients may be incoherent, and attend so little that it may be difficult to distinguish their level of consciousness. An atypical psychotic state may present in a confused, excitable condition. It may take a day or more to confirm the diagnosis, but the search for an underlying cause must not be delayed.

Treatment

Once the patient is recognised to have a confusional state, the cause must be sought at once. Often this is obvious. A 49 year old man was seen at home because of strange behaviour: appearing naked at the window, shouting and gesticulating. He was disorientated in time, although he recognised he was at home. It was difficult to hold his attention for more than 30 seconds. His mood was labile and ranged quickly from tears to anger. His temperature was 40°C and he had bronchopneumonia. It later emerged that he was a heavy drinker. He improved rapidly with an antibiotic, although for 24 hours he needed a small dose of chlorpromazine to control his behaviour.

Sometimes the cause is not immediately obvious. X-ray, blood count, urea and electrolyte levels, and hepatic functions reveal no abnormality. Investigations should then include a brain scan and electroencephalography.

In the meantime, *symptomatic medication* is often required. Clearly any drug likely to increase the patient's confusion must be avoided. Dosage should be kept to a minimum, but it is pointless to give so low a dose that it is ineffectual. When the delirium is due to infection say, or congestive heart failure, chlorpromazine is valuable and can rapidly calm the patient. With older patients, hepatic failure, or delirium tremens, a diazepine derivative – we use lorazepam – or chlormethiazole are useful, less likely to cause side effects and generally safer.

Good general management of the patient can frequently obviate the need for medication. Nurses must reassure him, speak to him by name frequently, explain where he is and why. He should have a radio and be allowed visitors. All too often in general hospital wards a delirious patient, particularly if difficult or unpleasant, is avoided. This increases his confusion, and difficult behaviour.

As he recovers he must be reassured and told what has happened. He will not remember the time of confusion.

21
Dementia

Between 5 and 10 per cent of the elderly show signs of dementia, the incidence rising progressively with age, reaching 20 per cent of those aged 80 and older. However, less than 5 per cent are in institutional residential care. They are cared for by devoted families, and not a few continue to live alone, helped by neighbours. This highlights the fact that the problems associated with dementia are not simply due to brain changes, but are coloured and modified by the basic personality of the patient, his or her physical health, and social factors.

Dementia is a diffuse, irreversible deterioration of mental functions due to structural changes in the brain. The onset may be acute and initially disguised by confusion, or slow and insidious. As in confusional states, symptoms are coloured by the basic personality of the patient.

Although dementia is generally irreversible, some improvement may be possible if the condition responsible for it can be removed; for instance, in general paralysis of the insane or myxoedema. If dementia occurs in childhood it is usually classed as mental impairment.

Symptoms and signs

Loss of memory for recent events, and particularly for names of people and places, is one of the first noticeable changes. At first this forgetfulness may be intermittent, and successfully disguised by the patient, even to the extent of confabulation. But sooner or later it becomes apparent. Sometimes it can appear suddenly, following a 'small stroke', or an acute infection associated with subacute delirium. Memory for distant events is retained. Most cases of dementia encountered today are progressive, and the loss of memory gradually extends backwards. A severely dementing individual may be unable to recall anything about himself, even his name. Loss of memory makes a patient unreliable in behaviour when alone. He or she can turn on the gas and think it is alight, switch on electric fires and start a blaze or burn himself, and turn on the bath, forget about it, and cause a flood. Money and other objects are put down and then lost. Paranoid reactions are common at this point, and angry or even violent accusations occur. When shopping he is liable to pick up goods and forget to pay for them, and may find himself in trouble with the law.

Learning becomes increasingly difficult, not simply because retention or recall is impaired, but also because his attention cannot be held for long. A serial 7s test will indicate this deficit. He is distractible. Concentration begins to fail in the early stages and may be an early complaint of the patient. He can no longer do his work efficiently, he is always fatigued, he can no longer show initiative and make decisions, for he is unable to grasp the nub of a problem. His judgment in consequence becomes increasingly faulty.

Initially he tries to compensate for his failing powers by withdrawing from activities likely to be too much for him. He develops an even more rigid pattern of behaviour; excessive orderliness, careful and repeated checking. At this stage, when asked to perform a task beyond his ability, he may react with *catastrophic* anxiety and break down into tears and childlike anger. His speech becomes full of clichés and lacks ideas and imagination. In time an increasing degree of perseveration appears and there may be dysphasia.

Depression and anxiety understandably are common in the early stages. Many patients quickly lose insight into their condition, but those who continue to recognise the deterioration are liable to attempt suicide, an action which often arouses both sympathy, feelings of guilt, and anger in relatives and professional helpers. But sooner or later, as dementia progresses, the dement appears to lose all understanding of himself and his situation. Mood then becomes labile and childlike, with evanescent tears, laughter and irritability. When frustrated he is prone to fly into rages.

Personality changes develop as control of emotional needs and appetites slackens. Sexual behaviour may run amok with disinhibited masturbation or exhibitionism in public places. Eating manners and habits become coarse. Rubbish is hoarded and the patient grows chaotic and filthy. Sleep is disturbed and sometimes reversed, so that the dement sleeps during the day and wanders about at night. In the latter stages there is often confusion, and consequently he may wander out of the house, seeking some 'old friend', perhaps with little or no clothing on him in the middle of winter. Inevitably he loses his way and is eventually found and returned home by the police.

Types of Dementia

1. *Senile dementia.* Senile dementia has an insidious onset. It may be noticed after an acute confusional episode. Depression in the early

stages is common and responds to treatment. Death usually occurs three to five years after symptoms first appear.

2. *Arteriosclerotic dementia.* Arteriosclerotic dementia is not necessarily associated with hypertension, although signs of arteriosclerosis can usually be detected peripherally. The onset may be apparent after a small stroke which causes temporary dysphagia and confusion, or is insidious. Memory loss is more patchy than in senile dementia. Emotional control declines but the finer feelings of personality tend to be preserved at first. Depression and anxiety reflect the patient's awareness of these changes, and lead to suicidal attempts. Later, as dementia increases, there are bouts of confusion and disturbed behaviour. It may be associated at some stage with arteriosclerotic Parkinsonism.

3. *Presenile dementia.* There are three main, comparatively rare forms of dementia developing before the age of 65: Alzheimer's disease, Pick's disease, and Huntington's chorea. Jacob-Creutzfeldt disease is a rapidly progressive dementia associated with visual, pyramidal, and often cerebellar signs, caused by a virus. There is no treatment for it and death occurs within about six months.

(a) *Alzheimer's disease.* There is little or no difference in pathology between this condition and senile dementia. The usual age of onset is between 40 and 60 years, but the condition can begin younger. Symptoms are the result of generalised atrophy of the brain. Fits occur in 25 per cent of patients, and the gait is stiff, slow and unsteady, rather like that of a clockwork soldier.

(b) *Pick's disease.* In Pick's disease atrophy is most marked in the frontal and temporal areas of the brain. Mood becomes fatuous and jocular. Loss of emotional control may lead to anti-social behaviour.

(c) *Huntington's chorea.* This condition is due to the effects of a single dominant gene, which manifests itself at any age from childhood onwards but usually between the ages of 30 and 50 years. Symptoms result from atrophy of the frontal lobes and basal ganglia. Memory is often well preserved, even after several years. The first symptoms are rapid jerky involuntary movements, most apparent in the face and upper half of the body. Speech is also affected after a time and becomes difficult to understand. The patient is often aware of the significance of these symptoms and suicide is not uncommon.

The course of the presenile dementias may continue for 10 or more years.

4. *Secondary dementias*

(a) *Brain injury.* Dementia can follow on from trauma.

(b) *Inflammatory diseases*: All forms of meningitis, encephalitis, and syphilis.

(c) *Intracranial tumour*, carcinoma of the bronchus, subdural haematoma.

(d) *Avitaminosis*, causing beri-beri, pellagra, Korsakov's syndrome, Wernicke's encephalopathy, and pernicious anaemia.

(e) *Endocrine disorders*, such as untreated myxoedema, prolonged and severe hypoglycaemia.

(f) *Prolonged anoxia*, such as occurs in carbon monoxide poisoning and prolonged cardiac arrest.

(g) *Toxic*, alcohol and the Korsakoff psychosis.

Differential diagnosis

Severe dementia offers no diagnostic problems. Early dementia may be mistaken for depression, particularly since depression may be present because of dementia. Testing of recent memory, attention and conceptual grasp will confirm suspicions of dementia. But in any case depression, when present, should be treated along the usual lines.

Diagnostic difficulties may also arise with patients dependent on large doses of barbiturates and other sedative drugs. However, when these are withdrawn the patient's mental functions improve rapidly.

A supporting history from a close relative or friend is invaluable, not only for dating the onset of the condition and for describing changes in behaviour, but also for giving an idea of the normal level of intelligence.

Hysterical pseudo-dementia (Ganser syndrome) is a rare occurrence (see p. 117).

Investigations

Every patient with dementia, unless the cause is perfectly apparent, should be fully investigated. This includes a thorough medical check of all systems, including serum B12 and folate levels; X-ray of chest and skull; EEG; brain scan; and EMI scan where possible. Angiography may be indicated when a subdural haemotoma or cerebral tumour are possibilities.

Psychological testing is only occasionally helpful. When there is clinical doubt over the diagnosis of dementia, all too often the results of intelligence testing are equally ambiguous.

Treatment

Much of the disturbed behaviour associated with dementia arises not so much from the brain changes as from the effect of the patient's surroundings on him. Indeed 95 per cent of demented patients can and do remain in their own homes. Dementia in fact may only become apparent when a patient has to live on his own or move to new surroundings, is socially isolated and perhaps lonely. Although secondary dementia improves or is arrested by treatment of the primary cause, no treatment arrests progressive primary dementias. In old people in particular every attempt should be made to improve nutrition, large doses of vitamins given, cardiac output improved, and so on. From time to time drugs are introduced which are claimed to improve cerebral circulation and metabolism, and therefore to help dementing patients, particularly those with cerebral arteriosclerosis. There is little convincing evidence that these drugs achieve much. Infection, physical debility, and depression should be treated energetically and sensibly. Depression responds well to antidepressant drugs, and sleep and behaviour improve as a result. Aggressive paranoid reactions can be reduced by means of a small dose of a neuroleptic. It is wrong to turn a difficult dementing patient into a cabbage, but it is equally bad to refuse to give drugs for fear of this.

The dement easily becomes disorientated and upset. It is important therefore that his surroundings should be kept as constant as possible. He needs regular stimulation, i.e. conversation with family and friends, his regular TV programme, a walk to the park, or even to the pub. It is essential that his physical and mental states are not exceeded, otherwise he is liable to become confused and difficult.

For the patient living alone and isolated, regular visits from the community psychiatric nurse are of immense importance. She can monitor his progress, and note any signs of deterioration, and act quickly and appropriately. The importance of calling the dement by his name, picking up his photographs, book, and other memorabilia, and talking about them reinforces his sense of identity and feeling of security. The community psychiatric nurse may be able to arrange for a home help, meals on wheels, luncheon clubs, outings with a group, visitors to call and so on. Attendance at a day centre or day hospital can provide greater stimulation and supervision. Occupational therapy, combined with music and simple games, is often of considerable value and prevents or minimises deterioration.

The strain on relatives who look after a dement is considerable and they need every support possible. The community psychiatric nurse or doctor supervising the patient's progress should discuss with the caring relatives any changes they may have noticed, their significance, and how they should best behave with the patient. Attendance at a day centre or hospital, apart from helping the patient, also allows the carers a breathing space during the day. It may also be helpful to arrange for the patient to come into hospital for a week or two from time to time, to allow the carers to go away on holiday, and generally give them a rest. It is of course essential to prepare the patient for such a move well in advance, to discuss the matter repeatedly, and perhaps for him to visit the ward or home and meet the people who will be looking after him.

Sooner or later the demented patient may become too difficult to look after at home, either because of changes in the carers' circumstances, or deteriorating behaviour on the part of the patient. Other arrangements must then be made. If dementia is not too advanced it may be possible to place the patient in a residential old people's home (so-called Part 3 accommodation). But supervision is sometimes perfunctory, and it is then necessary for the patient to go to a geriatric hospital.

Nursing in a geriatric ward is a difficult task, calling for considerable qualities on the part of the nurse. The patients frequently deteriorate, yet much can be done to preserve the core of the patient's identity, to give the patient maximum comfort and pleasure, and to maintain a patient's sense of self respect to the last. This is none too easy, but is possible if the nurse always continues to see the patient, however demented and helpless, as an individual, to address him by his name, to talk to him and relate to him, scold him at times no doubt, but without malice. All this is made easier by the nurse feeling part of the psychiatric team, by discussion, not only of the patient's progress and needs, but of the nurse's own problems if need be.

Psychogeriatrics

Old age officially begins at 65. More than 15 per cent of the population are 65 or more, and nearly 6 per cent are 75 or older, and these proportions will continue to rise until the end of this century. Women outnumber men, particularly single women living alone. About one-third of the elderly live alone, often on a low income in unsatisfactory housing conditions. Many are afraid, or due to physical disabilities, unable to go out alone. In consequence they live lonely, isolated lives.

Psychogeriatric assessment units

It is vital to determine the relative importance of physical, social and psychological factors in any elderly patient with a mental disorder.

Psychogeriatric assessment requires the co-operation of a team, a geriatrician and a psychiatrist, together with the patient's general practitioner, social worker, or community psychiatric nurse. Ideally a patient should be assessed at home or in the out-patient clinic, since admission to hospital itself may provoke anxiety and confusion in the elderly. However there are patients who need to be assessed in hospital. Psychogeriatric assessment units are being established throughout the country for this purpose. Patients are fully investigated, intensively treated, and a plan agreed upon within three to four weeks for their long-term care and treatment if necessary. If further in-patient treatment is required, the patient is transferred to the appropriate psychiatric or medical ward.

Psychiatric disorders are common among the elderly and neurotic symptoms are widespread. Depression can be a prolongation of a chronic state, present for many years before old age, often accompanied by manipulative behaviour. Circumscribed episodes of depression may have occurred before, or there may be a history of manic depression. But first attacks of depression can develop at any age, even in the 80s. Suicide is always a risk, for men especially.

> A man of 76 became severely depressed shortly after the death of his wife. In spite of supportive children and treatment from his general practitioner, he killed himself four months later.

Depression in old age is frequently precipitated by 'loss'; death of a spouse, retirement, moving home, or loss of health and mobility.

Depression must be carefully differentiated from dementia. The unwary may be misled by overlying signs of depression in early dementia, when the sufferer still has some insight into what is happening to him. But depressive illness may in turn mimic dementia. Apathy and withdrawal, inattention and poor memory with other depressive symptoms form a picture of pseudodementia. Depression understandably accompanies conditions such as Parkinsonism, and is sometimes a consequence of antiParkinsonian treatment. But a retarded depressed patient can also superficially resemble Parkinson's disease.

Manic illness is also seen in old age, sometimes for the first time. Treatment for depression and mania follow the lines set out on p. 205.

Schizophrenic symptoms become modified and less florid with time, and the aged chronic schizophrenic is usually emotionally flat and withdrawn. Aural hallucinations may still occur, but without much effect. Schizophrenia can develop around old age. It is usually of a paranoid kind. Occasionally symptoms develop acutely.

> A single woman of 67, living alone, became convinced that a neighbour was putting 'something' in her milk and waking her up at night by knocking on the ceiling. She complained to the police without effect. She woke one night to 'what felt like laser beams' on her body. She was both terrified and angry. She rushed upstairs and tried to break down the neighbour's door. The police were summoned and she was taken to hospital.

John Webster

John is an 83-year-old man who has been admitted for assessment. His immediate nursing problems are confusion and urinary incontinence. His initial care plan involves nurses preventing potential problems such as pressure sores (mobility) and accurate observation. There were ketones in his urine on admission which suggests that he has not been eating adequately and has been breaking down fat. The nursing care described for John involves orientating him in time and space (Reality orientation – see further reading list) while assisting him with activities of daily living.

As John progresses it will be necessary to re-assess his nursing needs while promoting maximum independence (Roper, 1976).

Although John is elderly the nursing team's aim should be to restore his ability for self care in order that he might return home. It is only if it becomes clear on medical diagnosis that he will be unable to do so, that this aim may need to be reversed.

Nursing Information Sheet

Hospital No: **Wards:** **Date of Admission:**

Surname WEBSTER **Forename** John Irvine

Address 7, The Hollys
Brenton, Middlesex

Likes to be known as: Mr Webster
Date of birth: 11.2.1901 **Age:** 83 **Sex:** M
Marital status: Widower
Religion: R/C **Nationality:** English

Relevant Psychiatric and General Medical History
Left leg below knee amputation in 1976 following a road traffic accident when he walked in front of a car

No previous psychiatric history

Is patient formal or informal?

Informal
Section

Next of kin: Mr Bill Webster (son)
Address: 16, Linocks Way, Daleby, Yorkshire

Tel. no.: Daleby 21964
Person to contact in case of emergency: (if different from above)

Address:
As/Above

Tel. no.: Work No. Daleby 21276

Occupation and past work history

Retired
Railway signalman for 40 years

Source of finance:
Old age and Occupational pension

Home conditions

Bedsit and bathroom in warden controlled accommodation. Lunch and supper taken in communal dining room

---

Community resources (CPNS voluntary agencies)
Distric Nurse

Significant persons in life
Son. Friend Mrs Elsie Smith who also resides in the Hollys

Patient's profile
Height 5ft 10 in
Weight 65 kg
Build Medium
Complexion Sallow/Pale
Hair–Colour Bald, small amount grey
Eyes–Colour Pale Blue
Marks and Scars False left leg below knee

T.P.R. T 36°C P 72 R 16

B.P. 125/90

Urine Ward urinalysis - ke tones present

Special nursing observation
Four hourly T P R
Urinalysis for microculture and sensitivity (form signed by Dr Reynolds)

Reason for admission:
Confusional state with urinary incontinence

For assessment

Referred by: **Accepted by:**
Consultant Geriatrician
G.P. **after a domicillary visit**
Tel No.: Senior Registrar Dr John Reynolds

Present Situation	Actual and Potential Problems (Level of independence/ dependence)
1. Maintaining a safe environment John is confused in that he does not appear to appreciate he is in hospital. He could be a danger to himself if he left the ward unaccompanied. John smokes 10 cigarettes a day	Not aware of his surroundings. Potential danger to himself if he leaves the ward un- accompanied. Risk of burning with cigarettes
2. Personal hygiene The warden at John's flat says that he is generally meticulously clean and strip washes every day - he does not like getting in the bath. At the moment he is dishevelled and does not appear to have washed thoroughly for some time, nocturnal eneuresis. John has dentures	Dishevelled - no evidence of regular washing. Nocturnal eneuresis
3. Special factors Ke tones in urine. Slightly raised temperature	Raised temperature Ke tones in urine
4. Care of clothing John's clothing is in good condition and he was neatly dressed on arrival	Potential problem - John may mislay his clothes due to confusion. He can dress alone
5. Co-operation in ward life John has been sitting in a chair by his bed since his arrival and looks anxious when approached by other people on the ward	John's disorientation may increase if a lot of people approach and try to talk to him
6. Attitude toward medication John is not on any medication at present	
7. Working and playing – social mixing John is unable to give a coherent account of his working and social life. He worked on the railway for forty years, was widowed six years ago and has been in sheltered accommodation for five. Likes television	Incontinence may cause social rejection

Aim of Nursing Intervention	Plan of Care
Tell John where he is and why. Do not allow him to leave the ward unaccompanied. Prevention of burning	S/N Smith will co-ordinate John's care and allocate a student to work with him in her absence. Orientate John to the ward and hospital by explaining where he is and why. Close observation to see that he does not leave unaccompanied. Allow him cigarettes but not in bed and observe closely
To maintain adequate personal hygiene	Strip wash with help whenever necessary - especially after nocturnal eneuresis. Observe skin for redness. Do not make him have a bath. Daily cleaning of dentures
To ensure no infection present. Collect urine as requested by medical staff	Collect middle stream of urine specimen for microculture and sensitivity - four-hourly T P R. Push fluids, See 12
To maintain independence while ensuring care is taken of John's clothing	Allow John to dress himself but encourage him to change his clothes and put them away safely as necessary. Send dirty clothes to the laundry clearly labelled. See 1
To orientate John to the ward	Do not allow a lot of patients to talk to John at once and encourage them to speak clearly and introduce themselves when they do
Reduce incontinence. To get him to join in ward activities without stressing him	See 3. Encourage John to watch television and go for accompanied walks in the grounds when he feels like it

	Present Situation	Actual and Potential Problems (Level of independence/ dependence)
8.	**Communicating** John answers clearly when spoken to. He says that he feels very tired and that talking is an effort. He would like to be left quietly alone. When asked where he is he replied 'in my childhood', when told he is in hospital he shook his head and held it in his hands	John can communicate clearly. He is tired and confused in that he says he is in his childhood
9.	**Perception** John says he is in his childhood, there is evidence of disorientation in both time and space. No evidence of delusion or hallucinations. Wears bifocal glasses all the time and has a hearing aid	Disorientation of time and space. Wears glasses and a hearing aid
10.	**Finance and budgeting** John has an old age and railway pension. His rent is paid by direct debit. Over the last six days since his confusion began he has become confused with decimal money and reverted to £.S.D. The warden has been helping him with this	Muddled about money - thinks we are working in £.S.D.
11.	**Mobility** Left leg below knee amputee, manages well when limb is fitted correctly. He has some difficulty putting his stump bandage on and restricts the blood flow if not helped. Norton score 12	Reduced blood flow to left stump. Instability if limb not fitted correctly. Pressure sore risk
12.	**Eating and drinking** John has been forgetting to go to meals. When given food and drink he eats and drinks without persuasion. He says that he is thirsty and loves hot sweet tea (two teaspoons)	Forgetting to go to meals. Thirsty
13.	**Eliminating** Incontinent at night for the last week. Small amount of incontinence in the day - John is aware that he wishes to pass urine but has difficulty in getting to the lavatory in time due to the fact he says he can't always remember where it is. No problems with constipation or faecal incontinence	Nocturnal eneuresis. Incontinence occasionally during the day
14.	**Expressing sexuality** John has been friendly with Elsie Smith who also lives at the Hollys; he goes old time dancing with her and thoroughly enjoys her company. Yesterday he upset her by calling her by his dead wife's name Margaret	Confusing his dead wife with a friend who is alive
15.	**Sleeping** John has been having Chloral hydrate at night for the last week and slept well. This has been discontinued in order to observe his sleep pattern for his first night	Sleep pattern may be disturbed

Aim of Nursing Intervention	Plan of Care
To communicate with John. Explain he is in hospital	Spend time each shift with John talking to him (See 9). Listen to what he has to say and report any evidence of confusion.
To orientate John to time and space. Ensure glasses and hearing aid are satisfactory	See 1. Show John the newspapers explaining what is happening, the year, current events, etc. See that John's glasses are clean, check when last sight test was done. Check battery of hearing aid and that it is working
To remind John about decimalisation	Point out what things cost to John - take him shopping for cigarettes, papers at the hospital shop and explain decimalisation
To ensure adequate circulation to stump and stability. Prevention of pressure sores	Assist with stump bandage while John is confused. See that limb is fitted securely. Change John's position two-hourly by encouraging him to go for a walk or turn him if he is in bed
Maintain adequate diet. Intake of 2000 ml fluid every 24 hours	Remind John to go to the table at mealtimes. Encourage fluids especially hot sweet tea. Fluid chart
Prevention of incontinence	See 3. Take John to the toilet every 2 hours, and ensure he passes urine before he goes to bed. Commode by his bed. Note the time when he is incontinent and take him to the toilet prior to this the next day
To reorientate John to the fact that his wife is dead and who Elsie is	Encourage John's son to visit and his grandchildren if possible. Remind John who Elsie is. Gently point out his wife is dead if he talks about her as if she is alive
To assess sleeping pattern	Close observation of sleeping pattern, i.e. when he goes to sleep, if confused at night, etc.

22
Epilepsy

Definition

Epilepsy is a paroxysmal and transitory disturbance of brain function, causing characteristic electrical discharges, which result in a disturbance of movement, feeling or consciousness.

Incidence

Between four and six people in every 1000 have epileptic fits at some time in their lives. The greatest incidence occurs during the first five years of childhood. About one-third of all epileptics have psychiatric difficulties.

Symptoms

Epilepsy can be divided into three types, all or any of which may occur in one patient.

1. *Grand mal (GM).* A full GM attack passes through a series of stages. Many patients feel irritable and depressed for some hours or even days before the fit occurs. The fit itself may be immediately preceded by an *aura*, lasting a second or two which consists of flashing lights and other visual disturbances, forced movements, or peculiar sensations and emotions; the aura can be intensely frightening.

The fit begins with a generalised tonic contraction of all voluntary muscles. Air is expelled from the lungs, resulting in a weird cry. Consciousness is lost. The tonic contraction lasts up to a minute and is followed by a clonic phase of alternating muscle relaxation and contraction. This phase may last several minutes and during it the patient may bite his tongue and be incontinent. Afterwards the patient has a headache, feels sleepy and may remain confused for some time. Repeated GM attacks in rapid succession are known as *status epilepticus.* The electroencephalogram (EEG) shows high-voltage fast waves or spikes.

2. *Petit mal.* Petit mal is less common. The attack consists of a sudden short interruption of consciousness. The patient breaks off a conversation or stops what he is doing for a second or so, then resumes where he left off. Sometimes muscle tone is suddenly lost

(*akinetic seizure*) and the patient falls. Continuous petit mal attacks are known as *pyknolepsy*.

The EEG shows spikes and waves occurring at the rate of three a second.

3. *Focal epilepsy* includes all epileptic phenomena, sensory or motor, in which the abnormal discharge remains localised to one part of the brain. From a psychiatric point of view the most interesting of these is *psychomotor* or *temporal lobe* epilepsy; seizure manifestations include automatic behaviour, visceral sensations, illusions and hallucinations, dreamy states, and memory disturbances. Symptoms manifest themselves in a variety of ways. The patient may become confused, paranoid or aggressive. Unpleasant emotions, particularly fear, make themselves felt. *Déjà vu* phenomena, hallucinations, unreality and depersonalisation feelings sometimes occur. During an attack the patient may behave as an automaton, subsequently remembering nothing. Abnormal symptoms of smell or taste are fairly common, as are auditory and visual hallucinations.

Psychiatric aspects

1. *Symptoms caused by epileptic activity interfering with mental functions.*

(a) *Directly related to the fits*:

(i) Depression and irritability may precede a fit by one or more days.

(ii) When consciousness is not totally lost, automatic behaviour, perhaps at variance with the personality of the patient, may occur. Violence however is rare. This *twilight* state can occur before, during or after a fit. Amnesia for the period of automatic behaviour is usually complete. Wandering (fugue state) can occur.

(iii) Delusions and hallucinations occur during *temporal lobe epilepsy* and may last several days.

(b) *Indirectly related to the fits*:

(i) *Schizophreniform psychoses* sometimes develop in patients with long-standing *temporal lobe epilepsy*. This is more likely in left-sided lesions.

(ii) *Epileptic personality* formation. The epileptic becomes egocentric, hypochondriacal, moody, touchy, and liable to outbursts of temper. This state, which is not common may be related to long use of anticonvulsant drugs, or more likely to the psychological disadvantages of epilepsy.

(iii) *Hysterical fits* are occasionally difficult to distinguish from true epilepsy, particularly when they develop in a patient known to have epilepsy (see p. 116). Attacks may mimic epileptic fits, but usually have a characteristic dramatic attention-seeking quality.

2. *Psychological effects of being epileptic*:

Epilepsy is still a social stigma, as well as a disability. Epileptics may not drive* and cannot take a job in which a fit is likely to have dangerous consequences. Although an epileptic can register himself as a disabled person many employers are reluctant to employ epileptics. In the public mind epilepsy is still mistakenly connected with crime, 'degeneration' and low intelligence. It is therefore hardly surprising that anxiety, depression and other psychological reactions are often seen in epileptics. There is, in fact, no consistent evidence that epilepsy leads eventually to intellectual deterioration or dementia.

Aetiology

1. *Heredity*. It is important to understand that any of us can have a fit if our brains are sufficiently stimulated. ECT does just that. Epileptics only differ in the fact that their brains have a low threshold for discharging. Hereditary factors are important in 'idiopathic' epilepsy.

2. *Brain damage* is found, during EEG investigation, in 75 per cent or more epileptics. Anoxia and trauma to the brain are believed to be responsible for many of these.

3. *Precipitating factors*. In young children, convulsions occur during fevers. Other precipitating factors are over-breathing, fatigue, emotional distress, over-hydration and hypoglycaemia.

Treatment and management

In the past, epileptics were sent to epileptic colonies. This is now considered to militate against their recovery, and the policy is to maintain epileptics in the community. However, about 2000 people still live in epileptic colonies and are unable, for one reason or another, to return to the community.

Treatment aims firstly to control seizures with the smallest dose of drugs possible, and without causing side effects, and secondly to help the patient deal with the social problems which may arise

* Since January, 1976 changes in the law on driving licences have taken effect. A licence can be granted to someone with a history of epilepsy provided that he has for at least 3 years been free of fits while awake, or if he does have fits, these only occur during his sleep.

from epilepsy. A number of drugs are available. Those in common use for the control of *petit mal* seizures are ethosuximide (250–1500 mg a day), and troxidone (300–1200 mg a day). For *grand mal* and *focal epilepsy*, phenobarbitone (60–180 mg a day), primidone (250–1500 mg a day), phenytoin (100–300 mg a day), sulthiame (200–600 mg a day) are recommended. Sulthiame (Ospolot) is mainly used in the treatment of temporal lobe epilepsy. Side effects, such as drowsiness, ataxia, headache, are common and require the dosage to be reduced. Psychotic reactions have also been reported. Carbamazepine (Tegretol) is also used in temporal lobe epilepsy as well as for trigeminal neuralgia. In practice, control is often best achieved by a combination of drugs.

Intravenous diazepam, 10–20 mg, is invaluable in controlling status epilepticus.

There are about 60 000 schoolchildren with epilepsy in England and Wales. Provided their intelligence is reasonable (about 10 per cent of epileptic children are mentally impaired), and fits are not too frequent, these children can attend ordinary schools. Even when fits are well controlled, the epileptic child is especially likely to have difficulties in learning and in making friends. Puberty and leaving school are periods of particular stress. Special residential schools exist for disturbed epileptic children.

Adults should understand what happens during a fit and the risks to be avoided in work and play. Severe epileptics may need to be assessed in a regional neurological centre, associated with a workshop and hostel accommodation. Marriage raises the question of epilepsy being transmitted to children, quite apart from the difficulties that an epileptic may encounter in marriage. No general rules can be laid down and the matter needs to be discussed fully with both partners.

Psychotherapy of a general sort is helpful in dealing with the anxieties and behaviour disorders that occur in epileptic patients. Parents, as well as their epileptic child, respond to explanation and encouragement. Temporal lobectomy may occasionally need to be considered, particularly when the epilepsy is associated with aggressive behaviour. However, it is never undertaken lightly, and although aggressiveness is frequently relieved, it is often replaced by serious depression.

23
Mental Handicap

The term 'mental handicap' is used to describe the condition of limited intelligence. Mental handicap is usually present from birth or early childhood due to arrested or incomplete development. Adults may become mentally handicapped after trauma or disease.

The 1983 Mental Health Act introduces the term *mental impairment* to replace that of mental subnormality used in the previous Act (1959). The 1983 Act defines two subgroups:

Severe mental impairment meaning 'a state of incomplete development of mind which includes severe impairment of intelligence and social functioning and is associated with abnormally aggressive or seriously irresponsible conduct on the part of the person concerned.'

Mental impairment meaning 'a state of arrested or incomplete development of mind (not amounting to severe mental impairment) which includes significant impairment of intelligence and social functioning and is associated with abnormally aggressive or seriously irresponsible conduct on the part of the person concerned' (MHA, 1983: 1–2).

It is important to be aware that both categories of impairment refer to 'abnormally aggressive or seriously irresponsible conduct' in the Mental Health Act. There are many people with limited intelligence who display neither of these characteristics. It is useful to differentiate by referring to those without severe irresponsible conduct or not abnormally aggressive as 'mentally handicapped' individuals.

It is necessary to recognise that an individual is usually labelled mentally handicapped, not simply because of a low IQ, but because of additional physical disabilities, difficult or disturbed behaviour, or because he lacks a proper home. The incidence of psychiatric and behavioural disorders is closely related to IQ level. Approximately 2.5–3 per cent of children have IQs between 50 and 70 and only 0.35 per cent of children fall into the category of an IQ below 50. It is recognised that mental handicap is associated with mood and behavioural problems.

Most children with IQ's of between 55 and 70 are not labelled mentally handicapped and only come to notice in school because of educational limitations. They are then moved to schools for the mentally handicapped: about one per cent of children of school age attend these schools.

On the other hand, if their behaviour is disturbed, until recently they were legally excluded from school and at that time termed mentally *subnormal.* Since April, 1971, under the Education (Handicapped Children) Act of 1970, the power to exclude such children from education ceased. Less than 0.1 per cent of schoolchildren come into this category.

After leaving school, the majority of mildly mentally handicapped individuals adjust well and become independent members of the community. Only a few mentally handicapped individuals, with additional personality problems, require admission to hospitals for the mentally handicapped.

Their parents are very mildly mentally handicapped mainly from social class 5. Many are capable of marriage and of having children, although the number they are likely to have per family is less than the national average. Individuals with an IQ of below 50 occur less frequently. Among English children aged 10–14, the incidence is about 0.35 per cent, Down's syndrome accounting for about a quarter of the cases. Most people with severe mental handicap require, at some time, assistance from the health service, either in terms of community support or hospital admission.

Causes of Mental Handicap

Although it is possible to discover changes in the brain at postmortem of severely mentally handicapped individuals, in most cases the cause is either unknown or doubtful.

1. *Genetic causes*

Harmful genes, dominant, recessive, or sex linked, are responsible for about 1 per cent of cases of severe mental impairment.

(a) *Dominant genes* are relatively rare. A single gene is transmitted by a parent to (in theory) half his offspring. Fresh gene mutations probably play an important part in dominant conditions associated with severe mental handicap such as *Epiloia* (tuberose sclerosis).

(b) *Recessive genes.* Both parents are carriers of the gene responsible for the recessive abnormality; they themselves are unaffected and fertile. Their offspring have a one in four chance of being affected. Recessive genes are responsible for such conditions as phenylketonuria, Wilson's disease and amaurotic idiocy. In recent years there have been considerable advances in screening and detecting heterozygous carriers of such genes.

Phenylketonuria is the result of an inability to convert phenylalanine to tyrosine, due to the absence of the enzyme phenylalanine hydroxylase. Phenylketonuric acid appears in the urine shortly after birth (identified by the ferric chloride test). Untreated, mental handicap is usually, although not always, severe. Provided a phenylalanine-free diet is started within the first few months, mental development, in terms of mental age, proceeds at a normal rate. The longer the delay in starting dietary treatment the more the brain is damaged. It is still uncertain how long treatment must continue.

2. *Chromosome abnormalities*

Cytogenetics is a rapidly advancing study. Autosomal abnormalities are nearly always accompanied by severe mental impairment. Sex chromosome anomalies can also cause mental impairment but to a less severe degree.

(a) *Autosomes.* Down's syndrome (Mongolism) is the best known condition associated with an autosomal defect. It exists in all races and is the commonest disease entity in mentally impaired populations. In hospitals for the mentally handicapped, Down's syndrome sufferers make up about 10 per cent of the population. The frequency of Down's syndrome at birth in London and the Home Counties is about one in 666, but falls off with increasing age due to the high mortality. Down's syndrome is related to maternal age. The incidence is less than 0.1 per cent below 35 but rises to 2.75 per cent at 45 and over.

Those with Down's syndrome have small round heads, slanting eyes, epicanthic folds, and often a convergent squint. Hands are square, with a single transverse palmar crease line, and there are characteristic dermatoglyphic patterns on palm and fingers. The little finger is frequently short and curved inwards. The tongue may be large, with transverse fissuring. Heart malformations are particularly common, but other organs are also abnormal. There is an increased incidence of leukaemia in young sufferers. Epilepsy and spasticity are unusual. These children tend to be friendly and cheerful. They enjoy jokes, particularly at other people's expense, and are often good mimics.

Over 90 per cent of Down's syndrome sufferers have 47 instead of the usual 46 chromosomes, the extra one occurring at chromosome 21 (trisomy 21).

(b) *Sex chromosomes.* Abnormalities of the sex chromosomes affect mainly the genital tract and do not generally reduce intelligence to a marked degree.

Turner's syndrome (XO) consists of dwarfism, sexual infantilism, and webbing of the neck.

In *Klinefelter's syndrome* (XXY), the extra X interferes with testicular development and affected individuals are sterile. They often have a eunuchoid appearance, with poorly developed secondary sexual characteristics. Their intelligence is usually, but not invariably, below average.

3. Acquired metabolic disturbances

(a) *Kernicterus* results if there is a large rise in unconjugated serum bilirubin in the fetal circulation. Usually this occurs in cases of Rhesus incompatibility or in severe prematurity. Choreo-athetosis, fits, deafness and mental handicap are likely to develop.

(b) *Hypoglycaemia,* which is only likely to happen in very premature infants.

(c) *Lead poisoning.* Most cases occur between 18 months and three years, usually in children from poor homes, from sucking or chewing objects with lead-containing paints.

4. Hypothyroidism

(a) Congenital absence of thyroid, unless treatment is begun within six months of birth, is likely to cause severe mental handicap. Even when treatment starts at once, intelligence is often below average.

(b) Acquired hypothyroidism can result from the injection of goitre-producing drugs such as phenylbutazone and para-amino salicylic acid.

5. Birth trauma

6. Prematurity

Severe mental handicap may be associated with a *very low* birth weight. Otherwise the suggested association between low birth weight and mental handicap is probably related to the common factor of social class 5.

7. *Infections*

These fall into two classes:

(a) Of the mother: such as rubella, toxoplasmosis, syphilis.
(b) Of the child: such as meningitis, encephalitis.

Clinical signs of mental handicap

Severe mental handicap may be obvious, or at least suspected within a short time of birth. The infant's appearance is abnormal, or the usual reflex reactions absent. On the other hand, mental handicap is sometimes not diagnosed until much later, perhaps after the child has started school.

When mental handicap is at all marked *all* developmental landmarks tend to be delayed. The retarded infant does not suck, does not smile until late, is late in holding up his head, in sitting, crawling, and walking, in talking and developing sphincter control. As the child grows, his educational difficulties become more apparent.

The mentally handicapped child lacks the curiosity and spontaneity of a child of average or above intelligence. Because of this he is often quiet and passive at home, and easy to manage. His speech develops slowly, his vocabulary remains small, and abstract or conceptual thinking is limited. In the majority of cases there is no impediment of the senses, memory seems to develop normally, and although he may be distractible, the child's attention can be held by what interests him.

The presence of deafness, poor vision, marked spasticity, or frequent epileptic fits, still further limit the child's intelligence. A high proportion of severely mentally handicapped children suffer from one or more of these conditions.

Diagnosis

Diagnosis depends on the clinical picture, the mother's account of her child and his development, intelligence tests at some stage, and full physical investigations including biochemical tests and chromosome studies. The history must include a search for possible factors from the child's conception until birth and later.

Sensory deficiencies, whole or partial, aphasia, states of minimal brain injury, autism and psychotic conditions must be excluded as primary causes of the child's difficulty. In older children specific learning or reading difficulties may be responsible for a child seeming to be backward.

Management and treatment

1. *Parental reactions.* Very often a mentally handicapped child's mother, particularly if she has already brought up other children, is the first to suspect that her child is abnormal. Frequently her worries and suspicions are at first ignored or ridiculed. Later, when the diagnosis is confirmed, she is not unnaturally resentful and distrustful of medical opinion. But in many cases the diagnosis of mental handicap is made even before the child's parents suspect, by a doctor or health visitor.

Parents should be told as soon as the practitioner is certain that the child has educational difficulties. Even when the diagnosis is plain at birth, it is still not exceptional for the mother to learn about her child through a casual remark by a nurse, or even from another patient in the ward who has overheard nursing gossip.

Except in a clear-cut condition such as Down's syndrome and even here there is considerable individual variation, it is unwise to make early long-term predictions about what the child will or will not be able to do. Rather, the parents should be told that their child will be slow in development, and lag behind children of his own age. Terms like 'mental handicap' should be avoided in general in the early stages. Most parents accept the diagnosis, and arrangements can then be made to follow up the child regularly and give support to the parents. Occasionally parents refuse to accept the diagnosis and argue aggressively against it. Not unnaturally, some degree of depression and guilt, particularly in the mother, occurs after learning that her child is abnormal. In some cases marital tensions, which may have been present beforehand, are exacerbated and brought into the open.

Parents may overprotect their child or continue to deny that there is anything wrong with him. Much less often they reject the child, and insist that he be kept in hospital or transferred to an institution. A sympathetic understanding attitude on the part of the medical staff usually helps to resolve these problems; aggressive over-reactions only make matters worse.

All too often there is failure to provide support and advice for the parents of mentally handicapped children. Problems which are particularly likely to arise at certain stages of development should be anticipated; schooling, sibling rivalries, sexual behaviour at adolescence, and so on. Marriage may be impossible for the severely mentally handicapped but it is not necessarily so for mentally handicapped men and women.

Genetic counselling may be required later.

2. *Treatment of the child.* A more enlightened optimistic attitude towards mental handicap has emerged in the past decade. It is now recognised that many severely mentally handicapped patients can be taught to read and write, and do relatively complicated tasks, provided such tasks are broken down into simple components, and they are encouraged and treated kindly.

The mentally handicapped child needs a prolonged period of dependency upon his mother or mother substitute. Institutionalisation is unsatisfactory but may be necessary if a child is severely mentally handicapped, with multiple associated handicaps, doubly incontinent, or overactive and destructive. In general, children brought up in large institutions are more retarded in emotional development, speech and verbal intelligence, compared to those who live at home. However, severely mentally handicapped children, as they grow older and more difficult to look after, and children with severe emotional disturbances who are causing the rest of the family to suffer, sooner or later require admission to hospital.

Most children with an IQ of above 55 are educable and can attend schools run by their Education Authorities. Children with an IQ of 70 and above, under the Education Act of 1944, are usually educated in ordinary schools. Those with an IQ of between 55 and 70 mostly go to special schools for those with learning difficulties. Before April, 1971, if a child had an IQ of less than 50, and was thought to be unsuitable for education at school, he attended a day training centre until 16. However, under the Education Act (Handicapped Children) 1970, the power to exclude such children from education has ceased. All children now come under the care of the Education Authorities.

It is of the greatest importance to deal with physical abnormalities as early as possible. Epilepsy should be controlled with anticonvulsants. A deaf aid, or spectacles, should be worn without delay. Hormonal deficiencies must be replaced, chronic infections treated, and suitable diets and vitamins given where necessary. Physiotherapy will help to relieve spasticity. If a child's behaviour is constantly destructive and upsetting a neuroleptic drug helps to control this.

Even the severely mentally handicapped child, when such additional disabilities are removed, can often be taught to speak, read and write, to do simple arithmetic. Occasionally mentally handicapped children and adolescents who have glaring physical deformities improve in mood and behaviour after suitable plastic surgery.

24
Nursing and Its Practice

There are widely varied definitions of nursing. Originally nursing meant suckling a baby but it has come to be associated with the role of people caring for the 'sick'. More recently the concept of nursing has embraced the promotion of health and encouraging individuals to be as independent as their health allows.

The most credible definition of nursing is that recognised by the International Council of Nurses. 'The unique function of the nurse is to assist the individual, sick or well, in the performance of those activities contributing to health or its recovery (or to peaceful death) that he would perform unaided if he had the necessary strength, will or knowledge. And to do this in such a way as to help him gain independence as rapidly as possible' (Henderson, 1960). It is suggested that nurses should initiate and control this function. In addition, the nurse has a role within the therapeutic plans organised by the multidisciplinary team for patients. Henderson lists the components of basic nursing on p. 294.

It has been established that nursing involves intervening to help patients meet their individual needs while promoting maximum independence. Nursing can be organised in a number of different ways; at either end of the spectrum are 'task allocation' or 'the process approach' (Fig. 24.1). *Task allocation* is the term given to the type of nursing where each nurse is given an individual task to carry out. For example, in the morning, one nurse may be asked to administer drugs, another to measure patients' blood pressure, and a third to give out breakfast.

The advantages of 'task allocation' include economy of time and avoidance of nurses becoming too close to patients, thereby provoking anxiety (Menzies, 1967). These advantages are the main reasons for the popularity of task allocation within nursing. The disadvantages include fragmentation of patient care, frustration amongst nurses bored with repeating tasks, and the neglect of individual patients' needs because of pressure of nurses 'to get the task in hand done'.

In recent years it has been acknowledged that the disadvantages of task allocation generally outweigh the advantages. This has resulted in the nursing profession embracing the concept of the '*nursing process*'. The nursing process is merely a simple problem-solving cycle with four steps: assessment, planning, implemen-

Components of basic nursing	*The Nurse considers both*	*Conditions always present that affect basic needs*
Assisting the patient with these functions or providing conditions that will enable him to: 1 Breathe normally 2 Eat and drink adequately 3 Eliminate by all avenues of elimination 4 Move and maintain desirable posture (walking, sitting, lying and changing from one to the other) 5 Sleep and rest 6 Select suitable clothing, dress and undress 7 Maintain body temperature within normal range by adjusting clothing and modifying the environment 8 Keep the body clean and well groomed and protect the skin's integrity 9 Avoid dangers in the environment and avoid injuring others 10 Communicate with others in expressing emotions, needs, fears, etc. 11 Worship according to his faith 12 Work at something that provides a sense of accomplishment 13 Play, or participate in various forms of recreation 14 Learn, discover, or satisfy the curiosity that leads to 'normal' development and health	↓ Formulates patients's care	1 Age: new born, child, youth, adult, middle aged, and elderly 2 Temperament, emotional state, or passing mood: a) 'normal' or b) euphoric and hyperactive c) anxious, fearful, agitated or hysterical or d) depressed and hypoactive 3 Social or cultural status: A member of a family unit with friends and status, or a person relatively alone and/or maladjusted, destitute 4 Physical and intellectual capacity: a) normal weight b) underweight c) overweight d) normal mentality e) handicapped mentality f) gifted mentality g) ability for hearing, sight, equilibrium and touch h) loss of specific sense i) degree of motor power

Table adapted from Henderson (1977) in Basic Principles of Nursing Care

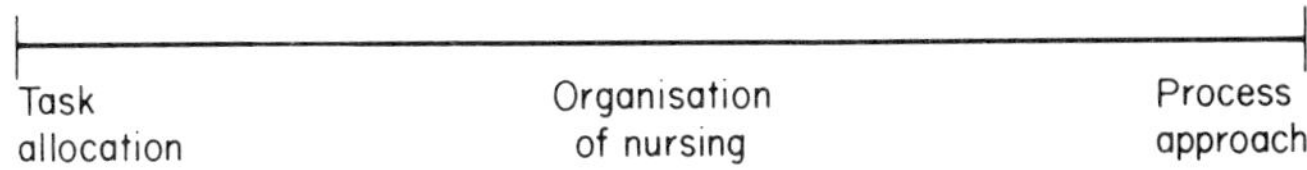

Fig. 24.1 The nursing spectrum

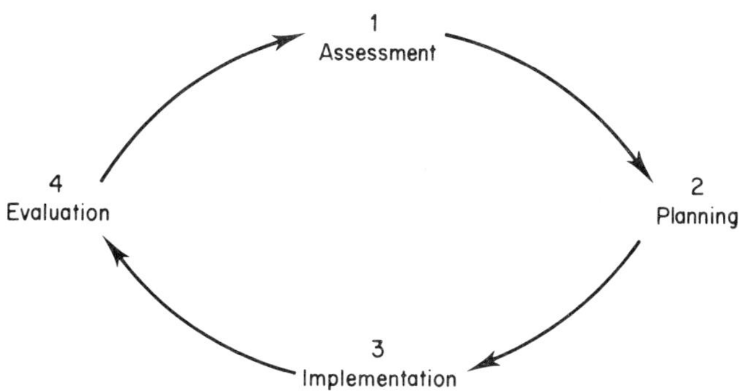

Fig. 24.2 A simple problem solving cycle

tation and evaluation (Fig. 24.2). The four stages in the cycle are inter-related and it is necessary to evaluate each stage. The problem solving cycle applied to nursing can be depicted with informal evaluation being utilised at all stages (Fig. 24.3). The nursing process requires defining the patient's actual (present now) and potential (likely in the future) problems. An actual problem is one that clearly exhibits, that is, the patient is displaying it or can describe it, such as rapid pulse or anxiety. A potential problem is one that nurses can define because of their knowledge. An example of the latter is the likelihood of 'anxiety', even delirium tremens, following withdrawal from alcohol.

The nursing process has been criticised for having a problem oriented approach, which overlooks the patient's own resources. It is important to identify what patients can do for themselves to regain maximum independence. For example, Mr Watson, an 86 year old man, has been depressed since his wife died. He has not been able to manage at home because his wife always did the shopping, cleaning and cooking. He, on the other hand, coped effectively with the family finances and was a union convener at his workplace. Any nursing care plan needs to highlight Mr Watson's skills with finance and union activities as well as his lack of skill in

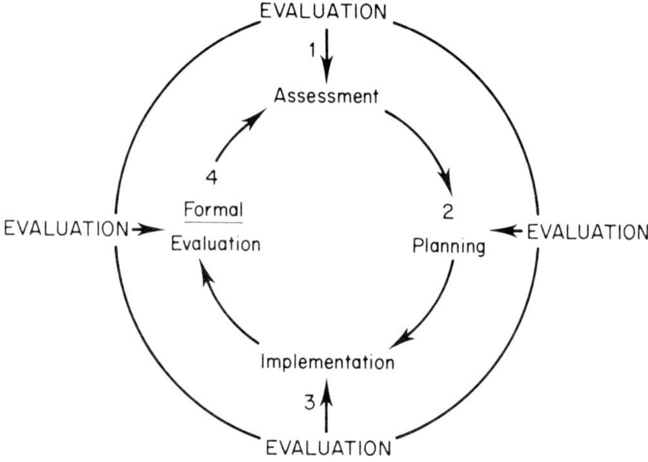

Fig. 24.3 Informal evaluation at all stages of the problem solving cycle applied to nursing

the household management sphere. The nursing process is an interactive process which involves the patient himself in decisions about his future (Fig. 24.4).

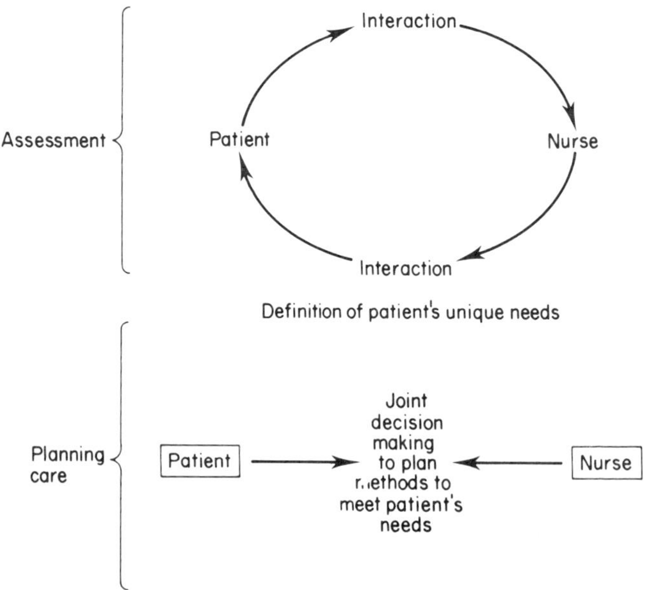

Fig. 24.4 The dynamic interaction involved in assessing patients' needs and planning intervention

The patient has a decision making role in all four stages of the nursing process. The term 'patient as partner' is sometimes used to describe this, the inference being that the patient and nurse are partners together in the patient's care. This partnership is not always equal. The nurse is more powerful than a patient who is detained in hospital under a Clause of the Mental Health Act 1983. An informal patient may decide to discharge himself – thus forcing the nurse to relinquish her part of the partnership. When patients are confused or severely depressed a nurse may have to make decisions concerning patients without their full co-operation. The important factor is for nurses to consider their patients' wishes as much as possible when making such decisions.

Each stage of the nursing process will now be examined separately.

Assessment

Nursing care can only be as good as the assessment technique. If the assessment fails to establish that a patient is contemplating harming himself, no strategy to prevent this can be planned. Alternatively a good assessment technique can give a detailed description of the same patient's state of mind; for example, that it is on wakening that the patient most strongly contemplates suicide. Night nurses can now be alerted and ready to be with the patient at this time.

Nursing models for assessment

The use of a nursing model can enhance the care of patients. Nursing models differ in form but are united in their assumption for goal directed individualised nursing care.

Selection of the appropriate model for the nature of the nursing required is important. One model of nursing will be used to highlight its use in assessment.

The most commonly used model in Britain is that developed by Roper *et al* (1985). This model is based on 'activities of living'. Roper (1985) states that the term 'activities of living' was selected in preference to that of 'basic human needs' as the word 'need' has a negative connotation, while the word 'activities' has a positive connotation even when a person requires help. Roper emphasises the need for nurses to consider the normal life style of their patients when they come into hospital. For example, a patient who normally has only a light breakfast should not be expected to have cooked breakfast in hospital.

The 'activities of living' suggested in this model of nursing include (Roper *et al.*, 1985):

Breathing
Communicating
Dying
Eating and Drinking
Eliminating
Expressing sexuality
Maintaining a safe environment
Mobility
Sleep pattern
Working and playing
Personal cleansing/dressing
Controlling body temperature

This model provides a clear concise framework for assessment that can be of particular value with the elderly mentally ill. It is, however, largely physiologically based and little allowance is made for an individual's mental attitudes and behaviour. There is no reason why these activities should not be added to Roper's (1974) original framework in order to enhance patient assessment. The majority of the care plans in the text involve this particular adaptation of this model.

Assessment skills

Nurses need to be skilled both in communication and observation techniques to assess a patient's state. It is important that a nurse obtains not only the information she needs but also the information the patient wants to give. In addition the nurse must observe

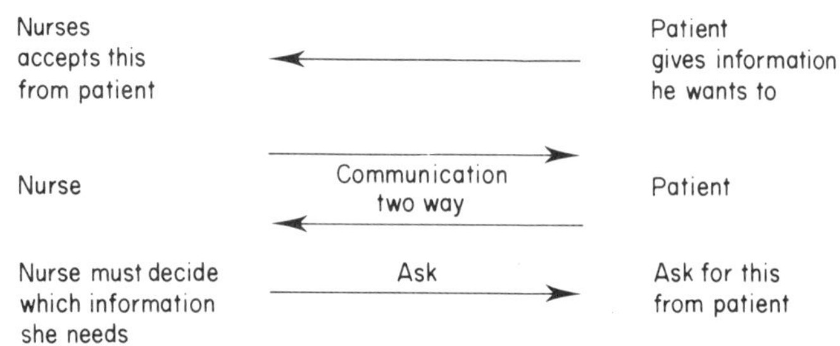

Fig. 24.5 Communication exchange

the patient, and it is at this stage that a nursing model can be especially useful. For example, what are the patient's body temperature, pulse, blood pressure, and attitude to being in hospital. A patient may say he feels 'OK' about being in hospital but have a pulse of 100, a normal temperature, a blood pressure of 140/90, be perspiring profusely, fidgeting with his hands and clearly anxious. Thus the nurse's observations here are in conflict with the patient's own words. Nurses will continue to assess patients throughout their stay in hospital and while they are seeing them in the community. When first seen, an 'assessment interview' is carried out.

Factors which enhance the assessment interview

Environment. It is important that adequate time and privacy is provided for this. A full assessment technique cannot be conducted in ten minutes in an open ward with other patients disturbing it. Ideally at least an hour should be set aside for the interview in a quiet well lit room without a telephone (to prevent interruption).

Answering patients' questions. The nurse should first introduce herself, and then be prepared to answer any questions a patient asks, and provide administrative details, such as the visiting hours on the ward and time of meals.

Tools for assessment

Tools such as Norton *et al.*'s (1962) pressure area calculator may be used at this time (Fig. 24.6).

Writing the History

It may be necessary for the nurse to write during the interview. If so this should be reduced to a minimum in order not to distract from the communication between nurse and patient. It can be worrying for patients to see that everything they say is written down. One method of overcoming this is to show the patient what is being written and ensure together with them that it is accurate. Some patients may volunteer to write down information themselves for the nurse. It can be helpful for the patient to describe his situation in his own words. Subsequently the nurse can clarify any ambiguities with him.

Ideally any written information taken at the interview should be

Physical condition		*Mental condition*		*Activity*		*Mobility*		*Incontinence*	
Good	4	Alert	4	Ambulant	4	Full	4	None	4
Fair	3	Apathetic	3	Walk/help	3	Slightly limited	3	Occasional	3
Poor	2	Confused	2	Chairbound	2	Very limited	2	Usual/Urine	2
Very Poor	1	Stuporous	1	Bedfast	1	Immobile	1	Double	1

After: NORTON, D., McLAREN, R., & EXTON-SMITH, A. (1962) *An Investigation of Geriatric Nursing Problems in Hospital.* National Corporation for the Care of Old People. Reprinted 1976 by Churchill Livingstone.

Nursing care

Score 12/14 = High Risk
Two hourly position change
Encourage chest physiotherapy
and passive leg exercises
Inspect dependent area –
recording state of skin

Score 14/18 = Moderate Risk
Four hourly position change
Otherwise as for High Risk

Fig. 24.6 Pressure sore risk chart

done in 'rough', so that the history sheet can be accurately completed at leisure later on.

Verbal Communication

A nurse should speak clearly and simply, and make sure that the patient both hears and understands her. It is important to *avoid 'jargon'*; for example, 'Have you ever had any nocturnal eneuresis?' is better phrased 'Have you ever wet the bed at night?' and 'Do you feel your heart pounding?' is better than 'Do you have palpitations?'

Information seeking skills

Nurses can use certain skills to encourage patients to give additional information. The following methods have been adapted from work by Bates (1979) and Miller (1981).

1. *Organisation of Questions*
These used should be asked in a form that is easy for the patient to understand. Questions should flow from the general to the specific.
e.g. Tell me about your problems
↓
Questions concerning the *specific* problems identified by the patient

2. *Open Questions*
These are questions that cannot be answered by just Yes or No. They require a comprehensive answer from the patient, which in turn give nurses detailed information.
e.g. What helps you go to sleep?
How long have you been feeling like this?

3. *Facilitation*
Facilitation can be verbal or non-verbal. Non-verbal techniques include silence, to give the patient time to clarify his thoughts and gestures such as nodding or smiling.

Verbal methods of facilitation include phrases like 'Do go on', 'I'm with you', or even 'umm'. These techniques are giving the patient license to continue talking.

4. *Clarification*
A nurse may not always understand what a patient is saying and needs to clarify it. For example a patient may say:
'You know what it's like to be unemployed'.
Nurse: 'What does it mean to you?', or 'Can you elaborate?'.
Patient: 'Well there's nothing to do all day. . . . .'

5. *Reflection/Echoing*

This involves repeating whole or part of a phrase that a patient has used in order to encourage him to continue.

Patient: 'I've been hearing these voices'.

Long silence.

Nurse: 'Voices?'

Patient: 'Yes, they keep talking about me'.

6. *Empathic Responses*

Empathy is the term given to 'feeling onself into' another individual's 'feelings'. For example, a patient may become very distressed as she explains how her son died. The nurse may respond thus:

'It must have been a difficult time for you'.

This gives the patient the chance to continue and explain what it was like for her.

The essence of an empathic response is that it demonstrates an *understanding* of another's feelings.

Sometimes moving closer to a patient or lightly touching them can convey the same message. It depends on the nurse and the patient whether this is appropriate.

7. *Confrontation*

Sometimes patients give an inconsistent history. It may be inadvisable to point this out to them, i.e. if a patient is acutely psychotic. Alternatively, a nurse may feel that she can usefully confront a patient, and establish the real facts. The following is an example:

John, a 24 year old Rastafarian, said that he had never taken any illegal drugs. The nurse was aware that the majority of Rastas smoke marihuana as part of their culture. The nurse felt it reasonable to say,

'Look, I know that most Rastas smoke ganja – are you truthfully saying you don't?'

8. *Questions about feelings*

Sometimes it is useful to ask patients how they feel about something such as the interview. For example, a patient who has not been altogether truthful may be asked, 'How do you feel about all these questions?'

9. *Closed questions*

These may help get specific information, e.g. 'Do you wake at 4 a.m. most mornings?'

Factors which hamper the assessment techniques

1. *Limited perception of the importance of the interview*
If the interview is not thought to be important by members of the nursing team it is likely to be hurried and inadequate. This of course results in an inadequate, if not positively misleading, assessment of the patient.
2. *Inexperienced nurses*
Junior nurses should sit in with experienced nurses to learn interviewing techniques.
3. *Anxiety, stress, fear*
If the nurse and patient are upset, whatever the reason, a good assessment is unlikely to be achieved.
4. *Culture/language barrier*
If the nurse and patient do not speak the same language it is obviously important to obtain an interpreter. Even so, an assessment tends to suffer. Some knowledge of the patient's culture is useful, if not essential at times. For example, a male Muslim's attitude to women was such that he refused to answer a female nurse; it was then necessary for a male nurse to take over the interview.
5. *Nurse's mental set*
Nurses must be aware of their own prejudices. For example, if a nurse believes all down and outs are 'layabouts', she may miss the vital signs suggestive of schizophrenia given by a tramp who has been admitted for assessment.

Information gathering from significant others

Information gathered from anyone other than the patient is often valuable, but takes second place to the patient's own account of himself.

Sometimes a patient is too confused or psychotic to give reliable information on admission. In these circumstances it is necessary to interview a relative, social worker, neighbour or friend to establish what has been happening to the patient. It is important to state clearly on the assessment form from whom the information has been obtained. As soon as practical, the patient should be interviewed himself, and contradictions between the earlier account and now should be noted.

Information sharing with the multidisciplinary team

The nursing process cannot be conducted in isolation from other health care workers. All information must be shared with members of the multidisciplinary team, just as nurses receive information from doctors, social workers, occupational therapists, etc.

Subjective and objective assessments

Every assessment, whoever carries it out, is subjective in some degree. It is the nurse's job to make an assessment which is as objective as possible. The nurse must be aware of her own prejudices and characteristic attitudes if she is to give of her best. Sharing data collected from other sources may result in a more objective assessment.

Collating the information collected

All the available information regarding an individual patient has to be integrated. A nursing model provides a framework within which to organise the information. Information can be usefully divided into that which is objective and measurable and that which is more nebulous and subjective. Examples of the former include temperature, pulse, blood pressure, urinalysis, height, weight, address, employment status and so on. Examples of the latter include family relationships, emotional states, general philosophy of life, etc.

It is useful to record this kind of information by including both the patient's opinion and the nurse's observation. For example:

1. John says he has a pain in his left shoulder.
   Nurse observation: John winces when his left shoulder is moved.
2. Sarah say she hears two voices which talk to one another about her in a hateful manner.
   Nurse observation: During conversation Sarah turns her head away and loses the thread of what has been discussed. At these moments she looks both anxious and confused.
3. Mr Jones says, 'My daughter is very busy with her own life – that's why she can't visit often – I understand.'
   Nurse observation: 'When Mr Jones' daughter telephoned he refused to speak to her.'

Another method of tabulating information about feelings is to ask patients to rate themselves on a scale of 1 to 10.

> Mr Fredricko states that he is anxious whenever he walks to work and returns home. The nurse suggests that he rate his anxiety on a scale of 1 to 10; 1 being hardly anxious and 10 being as anxious as he could possibly be. Mr Fredricko says that on his way to work he is anxious at '8' and on his way home at '4'. This information is easy to record and provides the nurse with some additional information, i.e. that he is less anxious after work than on the way there.

Nurses recording information must sign this with their full name and the date because of the accountability in nursing practice.

Planning of nursing care

In order to plan nursing care for a patient it is necessary to look at their assessment and consider the aim of the care.

Patient Assessment ⟶ Aim of Nursing Intervention ⟶ Plan of Nursing Care

The assessment should have accurately defined the patient's strengths and weaknesses. Now, in discussion with the patient and members of the nursing team, a plan of care can be organised. Pooling of ideas at this stage helps to ensure well balanced decisions about nursing care.

The planning stage begins by deciding which 'weaknesses' require immediate nursing intervention and which can be left to a later date.

Patient Assessment	*Aim of Nursing Intervention*	*Plan of Nursing Care*
Stress incontinence. Unable to reach toilet in time	Reduce stress incontinence	Observe at what times patient is incontinent. Record these and then take patient to toilet half an hour prior to this time in future
Able to dress herself unaided despite left-sided weakness due to cerebral vascular accident	Maintain independence in this sphere	Allow patient to dress herself even if this takes a long time. She can have her breakfast in her dressing gown and dress afterwards so that she does not feel rushed

Some patients may require more detailed aims of nursing intervention or 'expected outcomes' (McFarlane and Castledine, 1982). An 'expected outcome' is a statement of what the nurse and patient hope the patient will be able to achieve by a certain date.

The patient and nurse can measure the success of their plan against an 'expected outcome' thus using their plan as a tool for evaluation.

Patient Assessment	*Aim of Nursing Intervention (Expected Outcome)*	*Plan of Nursing Care*
1st. Dec. 1984 Gross Weight Loss Height 1.60 m Weight 35 kg	Weight gain of 1 kg/week for two weeks	3000 calorie diet as per dietician. *NO* fluids by her bed. Bedrest

There are four components to this aim.

Subject – the patient; *behavioural* – will put on weight; *condition* – bedrest; and *criterion* – 1 kg/week for two weeks.

An 'expected outcome' clearly defines a measurable aim and states how it is to be achieved.

Not all patients' weaknesses and problems can be so clearly defined and there are potential problems with stating a time limit by which goals should be achieved. It would clearly be silly to state that a depressed patient should 'smile twice a day by the third week in hospital', yet the aim of nursing intervention may be 'to elevate the individual's mood' by 'socialisation and discussion with a specific nurse about possible reasons for the depression'. It is important to establish 'Review dates' when nurse and patient evaluate together how successful the plan is, and change it if necessary. Such a method prevents the patient from the anxiety of failing to achieve.

In addition to planning intervention for actual problems, i.e. weight loss, it is necessary to look ahead to potential problems.

Some examples of potential problems are listed:

1. *Psychological*
   Suicide attempts due to depression.
2. *Sociological*
   Illegal drugs being brought into the ward for an addict by a friend at visiting time.
3. *Physiological*
   Pressure sores due to excessive weight loss coupled with bedrest.

Potential problems embrace all three spheres of the patient's needs: psychological, sociological and physiological.

Sometimes the best 'nursing interventions' are to allow patients to do something for themselves – even if it takes ages. Otherwise the potential problem of over-dependence will occur.

General principles when completing individual care plans

1. Encourage the patient to share in this, if possible.
2. Ask other nurses' opinions in order to enhance the care plan.
3. Always date and sign new plans of nursing action.
4. Enhance the patient's self-esteem by identifying his strengths as well as his weaknesses.
5. The nursing care plans are legal documents and so should be completed in ink. Merely draw a line through mistakes.
6. If a problem has an obvious cause, state this.
7. Encourage the patient's family and friends to participate in the care, e.g. taking the patient shopping.
8. Consider other disciplines involvement and act accordingly, e.g. that the occupational therapist teaches cooking on Thursday mornings and patients should attend.
9. If possible use 'expected outcomes'.
10. If it is felt the use of 'expected outcomes' may be detrimental, use 'aims of nursing intervention'.
11. Try to state nursing care clearly and concisely without using jargon, e.g. talk with the patient on a one to one basis for an hour on Tuesdays and Fridays; *NOT* one hour's psychotherapy with a nurse on Tuesdays and Fridays.
12. Try to agree common aims with the patient.
13. When utilising behavioural rewards other than verbal reinforcement check the reward is something that the patient actually wants, e.g. Mars bar, magazine, visit from a friend.

15. Always get a trained nurse to check care plans when they have been written.
16. Review and update patients' care plans regularly at a pre-planned time, e.g. in 24 hours, 3 days, 1 week.

Types of care plans

There are three main types of care plan, 'the patient's nursing needs orientated plan', 'the daily care plan' and 'the standard care plan'. The 'patient's nursing needs orientated plan' has been described in detail. The assessment and planning stages of this kind of plan can be seen at the end of each chapter with regard to individuals suffering from a specific illness.

The 'daily care plan' makes detailed statements about what a patient is expected to achieve at specific times of the day. It is suggested that this plan may be particularly useful with patients who have senile dementia, confusion states and memory disturbance. Such a plan needs to include any ward activities that occur, i.e., recreational music, therapy visit, ward housekeeping meetings.

It is sometimes useful to have a different care plan for every day of the week for long term patients who are relatively stable in order to include activities which only occur on a certain day. Alternatively a list of the day's activities can be pinned up in the ward with the relevant patients' names.

If the patient's condition changes the daily care plan will have to be altered. Alternatively some individuals respond so well to a clearly delineated organisation of their day that the plan can be in use for many months. It is *important* to get an accurate nursing assessment if long term care is planned.

This type of care plan can be especially useful in the community when constructed together with the patient's relatives. It provides relatives with the 'security' of a regime they can follow (Fig. 24.7).

Standard care plans

This is a type of checklist for certain circumstances. Its use is limited in psychiatric nursing because of the nature of mental illness. Schizophrenia rarely presents with identical problems in several patients, unlike appendicitis. A standard care plan can be used prior to electroconvulsive therapy because there are safety factors which must be met. Its use can reduce written work but care must be taken to establish that 'routine methods of nursing care' are not developed at the expense of an individual patient's requirements.

Daily Care Plan—Mrs P. Gillians	
Time	*Daily Activities*
6 a. m.	Usually awakes. Commode. Hands and face wash. Tea with two sugars
7 a. m.	Choose the clothes she is to wear for the day with her. Then take her to the bathroom, encourage her to clean dentures and wash. Use toilet
8 a. m.	Check that she has dressed correctly – if not give assistance. Breakfast. Medication
9. 30 a. m.	To the toilet and wash hands
10 a. m.	Volunteer to come to the ward and take Mrs Gillians to music therapy
12 Noon	Returns to the ward. Encourage her to use toilet and wash hands. Lunch. Medication
1.30 p. m.	Cup of coffee and rest in a chair chatting to others
2 p. m.	Take her to the toilet. Suggest that she join in ward activity, i.e., dominoes, knitting. Bath on Monday, Wednesday and Friday
4 p. m.	Cup of tea, then rest in day room, watch television if desired
6 p. m.	Take to the toilet. Supper. Medication. Visitors in day room
8.30 p. m.	Prepare for bed. Take to the toilet, wash.
10 p. m.	Likes to be in bed by 10 p. m. Commode by bedside, in case required

Fig. 24.7 Example of a daily care plan

Electroconvulsive Therapy Care Plan

11.30 p. m.	If desired give patient a drink and something to eat
12 Midnight	Nil by mouth until treatment completed
8 a. m.	Patient can have a bath. Empty bladder. Pre-medication if used
9 a. m.	ECT – Nurse to protect patient from hurting himself during fit
9.05 a. m.	Lie in left semi-prone position. Maintain airway. Observe breathing, colour and pulse. Have suction and oxygen available
9.30 a. m.	When patient fully conscious and orientated, return to the ward
9.45 a. m.	On return to ward make sure patient is warm and give a drink if desired or allow to sleep

Fig. 24.8 Care plan for ECT

Availability of care plans

Some patients may ask for copies of their care plans; generally there are no objections to agreeing. In certain circumstances the team may refuse; for instance, with a highly manipulative patient. Care plans should be kept in a readily available place on the ward. If they are not readily to hand relief nurses will not be able to maintain the highest possible level of care.

Implementation

This involves taking the nursing action required to carry out the plan to meet the patient's needs. The action should both provide for patient participation and maximum independence on his behalf (Fig. 24.9).

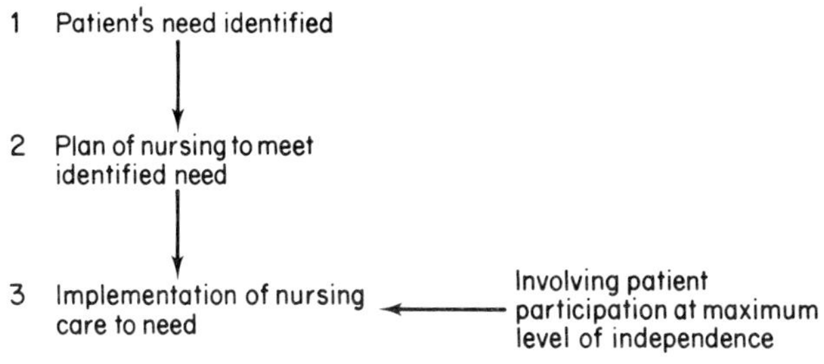

Fig. 24.9 The third part of the problem solving cycle – implementation

Roper's (1985) model has been described as a 'deficit' one, meaning that nursing care is needed when a person is no longer able to manage an activitiy when living alone. For example, a severely depressed patient may not wish to wash or dress. It is then up to the nurse to motivate the patient to do this. Once the patient can manage alone the nurse must then withdraw, thereby promoting maximum independence. Thus the nurse is intervening only when the patient cannot manage alone. It is important always to strengthen a patient's self respect and, within the limits of his ability, to encourage him to take responsibility for his own care. In the example above he should be encouraged to choose what clothes he is to wear, and to dress himself neatly.

The model defines three types of nursing intervention: prevention, comfort and responding to patients seeking assistance (Roper *et al.* 1985). She cites examples of preventative nursing actions as

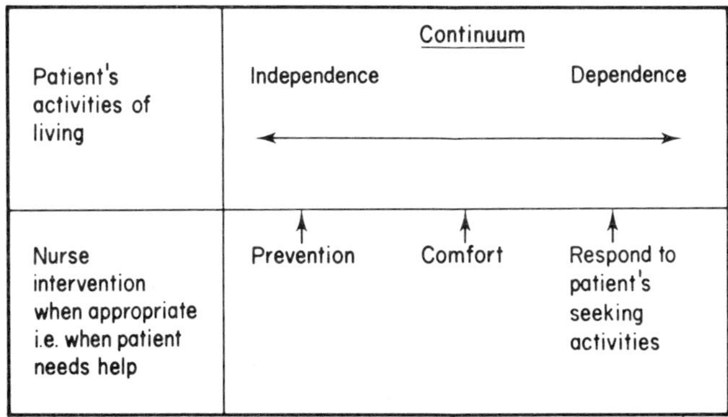

Fig. 24.10 Roper's (1985) model for nursing

those aimed at reducing deep vein thrombosis, and of comforting – placing a patient's locker within reach of his preferred hand. Those nursing actions which involve meeting a patient's seeking requirements could involve giving medication to a patient or taking crucial observation when they complain of pain. Another 'model' of nursing that can be usefully applied to psychiatry is that of Orem (1971) in the United States of America. This model concentrates on methods of delivery of nursing care and gives five levels of implementation. They are:

1. Acting for or doing for another
2. Guiding another
3. Supporting another
4. Providing an environment that promotes personal development in relation to becoming able to meet present or future demands for action
5. Teaching another

This type of nursing is described as a 'self help' model. The emphasis being placed on the patient/client helping himself with nursing support rather than nursing intervention being active and the client a passive recipient of care. For these reasons Orem's (1971) model should promote patient/client independence at an early stage, thus reducing institutionalisation of both patient and nurse.

A simple example of the use of this model in the implementation of nursing involving the giving of medication is given (Fig. 24.11). A plan of care defining *nursing actions* using Orems' (1971) model is given on p. 313.

It has been demonstrated that models of nursing can help nurses to define their actions when implementing nursing care.

The nursing skill at this stage needs to be threefold: determining the *level of intervention*, delivering the care in a *skilled manner*, and *co-ordinating* it. Mrs Janet Smith, an 86 year old, severely disturbed, confused lady, requires a bath. The nurse implementing this care must:

determine – how much help, if any, Mrs Smith requires to bath, i.e. whether she can run the bath, needs a hoist to lift her into it, can judge the temperature of the bath.
use skill – to ensure that the bath is run at the right temperature, the hoist is used with regard to health and safety and the procedure is properly explained to Mrs Smith.
co-ordinate – her actions, e.g. it is pointless to bath Mrs Smith if she is about to have an enema, go to art therapy, etc.

In:	*Patient needs Lithium Carbonate every morning*	*Plan of Nursing Care*	*Implementation Nurses & Patient Role*	*Orem Levels of Intervention*
WK 1	Out of touch with reality – very frigh-tened of taking medication	Ensure that Mary takes medication	*Nurse:* gives medication to patient *Mary:* swallows it *Nurse:* checks patient has swallowed it	(1)
WK 2	Mary's fright concerning medication is reduced but she forgets to collect it	Ensure that Mary takes medication	*Nurse:* re-minds Mary to collect medication	(2)
WK 4	Mary regu-larly collects medication at the correct time	Ensure that Mary under-stands why she needs me-dication and that she must continue to take it after discharge	*Nurse:* teaches Mary about need to take medication and asks for feedback *Mary:* ex-plains back to the nurse what she understands by the teach-ing session	(5)

Fig. 24.11 Orem model care plan for Mrs Jones, aged 27. Medical diagnosis – manic depressive psydiosis

The co-ordination of nursing care involves deciding priorities of care; for example, if Mrs Jones had been incontinent a bath would be more important than being late for art therapy.

When implementing nursing care it is sometimes necessary to consider individual needs in relation to other patients on the ward. This is a difficult task and one that few nurses relish. For example, Angus has broken a window and is still disturbing the whole ward. The nursing team believes that he would be better without any additional medication in that he will work through his aggression. However, he is written up for additional chlorpromazine. After several complaints from other patients the nursing team decides to give him some additional chlorpromazine, the reason for this being the 'common good' rather than the 'individual good'. Decisions like this should not be taken by individual nurses but after free discussion within the team.

Primary nursing

Primary nursing is defined as 'the distribution of nursing so that the total care of the individual patient is the responsibility of one nurse, not many' (Marran, 1974). If individualised care is practised utilising the nursing process then patient allocation must replace task allocation (Marks and Moran, 1978). Essentially patient allocation means that patients are allocated to a nurse for a certain time span; this can range from a matter of minutes to months.

It is an excellent method for 'implementation' of nursing care in that each nurse is well aware of what is expected of her. It involves nurses being given and accepting accountability for care. Each 'primary nurse' assesses her patients, plans their care and is responsible for ensuring that nursing actions are completed (i.e. implemented). This means that the primary nurse may plan care which she does not actually carry out. In general if she was on duty she would implement the care but if off duty she would be responsible for seeing that this work was completed in her absence. In some areas while leaving a prescription for care in her absence the primary nurse does not delegate an individual to do this but the senior nurse on duty distributes the work.

An increase in staff commitment and morale has been reported in psychiatric areas that have adopted primary nursing (Green, 1983).

The advantages of this system include continuity of care, accountability for care and the fact that patients can identify their own nurse. Some theorists believe that primary nursing is

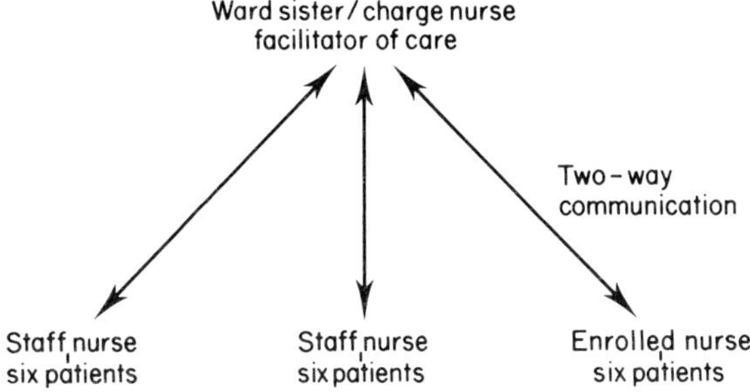

Fig. 24.12 Ward organisation using primary nursing

economic in nursing time in that patients do not pass information to or make demands from all the nurses, just their own.

In most areas it is normal for the primary nurse to work with at least one associate nurse. The associate nurse is either in training or a nursing assistant. The associate nurses are responsible for the delivery of nursing care in the absence of or together with the primary nurse.

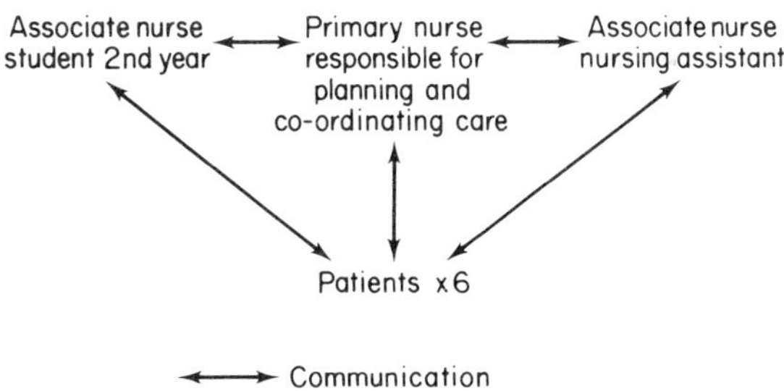

Fig. 24.13 Delivery of primary nursing care

In most instances a patient will be allocated to a 'primary nursing team' on admission and the patient's entire nursing care will be their responsibility. Sometimes this is not possible for a variety of reasons (i.e. patient takes an instant dislike to the nurse in charge or becomes very manipulative), and it is felt that a change in the nurses responsible for care would be beneficial. Similarly individual patients who require intensive nursing (i.e. suicidal individuals), may have to be nursed by other ward nurses for reasons of safety. If only one nurse from such a patient's team is on duty they must arrange via the senior nurse on duty for the patient to be cared for during absences at the nurse's mealbreaks, etc. The essential component within primary nursing is that the member of the patient's team is accountable for co-ordinating nursing actions.

It has been demonstrated that the use of a nursing model can help nurses to define the action they are to undertake when implementing care. The use of primary nursing can help to ensure that individual patients actually receive the nursing care prescribed to them. At all times nursing intervention should strive to include the patient as a partner and to promote maximum independence.

Evaluation

Evaluation involves testing the outcome of action against previously determined outcomes. The actions may be carried out by the nurse or by the patient supervised by the nurse. Thus an 'expected outcome' that the patient should put on 1kg of weight in one week can be used as an evaluation tool. The patient's weight can be clearly measured and the success of nursing intervention evaluated.

'Aims of nursing intervention' can also be used as tools for evaluation although they may not be so easy to measure. For example:

Aim of Nursing Intervention: That John's self esteem be strengthened.

Evaluation in this instance will involve the nurse making a *valued judgement* concerning John's self esteem on his *observable state*. Similarly John's opinion should be sought, i.e. ask him how he is feeling.

Thus if John has been observed by the nurse to 'offer help' to another patient and expressed a 'feeling' that he does not feel so worthless, the nurse could reasonably evaluate that the aim of nursing intervention was to some degree achieved.

Evaluation should be documented in the nurse's records as this clearly denotes that follow-up is being carried out. Such notes indicate both the patient's current situation and provide valuable information with which future care can be planned.

In certain circumstances evaluation can become a re-assessment:

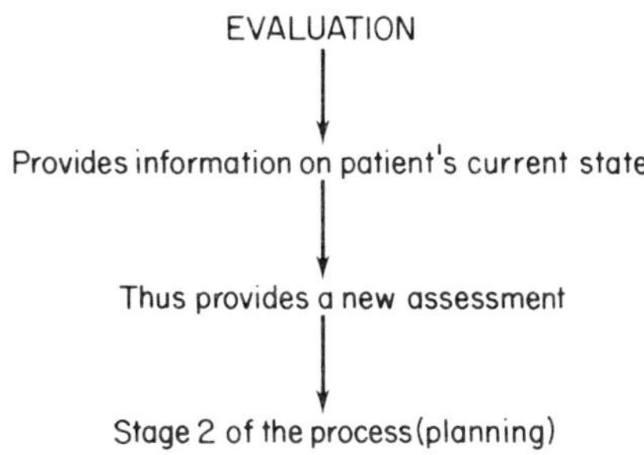

Alternatively evaluation may provide information that suggests while 'nursing intervention' is being successful the same plan needs to continue. This is particularly valid in patients with long term incurable illness such as dementia.

Sometimes evaluation will demonstrate failure of nursing intervention. In this situation it is essential to reassess the patient's situation, not merely change the care plan. The reason for this is that if the initial assessment is inaccurate changing the care plan will not be productive.

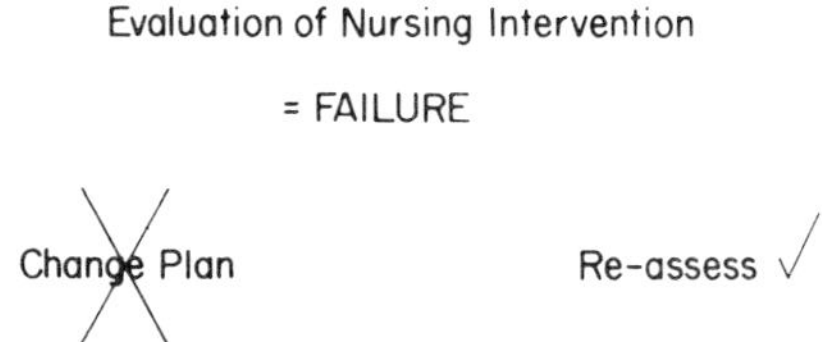

Nurses' meetings concerning evaluation of nursing intervention

These may occur at handover sessions or more formally within primary care team or ward team conferences. They have an especially important role within psychiatric nursing, as a multi-faceted evaluation is then conducted.

It is generally accepted that nurses should try to evaluate using only clearly observable signs, i.e. weight increase, improvement in dress. This is not always possible when a patient is suffering from psychiatric illness, the signs and symptoms of which are frequently difficult to observe behaviourally. Thus if nurses share together their opinions about the degree of change in a patient's situation, e.g. self esteem, affect, and communication skills, a more comprehensive evaulation will be formed. Frequently when sharing such opinions, observable behaviour is mentioned, e.g. a nurse says

'I think his self esteem is better because yesterday he said "I don't want to wear that tie with that shirt because it makes me look awful"'. In this situation observable behaviour can be linked to an increase in self esteem if previously the patient has not cared about how he dresses because he 'felt so worthless anyway'.

Frequency of evaluation

Evaluation may be short or long term. Short term goals may require evaluation as frequently as twice a day, while long term evaluation may be done monthly in some areas. It is important to decide when formulating a care plan, the expected time of evaluation, e.g. daily, weekly. In long term care unless the patient's state alters a tried and tested care plan may only require monthly evaluation. Alternatively in an intensive care situation a suicidal patient's nursing care plan may need to be evaluated on every shift.

25
Nurse-Patient Relationship

Nurses

There are many reasons why a person may wish to become a nurse. Medicine may be a family tradition. Perhaps her parents wanted her to be a nurse. Conversely, she may have taken up nursing mainly because her parents objected to the idea. Some girls play at 'nurses' from an early age, and probably identify themselves with their mothers as someone who 'nurses' the family. Others have a repressed curiosity about the human body which nursing satisfies. In addition nursing is recognised as a discipline in its own right and many people today, including graduates, enter it because of the career prospects. There are deep satisfactions to be derived from nursing. Nurses are held in high esteem by society. They form part of a respected group. It is gratifying to feel that a patient needs your help. It is satisfying to see patients recovering after serious illnesses as a result of good nursing.

It is not easy to be a nurse. Emotional conflicts often arise, especially among those leaving home for the first time. Anxiety is aroused by contact with suffering and death, human tragedy, excreta, sex, vulgarity and rudeness, and perhaps psychiatric illness. Contact with patients may arouse frightening sexual or hostile emotions which are difficult to control. Religious and moral beliefs may suddenly be lost. Anxiety may be so great as to interfere with the nurse's work.

Every nurse meets these problems. As a protection against excessive anxiety she must control her sympathy and feelings to some extent. She must be able to detach herself sufficiently from her patients to continue to nurse efficiently. But to be a good nurse she must also retain a reasonable degree of sensitivity and feeling for her patient. How these two requirements are met largely determines the sort of nurse she becomes. If she is too detached and suppresses all her emotions she becomes a cold, efficient, impersonal nurse, often better suited to administration than to practical nursing. The converse is the nurse who tends to become too involved emotionally with her patients. To overcome her anxiety she overworks and insists on doing everything herself, even when she is in charge of the ward.

During their first year of training nurses often become moody and irritable. Neurotic personality problems have to be faced. Most nurses resolve them satisfactorily but those who cannot often drop out during the first year. Menstrual irregularities are not uncommon. Some relieve anxiety by overeating. Anxiety may be reflected in off-duty behaviour. Excessive gaiety, drinking, smoking and sometimes promiscuity are more often than not due to inability to deal with anxiety in other ways.

In the wards where 'task allocation' is the method of nursing care the chance of becoming too emotionally involved with patients is reduced. Many students find that this lessens their anxiety. However the 'nursing process' method of organising patient care makes far greater emotional demands on all grades of nurse. It is important that students seek help from qualified staff members when worried or anxious about their feelings. With time, most nurses come to terms with such problems and learn to relate to the various types of patients they encounter.

Patients

Patients come from all walks of life. Each remains an individual, temporarily placed in the 'sick role'. Illness and death inevitably arouse fears and feelings of insecurity. And what frightens also fascinates. This is reflected in broadcasting, books and newspapers. Anxious people are liable to become irrational. They may deny they are ill, ignore symptoms until the disease is advanced, or refuse to enter hospital. But once in a hospital bed they may change completely and become childishly dependent on staff.

Anxious people also tend to distort and exaggerate what they hear. It is important for nurses and doctors to explain fully to each patient about his illness and treatment. Although there are instances when it is better not to tell the patient everything, in general, ignorance only increases anxiety.

Some patients regard illness as a sign of weakness. This is particularly likely with psychiatric conditions. Such patients frequently feel ashamed and guilty, that they are in some way responsible for their state. Consequently they may be resentful and hostile to those trying to help them, and nurses need to exert considerable self-control in trying to understand them. Hostility on the part of the nurse only serves to confirm the patient's fears.

Sometimes the patient's anxiety is related to his work or his family. He may have a one-man business and face ruin as a result of a long spell of hospital treatment. Or the mother of a young family may have no one to take her place while in hospital. Less often, patients welcome the idea of entering hospital. These are usually lonely old people, to whom the security, warmth and friendship of the ward appeals.

Special problems arise with children and old people. A child is often terrified at leaving home, even when old enough to be given an explanation. His mother may be as anxious as he. In consequence she annoys the nurses by her questions or demands. Provided nurses remain sympathetic and tolerant she gradually becomes more reasonable and trusting.

Old people may be unable to adapt to the change of coming into hospital. They become confused and disorientated, particularly at night, and develop paranoid ideas (see p. 271). Some old people value their independence as highly as life itself. They fear that hospital is the first step towards being put into an institution, and they are suspicious and resentful of the hospital staff.

Regression may occur. Behaviour becomes childlike. There may be tempers and scenes, refusal to co-operate, or alternatively a childlike dependence on the nurses. As with children, affection and reassurance are sought. Generally, the more ill the patient the greater the degree of regression. Most children regress to some extent. A boy previously dry at night may now wet the bed nightly. A child who fed himself easily may refuse to eat unless spoonfed by his nurse.

Patients may come to rely on their nurses for emotional comfort as well as physical help. A nurse is then transformed in the patient's eyes, into a parent figure. She becomes a symbol of love and safety, to whom the patient must cling to at all cost. This recreation of childhood emotional feelings and behaviour is known as transference (see p. 66).

Transference can occur with either sex and in varying intensity. Difficulties may be created by a patient developing such feelings for a nurse, particularly if the nurse is herself attracted to the patient. Transference situations may occur in the opposite direction, from nurse to patient. Such a situation is dangerous emotionally unless handled skilfully. This is one example of the potential hazards of working closely with patients. As long as nurses are aware of such conflicts within patients this kind of situation can be used constructively to help the patient gain insight and tackle his personality problems.

Recovery and convalescence

As the patient recovers his feelings of dependence fade. Sometimes a 'positive transference' gives way to negative hostile feelings. The patient for whom you have done so much leaves hospital without a word of thanks.

Most patients are ready to leave hospital. But lonely people, who have little to go back to, may cling to their symptoms. Encouragement and help from a sympathetic nurse or doctor can sometimes work miracles. Symptoms from which the patient gains something may persist despite adequate treatment, and should be viewed sympathetically by the medical staff. It is unforgivable to denigrate a patient, whether deliberately or from stupidity.

One method of helping a person to face the loneliness that may occur on discharge from hospital is to arrange for him to attend a day centre. A day centre provides company and recreation for people who otherwise have little social contact.

All too often patients are discharged from hospital into a community setting that lacks adequate resources to help them rehabilitate themselves. Many return repeatedly to hospital only to be discharged back to the same therapeutic wasteland. This is sometimes referred to as the revolving door syndrome (Fig. 25.1).

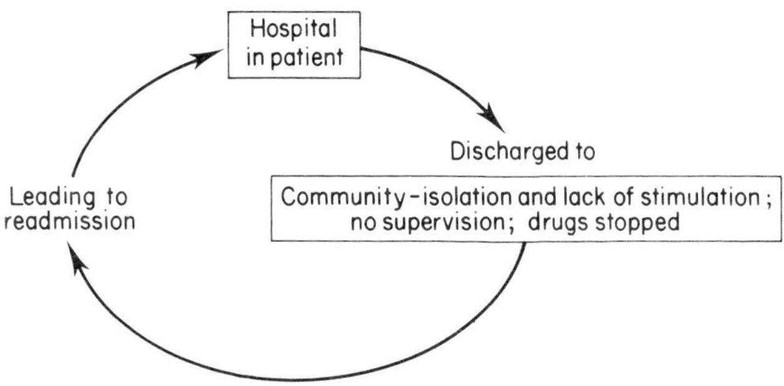

Fig. 25.1 The revolving door syndrome

Psychiatric nursing

That psychiatric nursing differs widely from other branches of the profession is a commonly held view, especially by psychiatric nurses themselves. This is not altogether so. It is different only in so far as the *main* object of effort is directed towards care of the mentally rather than the physically ill, and the nurse is required to develop a fuller understanding and relationship with her patients. Over 80 years ago a psychiatrist, David Yellowlees, criticised the practice of appointing general hospital nurses as Matrons of mental asylums: 'An asylum trained nurse', he said, 'must learn to do much more – in addition to the hospital nurse's duties she has to deal with all the patient's vagaries of talk and conduct, to calm the restless, to guide the perverse, to rouse the apathetic, to comfort the desponding, she must be constantly alert and observant, act on her own judgment and responsibility' (Walk, 1961). Treatment of the mentally ill has changed greatly since then, but not the essential role of the psychiatric nurse.

Before examining more closely what the psychiatric nurse actually does, it is relevant to mention here that there are two major factors which, because they affect the actual role of these nurses and other people's attitude towards them, are becoming of increasing importance.

The first is that the work of psychiatric nurses is no longer confined to the hospital environment. Slowly, along with the established district nurse and health visitor, they are taking their place in the community as specialists in their own right.

The second factor stems from the realisation that nursing in any field involves the care of the whole person, and that all patients who are hospitalised need some psychological as well as physical care. As a result, all nurses now receive some instruction in psychiatric nursing during their basic training.

Attitudes do not change overnight. There are still many people who regard mental illness as a frightening, hopeless phenomenon. They see the mentally ill as violent and dangerous, unreasonable and unreasoning, and therefore unacceptable to society, to be kept behind locked doors. In fact (except in special institutions like Broadmoor), the locked door is now the exception rather than the rule. If it is used at all, it is usually to prevent the elderly, confused patient from wandering away.

Patients' symptoms are no longer simply tolerated and contained, which was the old custodial approach. Nursing care now depends on understanding the reasons for a patient's behaviour and reacting to him in the light of such understanding. Nurses have to learn to meet the patient on equal terms, to be a person as well as a nurse to him. Some hospitals have abandoned uniforms for this reason, believing that it is not the nurse's outward appearance but her attitude which matters.

It is a stimulating, challenging time of change for nurses. Most of them are unaccustomed to being questioned at a personal level. Like doctors, they have tended to enjoy the privilege of trust in their near infallibility. Alas! This is fast disappearing in all fields of nursing, but particularly in psychiatry. Not only must the psychiatric nurses be willing to be challenged as an individual, but they must actually encourage such confrontation. In this way, the psychiatric nurses' role is very different, and they are subject to much greater stress than nurses working in other fields.

Because every nurse is an individual, her own personal contribution to each patient's treatment programme contains something unique. Although she works according to guidelines indicated by medical staff, she has the opportunity to use her own skills and talents. Once she has developed insight into her own emotions and behaviour, she is in a position to broaden this understanding and extend it to her patients.

An important aspect of psychiatric nursing care is consistency of approach. To achieve this nurses must understand their reactions to each patient. One way to achieve this is to discuss their feelings with a more experienced member of the treatment team, in a staff group discussion. As confidence grows they are able to talk with the patient himself about the feelings he has aroused in them. A remark, 'You make me feel angry when you do that', can set off a discussion which results in increased understanding for both nurse and patient.

Psychiatric nurses in a ward may appear to an outsider to be doing little. But in fact they are intensively busy. A game of Scrabble is started by one nurse to activate a retarded depressed patient, or to make contact with a withdrawn schizophrenic, or to show her friendliness to a paranoid patient. Scrabble is a slow moving game, so that during it the nurse can observe the behaviour of other patients, not simply the one she is with, in an unobtrusive way. Later, she relays her observations to other staff members, doctors, nurses and occupational therapists, for it is important that all information is shared.

How should a nurse/patient relationship develop?

Some psychiatric nurses believe that they should act towards the patient in a totally spontaneous and natural manner, implying that there is little or no difference in status between patient and nurse: both are passengers on the same seat of the Clapham omnibus! This may be acceptable when dealing with patients with personality disorders. It is far from so when nursing patients who are seriously ill, who require a sympathetic understanding approach that allows them to feel that they are cared for and safe. An experienced, mature nurse can naturally vary her behaviour from patient to patient, but even she may encounter difficult situations at times, when she is unsure of her feelings and how to react. However friendly a nurse or doctor may be towards a patient the friendship can never be a straightforward one, certainly not until the patient has fully recovered and treatment is over. The nurse is invariably in a 'superior' position, since she represents authority, the hospital or the psychiatric department. This applies even to the most junior student nurse. A patient's attitude towards authority distorts the way he perceives those looking after and wanting to help him. He may be 'agin all authority' and delight in upsetting the nurse, being so obstructive and unpleasant that it is an effort for her to contain her dislike. He may derive pleasure in playing off one nurse against another, skilfully manipulating inexperienced staff towards increasing dissension and impotence. Or he may reflect the other side of the coin and do everything he possibly can to please the nurse and gain her love and approval. These are extreme instances, but such childlike behaviour – it may usefully be looked upon as persistent remnants of childhood attitudes – will be recognised at times by the percipient nurse in most of her patients.

The psychiatric nurse faces a complex, fascinating and at times threatening world. We are not concerned here with patient violence – which is rare – but with threats that arise from within the nurse herself out of her own imaginative needs and anxieties. Then her emotions become too great, threatening her peace of mind and distorting her judgment and professional behaviour. Circumstances like this usually develop when nurse and patient become overinvolved and their relationship becomes dangerously out of control.

One way of insuring against such occurrences is to use a nursing model as a framework. For instance, consider the example of Mrs Jane Smith, severely depressed following her husband's death three months earlier.

> On her admission she is incontinent and dehydrated. Her nursing care is planned as follows using Orems' (1971) model of nursing (see p. 312).

1. Assist her to increase her fluid intake.
2. Guide her to the lavatory at two hourly intervals, to prevent incontinence.
3. Support her during her stay in hospital; encourage her to talk about her grief; verbally reward each step she takes towards greater independence.
4. Provision of environment: ensure that Mrs Smith has some time to herself, but she also mixes and socialises with others.

5. Teaching: encourage Mrs Smith to participate in activities that can help her to become more outgoing on return home. Teach her tasks that her husband always dealt with: to change an electric light, pay the electricity bill, or read the meter.

From this 'care plan', the nurse has clear guidelines on which to base her relationship with Mrs Smith.

Individual nurse/patient relationship

Primary nursing implies that a nurse has special, or primary, responsibility for a small group of patients. She is responsible for planning their care, and must leave clearly defined 'care plans' for use in her absence for other nurses. This kind of nursing inevitably means that a nurse develops a more or less close relationship with her patients. There is then always a risk that this may place unreasonable strain on the nurse. Indeed Menzies (1970) suggested that one reason for nurses practising 'task allocation' was to protect themselves from the anxieties produced from 'intimate relationships' with patients.

Can we practise psychiatric nursing without getting involved at some level with our patients? Very unlikely, but this is a question all nurses must ask themselves at some point. The very nature of psychiatric nursing requires a nurse to listen to patients and encourage them to explore their doubts and fears. This cannot be done well in the absence of emotional warmth and a good rapport. Without this, nursing care can only be 'custodial', or at best 'non-damaging'.

How should a nurse cope when she feels that she is getting overinvolved with a patient? The answer some people might give is for the nurse to arrange for someone else to take over the patient's care. This may indeed occasionally be necessary, but in most instances it can and should be avoided for several reasons.

1. If the nurse terminates the relationship she will not learn through her mistakes, and may repeat them next time.
2. The patient will be upset and feel rejected. Many psychiatric patients are dealing with just this problem, and such action is likely to reinforce their sense of rejection and increase their difficulties.
3. The problem may have arisen because the patient has made unreasonable demands on the nurse. If this is so it is important to point this out to the patient and what can reasonably be expected of the nurse.

4. It is possible that the patient is being deliberately manipulative and changing nurses may not be therapeutic.

The best action a nurse can take when she feels she is becoming overinvolved with a patient is to ask for help. Who she goes to for help will depend to some extent on her status. A nurse learner may seek guidance from a Staff Nurse or Tutor. The Staff Nurse may ask the Ward Sister or Nursing Officer. The Ward Sister may ask her nursing officer, or a colleague from another discipline. It is important to remember that a 'multidisciplinary team' exists and there is no reason for nurses to seek help only from within their own discipline.

The following examples describe how nurses coped in various situations:

Anne, a Ward Sister, was worried that she was too protective to Helen, a 13 year old girl on the ward

Helen had been there for nearly six months and was one of the most difficult patients that Anne had ever nursed. She had a long history of eating problems and had been admitted after a series of admissions to an Intensive Care Unit. A new Staff Nurse had recently come to the ward and inferred that Helen was getting a disproportionate amount of nursing attention.

When Anne was honest with herself she knew this to be true, but at the same time felt angry with the Staff Nurse. Anne knew that the reason for her anger was that the Staff Nurse had not been on the ward during Helen's most difficult time. During this time Helen had bitten Anne and frightened her by her constant headbanging. The Junior Doctors had recently changed, and Anne felt unable to discuss this matter with their replacements. She shied away from confronting the Staff Nurse as she was afraid of the strength of her own anger. But Anne recognised she needed support and advice. She decided to ask the Consultant Psychiatrist, John, responsible for Helen, to help her. He was happy to listen to Anne and commented on how well he thought Helen had been nursed through her difficult stage. Anne volunteered that maybe it was time to give Helen more responsibility for herself. John agreed. Anne then discussed the best way of doing this and it was decided that they should plan for Helen to go back to school from the ward.

As a result of this discussion, and John's approval for the nursing care given so far, Anne felt able to stand back and encourage greater independence in Helen. Anne was also able to tell her Staff Nurse how pleased she was that she had raised the issue of Helen's care with her. During their conversation the two became much easier with one another and were able to be honest and open about their previous hostility for each other. Thus Helen's care benefited and Anne and the Staff Nurse developed a better working relationship.

It must be said that this was not easy for Anne. It was painful for her to have to face up to the fact that she was in the wrong. But she showed courage and self awareness, and she dealt with the problem correctly, with all round benefit.

Jane, a second year Student Nurse, approached Sally, the Ward Sister, because of her problems about Simon, a 22 year old admitted for treatment of drug addiction. She explained that she found Simon disturbingly attractive sexually, and was aware that this was undesirable.

During discussion Sally learnt that Jane had recently split up with her boy friend of two years' standing. Jane said that she had been asked to sit with Simon and his visitors to ensure that no drugs were being smuggled to him at visiting time. Sitting there and seeing Simon flirting with a girl of her own age, she had recognised how good looking he was.

Sally asked Jane how she thought the staff could help her. Jane replied that she would like to change wards. Sally pointed out the difficulties of such a move, and added that if Jane were to leave, this would not stop a similar situation arising in the future. Jane could see this and was willing to stay when she saw that Sally understood and was prepared to support her. Sally suggested that Jane should continue her relationship with Simon and sit with him at visiting time, and that at the end of each shift Jane would discuss her feelings over Simon with Sally or the nurse in charge. Jane did this and over the next two weeks regained her composure when with Simon and no longer found him sexually attractive – although no one, she declared, could deny that he was good looking!

The important points to note here are that Jane felt able to approach Sally before a serious problem arose. Sally was not condemning and was prepared to help Jane. Jane showed common sense and understanding in the way she tackled this problem.

The problems which arise when nurses grow too fond of their patients are unlikely to become serious when nurses are honest with themselves and open with other members of the team.

The problem of the unpopular patient

Most nurses can think of at least one patient who has consistently irritated them. If the nurse has difficulty in coping with her feelings then the most sensible course is to discuss the matter with a colleague, in the way just described. Occasionally it may be better to switch the patient to another nurse, less irritated by him. But before deciding on such a move it is necessary to understand why he is so irritating. Is it because the nurse herself cannot stand his particular manner and habits, or does he irritate everyone on the team?

If it is an individual matter, affecting only this one nurse, it may well be advisable for senior staff to support her while she continues to nurse the patient. At the same time it is important that her feelings are explored and the deeper reasons for her intolerance revealed to her. Only then can she be helped to develop into a good nurse.

If everyone on the team is irritated by the patient it is reasonable to tell him of this. The manner in which this is undertaken will naturally depend on his diagnosis. To tell a psychotic patient that he is irritating everyone can have destructive consequences, while telling someone with an anxiety neurosis or a personality disorder may be constructive. The friends and relatives of such people may have buried their heads in the sand and never expressed the irritation they have long felt. If telling such a patient the truth about himself can have good effects, the nurses should not hesitate to do so when the occasion is appropriate.

It is important that an individual nurse should not have too many patients of this type at any one time, for they can be very exhausting.

Stockwell has studied the unpopular patient in a general hospital, and her conclusions apply as much to psychiatric as to general nursing. She demonstrated that the unpopular patient was usually the anxious patient. She suggested that by going to the patient promptly when he asked for help his anxiety was rapidly decreased and, in consequence, the amount of nursing time he demanded was reduced. This is a useful fact to remember.

Unpopular patient demanding → Nurse gives time promptly → Patient less demanding

Mrs Watson is an 82 year old lady with depression. She also has a urinary tract infection and requires to be nursed in bed. Every time Mrs Watson is approached she asks to be taken to the toilet, and then, more often than not, is unable to pass urine when she arrives there. Apropos of Stockwell's findings, it is important for Mrs Watson to recognise that she has a bell by her bed and that she must ring immediately she wishes to go to the toilet. A nurse will come as soon as she rings. It is of course essential that the nurses do just that and come quickly, otherwise Mrs Watson's anxiety will continue to increase.

The unpopular patient can usually be nursed well on any ward as long as nurses understand the problem and tackle it along the lines described. Danger arises when the problem is not discussed among the staff and the patient is avoided or ignored at the expense of his nursing care. Every patient has the right to expect the highest quality of nursing care that can be provided within the constraints of the environment. Nurses cannot unequivocably provide this unless they recognise the psychological problems of their patients, irrespective of what is organically wrong with them.

It is important that a nurse be as honest as possible with patients, so that maximum trust exists between them. She must also respect her patients' sense of dignity. She should not discuss the patient with anyone in a derogatory manner, and should show the patient the same respect as she expects for herself. The psychiatric nurse inevitably meets people who have been labelled by their society as misfits and failures. She must recognise and deal with her prejudices and never forget that they are human beings asking for help.

How should a patient be addressed?

The nurse should ask a new patient how he or she likes to be addressed. Some like to be called by their first name, others prefer to be known by their surname. The latter may be angered if addressed gratuitously as Fred or Susie. Problems sometime arise when psychotic patients expect to be addressed in a grandiose manner, Your Majesty or some other title. Here the nurse may have to override the request!

Ward and group meetings

In most psychiatric units it is now usual for patients to decide and enforce the rules necessary to control their own small and specialised community. Ward meetings of staff and patients are frequently held to discuss the daily problems that arise. Patients are encouraged to feel responsible for their own behaviour and that of their fellows. If the community as a whole has decided on a particular rule, which one patient ignores, it is more likely to be the other patients who take him to task rather than a staff member. In some therapeutic community settings the group elects a weekly chairman, who may be patient or staff. Topics for discussion include how facilities can be improved or meal services speeded up, staff attitudes, why one patient always tries to dominate the meeting, why another patient resents a particular staff member or patient, or how occupational therapy can be made more interesting.

Both new patients and nurse learners often feel too shy at first to speak at group meetings; the nurses particularly are conscious of their inexperience and lack of knowledge. It requires confidence to question the view of a doctor or other senior staff member and this can only be gained if the student nurses are made to feel that their observations and ideas are valued. It is often useful for the staff to meet on their own after ward meetings, perhaps over a cup of coffee, to discuss the meeting and what occurred there.

Ward rounds/meetings

Psychiatrists rarely do ward rounds; it is unusual for their patients to be in bed. Ward meetings are held regularly to discuss each patient's progress and whether a change of treatment is indicated. At these meetings all staff involved with patients are present. These include nurses on the wards, the CPN, if a patient is about to be discharged home, social workers, occupational therapists and so on. At times a patient's relatives may be invited to attend and contribute to out-patient management. Meetings are run more or less on egalitarian lines. Participants give their observations and opinions. Everyone agrees, for example, that a patient has a depressive illness following bereavement. A nurse describes her disturbed sleep and appetite. The occupational therapist comments on her inability to concentrate. The social worker sees the patient as an isolated housewife whose whole life has revolved around her husband. In this instance all the staff contributions tally. But this is not always so. Meetings sometimes turn into hotly contested debates!

> A nurse feels that another patient is being manipulative in order to lengthen her stay in hospital, but the social worker says that her life outside is so depressing that she should only be discharged when alternative accommodation has been found.

> The doctor is sure that his patient has a schizophrenic illness. The social worker, on the other hand, believes the patient is 'well' but that the religious beliefs the patient holds are incompatible with British society.

Normally such debates are eventually settled with mutual agreement. Occasionally the Consultant Psychiatrist will make a decision in the absence of consensus. Although this may cause annoyance to some team members, ultimately the doctor is responsible for his patient, and must stand by his own opinion. It is usual for patients in turn to come to the meeting and contribute their views on themselves and their proposed treatment, to ask if they can go home for the weekend, or to have their medication altered.

Staff meetings

There are various types of staff meetings and they may be multi-disciplinary or for one discipline only. The meetings exist to exchange ideas and information, or for staff support. Staff support groups are most easily described by means of an example.

> Ward 2 has regular weekly meetings for all nursing staff, and they are normally conducted on an informal basis. All members are encouraged to discuss any negative and positive feelings they may have about their work. Nurses who feel out of their depth emotionally, or otherwise in need of support and advice, are helped and encouraged by the rest of the group. The meeting lasts for an hour. Topics which do not directly relate to the work setting are discouraged, unless there is a direct consequence for the unit. Problems concerning a nurse's relationship with one or more patients, or with other members of staff, are frequently discussed, and ways in which they may be resolved explored. The theory behind this type of group is based on humanistic philosophy (Rogers, 1967).
>
> Further reading about these methods may be useful.

Ward routine

The principles of psychiatric nursing are essentially the same whether they are practised in a short-stay unit of a general hospital, an admission ward of a psychiatric hospital, a long-stay rehabilitation ward or a psychogeriatric ward, but the routine may vary considerably.

Each ward is run according to the needs of its patients. In a *psychogeriatric* ward the routine is geared to the patients' physical as well as psychological needs. Elderly patients need a safe, homely environment where the pace is relaxed but the atmosphere still stimulating. Confused, disorientated patients require a simple, ordered ward routine with opportunity for as much activity as they are capable, and some entertainment. It is important that the elderly are kept in touch with the outside world, even though they may be destined to spend their last days in hospital; television, radio and daily newspapers thus play an important part. However, while radios and television should be available whenever possible, they should not be allowed to become a substitute for human contact. It is not unknown on a very busy ward for patients to be stuck in front of the television for most of the day or for the radio to be left on loudly and continuously. This can increase the confusion of elderly patients, particularly if they are hard of hearing and cannot actually hear their neighbours or staff speaking to them because of background noise. Nurses must always anticipate and think ahead. If an old person is given a magazine or newspaper to read the nurse must ensure that she has her reading spectacles to hand. There is a moving book about this subject which is well worth reading (*Sans Everything*, Robb, 1960).

In a *rehabilitation ward* many of the patients leave the ward each day to attend occupational or industrial therapy units, sheltered workshops or employment in a nearby town. The nurse rouses her patients early and encourages them to make their beds, and perhaps gets them to help prepare breakfast. She reminds a patient starting work for the first time to make himself a sandwich lunch, persuades another to have a haircut in readiness for an interview, encourages a third to smarten himself up. She may then accompany some patients to occupational therapy and work alongside them, observing how they react to this new department.

On an *admission* ward there are new patients for the nurse to meet, most of whom have never been in a psychiatric unit or hospital before. Many people still have preconceived ideas that psychiatric wards are horrific and patients and relatives may both need to be reassured that this is no longer so.

The way in which the admission procedure is carried out is particularly important, as first impressions are lasting. One nurse should be allocated to admit the patient and all formalities. All formalities should be completed with as little fuss as possible. If the patient is reluctant to provide the nurse with the necessary information about himself he should not be pressed. This can be obtained later when he is more settled. The nurse should tell the patient what is going to happen, such as a routine physical examination, and give him general information about the time of meals, location of the bathroom and any ward rules which he will be expected to obey. Since the patient is an unknown quantity at first, he should be kept under strict observation. Observations in the acute stage of the patient's illness are, in any case, often of great diagnostic value to the doctor.

It is a good idea to introduce new patients to one or two others who have already settled in, as new patients are often mistrustful of staff at first. In this way no pressure is brought to bear on the patient, and the nurse has an opportunity to see how he reacts to other people. To force a new patient into long discussions about himself, or to make him join in group activities immediately, gives him no time to adapt to his new surroundings.

As well as receiving new patients the nurse on an admission unit is also looking after patients in various stages of treatment.

Some admission wards are often also called *observation* wards, mainly because observation and the reporting of these observations constitutes the main duty of the psychiatric nurses working in these types of units.

Community psychiatric nursing

The role and working of the community psychiatric nurse is discussed in detail in Chapter 26. It is important however to remember that her relationships with patients differ from those of the ward nurse. There are two main reasons for this; firstly because she is a 'guest' in the patient's home and secondly because the relationship is generally on a one to one basis. Thus the relationship between nurse and patient is a more equal one in many instances than in a ward situation.

26
Community Care

The last twenty years have seen a shift in emphasis on delivering care for the mentally ill away from the mental hospitals to more convivial settings in the community. Many areas have small psychiatric units attached to general hospitals for acute admission and patient assessment. Although long term in-patient beds for the elderly and chronically mentally ill exist, these are steadily reducing. Instead it is envisaged that eventually most patients/clients will receive psychiatric care without long term admission.

In order to achieve this, it is essential that the system is able to provide supervision, day hospitals, hostels, sheltered workshops and community nursing services for patients. The health authorities are bound to provide some day hospitals and community nursing services; local authorities should organise the majority of other services but they are not obliged to. There is a potential problem in that as health authorities cease to admit patients there may not be a safety net provided by local authorities in the form of housing, etc. This is already evident in some areas wnere the mentally ill are to be found sleeping rough four or five to a room in common 'doss houses'.

Similarly, caring for a patient at home can sometimes result in considerable hardship for a family and, unfortunately, it may be necessary to admit him or her to hospital for the sake of the relatives. Recently, the National Schizophrenia Association has argued that too many patients are being cared for in the community without adequate resources. On the other hand, MIND firmly believes that patients should be cared for in the community for as long as possible. Some of the systems provided by local authorities are described below:

1. *Hostels and sheltered residential accommodation.* A period of residence in a *half-way house* or hostel may help the patient who is discharged after a long-time in hospital to adjust to the responsibilities of everyday life before emerging fully into the community. He is able to go out to work, knowing that his general needs will be looked after. Residential accommodation is also needed for elderly patients who are not capable of living alone or in small families, but who do not yet need care in hospital. Hostel accommodation may also be required for mentally impaired

children whose homes are situated a long way from a training centre.

Residential accommodation is also provided by the Mental After-Care Association.

2. *MIND* is the National Association for Mental Health and is the leading mental health organisation in England and Wales. It has 190 affiliated local associations, six regional centres and a central London office.

The aim of MIND is to improve and develop mental health services in response to the needs of people who use them. They have a Legal and Welfare Rights Department who fight for the rights of people with mental disorders. MIND played an important part in the development of the 1983 Mental Health Act, representing the mentally ill.

3. *Therapeutic social clubs and centres*, which help to offset the bad effect of loneliness.

4. *Day Centres and Day Hospitals. Night Hospitals.*

Patients not needing or unwilling to accept complete hospitalisation, but requiring more intensive treatment than an ordinary out-patient clinic can provide, benefit from treatment in a day hospital. Day hospitals cater ideally for between 20 and 30 patients at a time, attending five days a week between 9 a.m. to 4 p.m. All forms of treatment are given, and all types of patient treated there. Group therapy is particularly useful in such a setting. Close co-operation is required between nurses, occupational therapists and doctors. Early treatment in a day hospital reduces the admission rate of patients to the parent hospital. Day centres are oriented towards caring for rather than actively treating people. They are particularly useful for elderly patients who cannot be left alone while their relatives work.

Patients who are capable of working, but are too disturbed for ordinary family life, often improve slowly if they can continue to work. This is sometimes possible in the absence of a halfway house, by arranging for them to return from work to a *night hospital.*

5. *The Disablement Resettlement Service* helps registered disabled persons to obtain and keep suitable work. All employers of twenty or more people must employ a quota of disabled people, and certain jobs such as lift and car park attendants are reserved for them. A *disablement resettlement officer* (DRO) is attached to each labour exchange. He helps in one of four ways:

(a) By finding a suitable job.

(b) By organising *sheltered* employment for the chronically sick; special facilities, for instance, exist with non-profit making firms, such as Remploy Ltd.

(c) By arranging for a course at an *Industrial Rehabilitation Unit.* There the patient is gradually reconditioned to the stresses of industrial life.

(d) By arranging *vocational training* at a Government training centre.

(NB – There are 800 000 registered disabled people, of whom 74 000 have psychiatric disorders.)

Facilities provided by Health Authorities

1. *Core and cluster services*

A new idea for community care involves a small in-patient unit for assessment of patients with houses 'clustered' in the local community for the aftercare and supervision of discharged patients. The advantages of this system are:

(a) The patient is cared for by the same team of staff both as an 'in' and 'out' patient.
(b) It is run by the health authority and is thus funded on a long term basis (rather than local authority funding which may fluctuate depending on the politics of the council)
(c) Both admission and discharge should be conducted quickly when necessary.

It will be necessary to evaluate the effectiveness of this type of care when it has been functioning for a period of time.

2. Community teams of psychiatrists, psychiatric social workers and nurses exist in some health authorities to provide accurate assessment of patients' needs. These will need to be developed further if the community care system is to be fully adopted. The subject of whether they should be employed by health or local authorities will also have to be considered.

3. General practitioners play a vital part in the community care services. They are well placed to diagnose and treat early psychiatric illness. Frequently the entire burden of looking after discharged psychiatric patients falls on them, and they are not always able to meet all their patients' needs. The advent of community psychiatric nurses is reducing this risk and enhancing the care of discharged patients.

4. *Community Psychiatric Nursing*

The community psychiatric service is now well established in most areas. It first commenced in the 1950s and its role has developed significantly in the last ten years.

Most psychiatric nurses who work in the community are employed in the grade of sister. They have usually gained considerable earlier experience with the mentally ill in hospital before moving to community nursing. There is a move towards making a post basic course in psychiatric nursing mandatory for practice in the community, as with District Nurses.

At present 40 per cent of community psychiatric nurses have completed a course which is approved by the relevant National Board for Nursing, Midwifery and Health Visiting. The majority are full time courses, last for an academic year and are organised by colleges of further education or polytechnics. Recently, a modular course has been approved which will run over a period of two years; technically this course could be run by a school of nursing. It is envisaged that this method of training may be especially useful for experienced staff who will move into the community to work as large mental hospitals are reduced.

It is unlikely that mandatory training will be introduced in the immediate future for several reasons. Firstly, because of the expense involved in training; and secondly, because there is such an increase of patients to the community that it would be impossible to train all the nurses required to work in the area quickly enough. At present the majority of nurses have a caseload of approximately 40, some of whom need intensive surveillance, while others only require a watchful eye on discharge from hospital.

Community psychiatric nursing (CPN) involves four main areas of responsibility: assessment, support, medication administration and treatment. There is evidence to suggest that the job also regularly involves liaison with other disciplines, counselling, administering physical treatment, delivering messages and advising relatives (Skidmore and Friend, 1984).

Increasingly patients are being supported at home by community psychiatric nurses and thereby avoiding admission to hospital. This is normally preceded by a hospital out-patient or domicillary visit from a psychiatrist to assess the situation. Sometimes the medical supervision is provided by the General Practitioner alone. Obviously, the back up of the Social Services is often needed; for instance a home help or meals on wheels.

The patient who has been discharged from hospital is often referred to the psychiatric community nurse, who visits him at home or arranges for him to visit her.

Home visits from a nurse are an extremely valuable development for both patients and nurses alike. Often it is impossible for the hospital doctor or nurse to gain a clear picture of the home environment of their patient. The psychiatric social worker takes a history from the patient and his relatives concerning the family circumstances, but this may merely represent the picture they wish to present. First-hand impressions gained by a visiting nurse can be far more enlightening.

It is easier to judge a person in the setting of his home than in hospital. Relationships between the patient and other family members soon become clear, particularly as they come to accept the nurse's presence. The community psychiatric nurse who visits a patient after discharge often learns more about the psychodynamics underlying his symptoms and difficulties than the hospital staff were ever able to do. Armed with this knowledge the nurse is strongly placed to prevent relapse and readmission to hospital. She is in a position to assess the extent of his recovery and what further treatment he may need. Much of the work of the community nurse consists of counselling and support, not only the patient but also his family. Relatives have a vital role to play in the patient's rehabilitation. The community nurse must enable them to understand the nature of the illness and how they can best help the patient. Many patients need to continue with medication after leaving hospital and it is vital that they and their families understand the reasons for this.

Behaviour modification treatment programmes initiated in hospital may be continued at home by the community nurse. Only if she meets some unforeseen difficulties requiring advice or help from the specialist team need she directly involve them. Normally she reports back to the multidisciplinary team about all her patients at regular intervals.

An important advantage of a community psychiatric nursing service is that it provides the vital link with hospital which a patient so often needs after his discharge. Many patients are frightened and sometimes openly reluctant to be discharged, apprehensive at the thought of having no doctor or nurse on hand. Hospital nurses sometimes receive invitations to visit a patient's home. Usually these invitations are extended under the guise of gratitude for what the nurse has done for the patient. In reality, of course, what the patient is really saying is that he is frightened to leave the safe hospital environment. Sometimes seeing the community nurse will reassure a patient of support after he leaves the hospital.

In addition to the support and care of patients discharged from hospital, the community nurse has an educative role within the community. Despite the common acceptance of the role, research has demonstrated that community psychiatric nursing is progressing on a 'hit and miss basis with little evidence of role evaluation or intervention assessment' (Skidmore and Friend, 1984). If the community nurse utilises the nursing process and evaluates each visit she makes for its usefulness she can begin to organise her workload in a methodical fashion.

Support is an essential part of the community psychiatric nurse's role. The person most frequently in need of support is the patient who was originally referred to the nursing service. In addition, relatives, friends and workmates may be supported by the CPN. Support may be required in the short and long term.

Short term support may involve encouraging the patient to return to work after a depressive illness. For example: Mr John Tang is a twenty six year old cashier in a high street bank. He has been on fully paid sick leave for four months with depression after his girlfriend broke their long standing relationship. John had been very distressed as he had been saving up to get married. Prior to going sick, he had begun to arrive late at work and had become careless, having previously been punctual and meticulous. His manager was concerned about him and advised him to seek medical help. As a result John was referred to a consultant psychiatrist who arranged for treatment by psychotherapy and group activities in a day hospital. The community psychiatric nurse, Sally, was actively involved in a 'social skills group' and John joined this in order to regain confidence in social situations, especially in the company of women.

John responded well to treatment and began to understand the reasons for his depression. The team at the day hospital felt that he was ready to consider returning to work, having first made sure that the bank was prepared to give him every help and encouragement in re-establishing himself. Sally was given the task of supporting John until he was securely settled, which she duly undertook. This example demonstrates the 'planning' stage of supportive nursing intervention.

In addition nurses in the community are frequently involved in the administration of long acting intramuscular phenothiazines (Modecate, Depixol). Community psychiatric nurses give these at regular intervals and at the same time can assess the patient's needs and provide extra support if necessary. This service is invaluable to the patient who is working, as it does not necessitate taking time off. Most community nurses organise their workload so that injections can be given outside a patient's working hours. CPNs need to liaise with other disciplines in the community to enhance patient care (Figs. 26.1, 26.2). The roles of other nurses are briefly discussed:

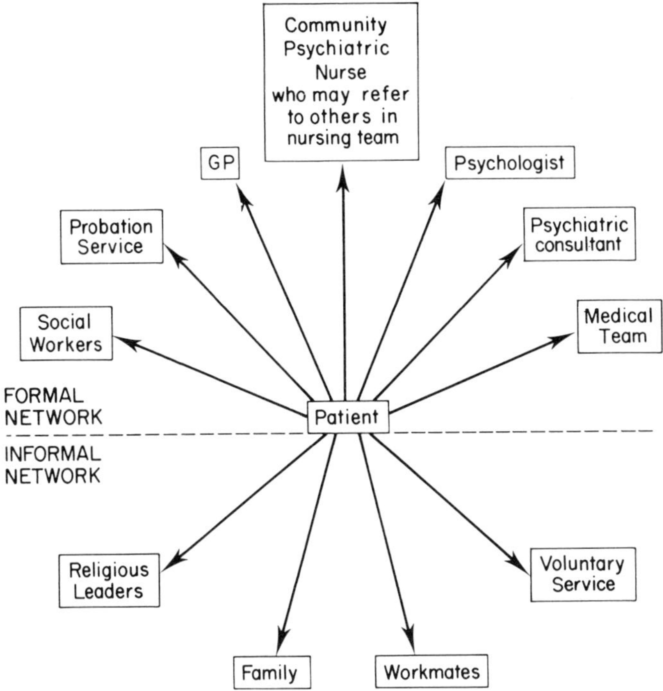

Fig. 26.1 A patient may come into contact with all these people during his period of illness and rehabilitation

The health visitor is primarily responsible for health care screening and prevention of illness in children under five years of age. Some are specifically appointed to promote health within the elderly population.

The midwife is responsible for pre- and antenatal care for pregnant mothers. She has a statutory right of entry to the home to ensure that babies are well from the age of 1–10 days. **NB** No other community nurse has right of entry.

The district nurse is responsible for 'nursing care' delivery to patients with physical illness, and has an educative and preventative role also.

Very few *community mental handicap nurses* exist at present. Their role is similar to the community psychiatric nurse, but involves working with mentally handicapped children and adults.

Assessment for the CPN involves establishing a patient's needs and deciding whether nursing intervention can be useful. The skill is a

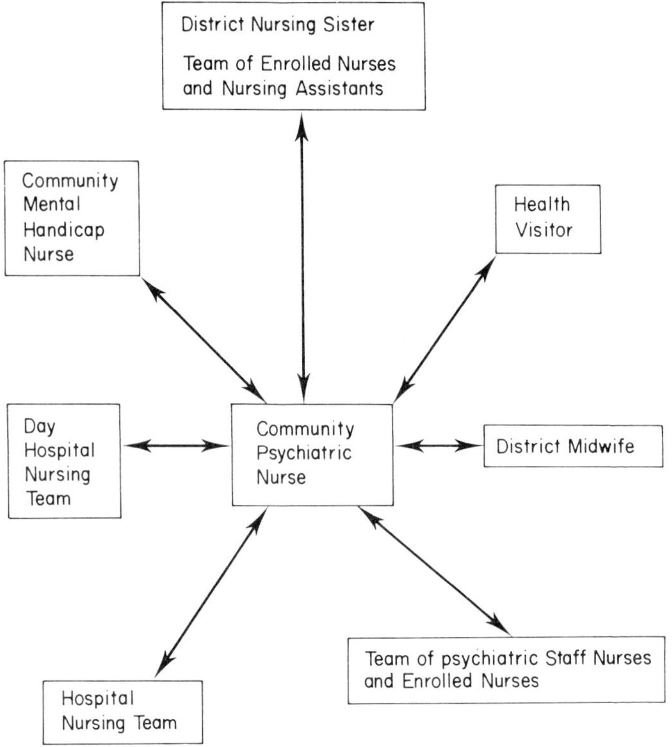

Fig. 26.2 The community psychiatric nurse may consult or refer to any of the nurses in the health authority

difficult one to acquire but is essential if caseloads are to be kept manageable. Three nursing histories are described to demonstrate this:

Mrs Jenkins

Mrs Jenkins, a 64 year old widow, is referred to the community psychiatric nurse by her general practitioner because she is depressed. On assessment, the C P N concludes that Mrs Jenkins is lonely and isolated and that nursing intervention is not appropriate. The C P N discusses with Mrs Jenkins how she may usefully fill her day. Both agree that Mrs Jenkins will answer an advertisement for voluntary help in a local charity shop. The community nurse must now decide whether to continue visiting Mrs Jenkins. She may decide that one more visit is justified 'to establish that Mrs Jenkins is now motivated to seek a better social life'. If the C P N's motives are to 'visit Mrs Jenkins' merely because she was referred, this demonstrates an inability to manage a 'caseload efficiently'.

Mrs Jones

Mrs Jones was a 76 year old widow who lived in a council house with her spinster daughter of 48. Mrs Jones became increasingly confused and forgetful. Her daughter finally called the G P when her mother was incontinent of urine and faeces.

The G P believed that Mrs Jones had a urinary tract infection, coupled with senile dementia. He suggested that with treatment of the infection, Mrs Jones might improve sufficiently to be left alone while her daughter went to work. The daughter was reluctant for her mother to be admitted to a psychogeriatric unit for assessment because this was twenty miles away and it would be difficult for her to visit.

The community psychiatric nurse visited and organised a supply of incontinence pads and a commode. She also helped Miss Jones bathe her mother, and explained the importance of getting her out of bed and moving regularly and the need for plenty of fluid. The daughter said that she had given her mother only minimal amounts to drink recently in order to stop her being incontinent. She also added that she hoped her mother would soon be well enough to be left alone otherwise her job might be in jeopardy.

The nurse visited twice a day for three days. On the fourth day she arrived to find Miss Jones huddled in a chair crying and her mother sitting in a sodden bed. Miss Jones was in despair about her job and could see no prospect of an early return to work. That morning she had telephoned her brother to ask if either he or his wife could come to stay for a few days. Her brother had replied that this was impossible and that their mother should go into hospital. The C P N contacted the G P, who arranged for a domiciliary visit by the psychiatrist. He agreed that Mrs Jones needed admission for assessment, and Miss Jones acquiesced reluctantly.

After her mother had left for the hospital, Miss Jones talked freely to the C P N about how badly she felt about her mother having to leave home. The nurse pointed out that her mother would get excellent care and might be able to come home later. She also agreed to accompany Miss Jones on her visit to the hospital as Miss Jones was fearful of this.

Miss Jones was gratified to see how well and content her mother seemed in hospital. In time it became increasingly apparent to her that her mother's mental state was not going to improve enough for her to return home. This case history shows that admission became necessary through no fault of the family or community services, and that it was in the best interests of Mrs Jones.

Mrs Fitch

Mrs Fitch was a 27 year old woman – previously the manageress of a large department store – who developed a post-natal depression after the birth of her first child, Sarah. Her husband was a self-employed mechanic whose garage was in the garden of their house. Both his mother and his wife's mother lived nearby.

A consultant psychiatrist visited Mrs Fitch at the request of the general practitioner, diagnosed post-natal depression and prescribed an anti-depressant drug. A community psychiatric nurse subsequently saw Mrs Fitch. Together they agreed that Mrs Fitch needed help in looking after the house and Sarah. After a family conference, it was arranged for Mrs Fitch's mother to do the washing and ironing and for her mother-in-law to do some light housework.

Mrs Fitch was encouraged to look after Sarah, and to show her off to the neighbours. Her social confidence was steadily built up as the C P N arranged for her to undertake activities which called for increasing initiative and independence. Over the next weeks Mrs Fitch's confidence with Sarah improved, reinforced by repeated assurances from the C P N that she was coping well. Mr Fitch, delighted with his wife's improvement, readily acquiesced to the suggestion that he take her shopping for new clothes, and to have her hair done. Mrs Fitch's mother arranged to have Sarah for the day and it was an enormous success all round.

Over a period of six months Mrs Fitch gradually took over full responsibility for Sarah and the house. She and her husband were both relieved that she had been cared for at home and avoided admission to hospital. Indeed, this seemed to play an important part in her recovery; on more than one occasion she commented, 'I was not ill enough to have to go to hospital you know'.

It was relatively easy to manage this young woman in the community because of the social support available from the family, and the fact that at no time had either Mrs Fitch or Sarah been considered to be 'at risk'.

Choice of nursing model for community work

The systems model depicted by Roy (1974) is a complex one (stress adaptation). It revolves around the stability or adaptation of the client. The nurse's role is seen as assisting the client to remain in, or return to, an adaptive state. This model views man as a bio-psycho-social being who is in constant interaction with the environment (McFarlane, 1980). Nursing focus is on man in relation to his position on the health–illness continuum. If man is 'healthy' nursing intervention may not be necessary, if he is ill it may. This model suggests that man will move along the continuum in relation to his ability to adapt to stimuli that confront him. Three types of stimuli are described: (1) focal stimuli which confront the person and to which he makes an adaptive response, (2) background stimuli which contribute to the persons's behaviour caused by focal stimuli and (3) residual stimuli which arise from the person's past experience (Roy, 1974, cited in McFarlane, 1980).

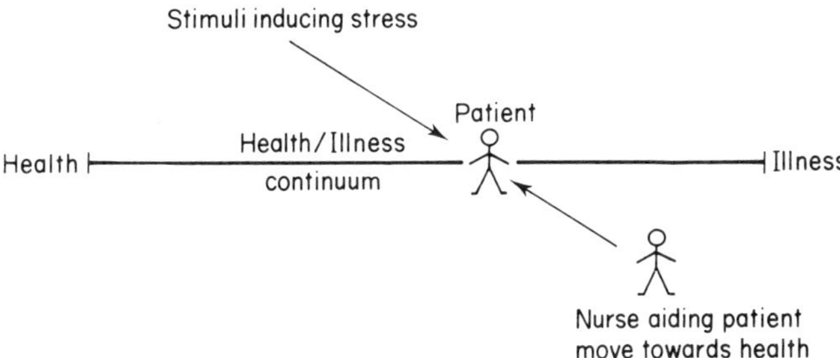

Fig. 26.3 Nurse helping patient adapt to stress (Roy, 1974)

The stimuli may evoke a negative or positive adaptive mode. The modes of adaptation conceptualised by Roy (1974) are physiological, self concept, role function and interdependence. The self concept and role function modes interact in the environment to influence each other, and this is the interdependence mode referred to.

A simplified version of this model could provide nurses with a good framework for the care of patients in the community. The role of the nurse is that of helping patients to adapt to stimuli and move them from illness towards health on the continum.

For example a client who is stressed by the birth of a new baby (*stressor*) may be helped by the nurse to reorganise her day to reduce stress (i.e. adapt to the situation).

Future Developments

Community care services for the mentally ill are developing rapidly and vary from area to area. A reading list is included in the Appendix to give further information about individual projects.

27
Treatment

Over the past 30 years tremendous advances have occurred in the treatment of psychiatric illnesses. These, combined with changed social attitudes, have greatly altered the outlook for psychiatric patients.

Insulin coma, convulsion therapy and leucotomy were introduced between 1930 and 1940. Electro-convulsive therapy is still the most effective treatment for serious depression, but treatment by insulin coma is now virtually never used, having been replaced by phenothiazine tranquillisers.

The last three decades have seen the rise of psychotropic drugs, drugs which influence mental states and behaviour. Tranquillisers and anti-depressant drugs have multiplied and further advances can be expected in the future.

Psychiatric illnesses are now treated at an early stage, and vicious circles and bad habits are prevented from forming. But effective though these treatments are, they have their limitations. Often they only relieve symptoms rather than bring about a permanent cure. In the case of depressive illness, which usually 'lifts' spontaneously after a time, treatment may need to be continued until this occurs. But in some cases of schizophrenia there is no spontaneous remission, and drugs may have to be taken for many years, in the same way as a diabetic has to take insulin.

Each patient must be assessed individually. The majority need some form of psychotherapy or support. Physical factors, such as weight loss and/or vitamin deficiencies must never be overlooked.

After treatment, many patients require help to find a suitable job. Adequate *community mental health services* are essential at this stage otherwise the relapse rate will be high.

The following methods of treatment and care are described below:

1. *Drug therapy*:
   (a) Major tranquillisers or neuroleptics
   (b) Minor tranquillisers, sedatives, hypnotics
   (c) Anti-depressant drugs
   (d) Miscellaneous

2. *Electro-convulsive therapy* (ECT)
3. *Behaviour therapy*
4. *Non-physical treatments*:
   Psychotherapy and analysis; Group therapies
5. *Prefrontal leucotomy*

Tranquillisers

A *tranquilliser*, by definition, has a calming effect on disturbed behaviour, without causing drowsiness. The term was first applied to the action of chlorpromazine.

Major tranquillisers, or neuroleptics, are those drugs which are effective in the treatment of psychotic disorders. They act predominantly on subcortical structures and functions. Biochemically, all neuroleptics block dopaminergic systems in the CNS (see p. 251).

Major tranquillisers (Neuroleptics)

Phenothiazine derivatives. There are nearly twenty different compounds. In their molecular structure they all share the phenothiazine nucleus (Fig. 27.1). They fall into three groups, depending on the nature of the side chain substitution on the nitrogen atom in the middle ring; chlorpromazine has a dimethyl amino propyl side chain, thioridazine a piperidine side chain, and trifluoperazine a piperazine side chain. The most marked effect on the CNS occurs when the nitrogen substituted chain contains three methyl groups; all the effective antipsychotic phenothiazine derivatives have this structure.

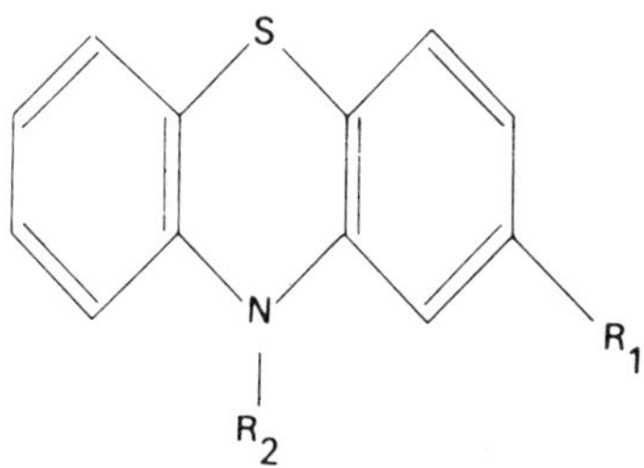

Fig. 27.1 Phenothiazine structure (R = side chains)

It was quickly recognised that patients with acute schizophrenia treated with chlorpromazine recovered more rapidly and in many cases were able to leave hospital after quite a short time. But it soon became apparent that this improved rate of recovery and discharge from hospital was followed by an increased rate of relapse and readmission. Research into this showed that recovered schizophrenics relapsed when they stopped taking their phenothiazine. The majority of recovered schizophrenics must continue phenothiazine medication, perhaps indefinitely, if they are to avoid relapse and deterioration. The introduction of long-acting phenothiazine preparations, such as fluphenazine decanoate (Modecate) and flupenthixol decanoate (Depixol) has made this task easier. Regular injections obviate drug defaulting and ensure that the drug is fully absorbed. Recent studies, comparing the effect of long-acting neuroleptics with placebo in severe chronic cases of schizophrenia, confirm the protection provided by these drugs.

How long phenothiazines need to be continued depends on many factors. It is important to recognise that neuroleptics do not simply control a patient's symptoms. They also enlarge his emotional life by protecting him from emotional stresses. Without the help of neuroleptics, patients withdraw into themselves. With these drugs patients are better able to function socially. And the strain on the relatives with whom they live is considerably lessened. A minimum of three years' maintenance treatment in most cases of schizophrenia is advisable, and the drug is only stopped then if the patient has remained free of symptoms for at least a year.

Acute schizophrenia almost invariably needs to be treated in hospital. A minimum of 150 mg a day of chloropromazine, or 15 mg trifluoperazine are required. ECT may be given concomitantly, particularly when depression is present.

Extrapyramidal side effects develop from the action of neuroleptics in blocking dopamine and are dose related. Those neuroleptics with the strongest anticholinergic properties, such as thioridazine, are less likely to produce Parkinsonism. The piperazine derivatives are the worst offenders. There is no evidence to substantiate earlier claims, still sometimes made, that the antipsychotic and extrapyramidal effects of the neuroleptics go hand in hand.

Parkinsonism and akathisia are the most common extrapyramidal side effects, dystonic reactions the most frightening. Dystonic reactions usually develop within two to three days of starting treatment and are most likely in young patients. Tardive dyskinesia, affecting usually the mouth, tongue and face, develops when neuroleptics are given over long periods – although it has occurred after a few months – in high dosage, particularly when a patient has pre-existent brain damage. It is not possible to anticipate which patient is liable to develop tardive dyskinesia; it is important always to be on the watch for signs of it. Dyskinesia often becomes worse when the phenothiazine is stopped, and may in fact be first noticed at this time. Most patients lose their symptoms slowly when the drug is stopped, although this can take up to a year. In some cases, however, the condition persists and it may be necessary to go back to the neuroleptic responsible.

Anticholinergic and alpha-adrenoceptor blocking effects are responsible for such side effects as dry mouth, constipation, blurred vision, tachycardia and postural hypotension. Allergic reactions include photosensitivity, particularly common with chlorpromazine, skin rashes, agranulocytosis and cholestatic jaundice. Jaundice occurs in about 1 per cent of patients treated with chlorpromazine, and usually develops in the first six weeks. It resolves spontaneously when the drug is stopped. Other effects of long term treatment, or of using large doses, are pigmentation of the exposed skin, and fine brown deposits on the anterior lens capsule. Retinitis pigmentosa is particularly likely to develop with high doses of thioridazine (over 600 mg a day). Epileptic fits may be provoked, particularly when large doses are first given, or if the drug is suddenly stopped.

Depression can develop with any phenothiazine; between one-third and one-half of treated schizophrenics show signs of depression at some time. Long-acting phenothiazines like Modecate have no greater tendency to cause depression than other phenothiazines. Earlier reports that they did so were biased by selection.

With so many available neuroleptics, how do you decide which to use and when? The phenothiazines are first choice in the treatment of acute schizophrenia. When a patient is agitated and difficult to manage, chlorpromazine is indicated. Dosages of up to 1200 mg a day may be required for a time. In paranoid schizophrenia, or when a patient is apathetic, one of the piperazine phenothiazines such as trifluoperazine is a better choice. The dosage ranges from 15 to 45 mg a day. For most patients who need long-term maintenance therapy, either Modecate or Depixol is preferable. A dose of 25 mg Modecate is approximately equivalent to 40 mg Depixol. There is considerable individual variation both in dosage and the interval between injections. Over a period of time, for any one patient, both may need to be varied. Depixol seems to have some antidepressant effects, or perhaps less depressing effects, and is probably preferable to Modecate in depressed schizophrenics. Modecate is a better choice for elated or aggressive patients. However, some patients dislike intramuscular injections, and also complain of feeling over-sedated for some days after the injection. Provided they can be trusted to take the drug, it is reasonable to continue phenothiazines orally.

Chlorpromazine was used routinely at one time in our psychiatric unit for the treatment of anorexia nervosa. The disadvantages of the drug are its side effects, particularly its ability to provoke fits in about 10 per cent of these patients, and dystonic reactions. Today, with good nursing, only about 10 per cent of our patients require chlorpromazine.

Promazine (Sparine). Some clinicians fear that chlorpromazine may cause jaundice and fits, and do not like to use the drug in the treatment of alcoholism. They therefore use promazine, which is not hepatotoxic. It has only about a third of the potency of chlorpromazine, and is *not* an adequate substitute in schizophrenia. The dose varies from 75–1500 mg a day, depending on the patient's condition. It is also a useful hypnotic, in a dosage of 50–100 mg, particularly in old people.

Thioxanthene derivatives

The thioxanthene derivatives are closely related to the phenothiazines in structure and derivatives (Fig. 27.2). They are not as potent as phenothiazines in the treatment of schizophrenia. Flupenthixol is the only one of the series that is widely used. In small doses orally, flupenthixol acts as a tranquilliser. Flupenthixol decanoate (Depixol) is an effective, long-acting neuroleptic; 40 mg is approximately equivalent to 25 mg of fluphenazine decanoate (Modecate).

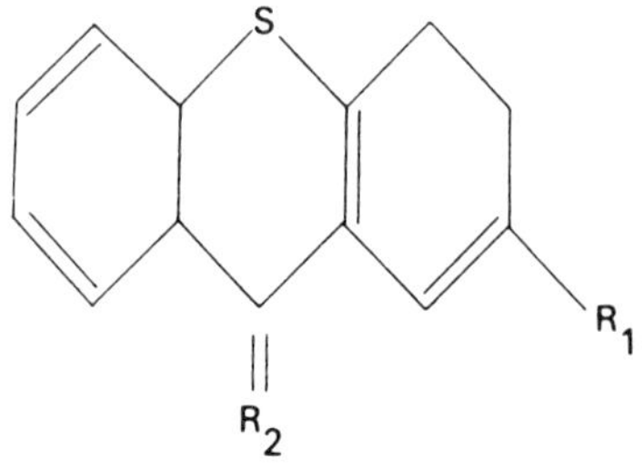

S

R_1

R_2

Fig. 27.2 Thioxanthene structure

Butyrophenones

Haloperidol is the prototype. All are potent inhibitors of dopamine. They have little or no anticholinergic or adrenoceptor blocking effects. Haloperidol is rapidly absorbed from the gut, and reaches a peak concentration after about 6 hours. Excretion is slow and not more than two doses a day are required. The drug can be given orally, intramuscularly or intravenously.

Haloperidol is used to control mania and hypomania, catatonic excitement, and acute delirium tremens; indeed any seriously disturbed behaviour. In these conditions treatment starts with 10 to 15 mg a day or more orally, and is increased until the patient's behaviour is controlled. Up to 100 mg or more a day may be required for a time. As the patient improves the dosage is gradually reduced.

Chronic schizophrenics, resistent to phenothiazines, provided they are not emotionally deteriorated, may respond to high dose therapy, with up to 200 mg haloperidol a day. This dosage is reduced once improvement occurs.

Small doses of haloperidol, 1 – 3 mg a day, are useful in anxious or agitated old people; 1.5 mg are a safe and useful hypnotic.

Claims have been made for haloperidol in the treatment of motor tics, including Gilles de la Tourette's syndrome, stuttering, and childhood behaviour problems.

Side effects are minimal apart from extrapyramidal ones, and the incidence of these is much the same as with the piperazine phenothiazines. Anti-Parkinsonian drugs are required in about 50 per cent of patients on medium dosage, but high dosage and parenteral injections rarely cause extrapyramidal side effects. The drug is remarkably safe, but tardive dyskinesia must be watched for when treatment is prolonged.

Other drugs in this group include:

Pimozide. This has the advantage of only needing to be taken once a day. The daily dosage ranges from 20 mg in the treatment of schizophrenia to 2 mg in neurotic disorders. Side effects are few, but skin rashes sometimes occur.

Penfluridol. Given orally 30 mg is effective for a week. The drug enters and leaves the brain slowly and is not metabolised there.

Fluspirilene. Between 1 and 10 mg is given intramuscularly, and has a duration of action of about a week, with a peak effect after two days.

These drugs are used in chronic schizophrenia, unresponsive to phenothiazines and other neuroleptics, or particularly sensitive to extrapyramidal side effects.

Minor tranquillisers (anxiolytics), sedatives, and hypnotics

Barbiturates. The barbiturates have been in use since the start of this century. They reached their prescription peak about ten years ago. They exert a generalised depressant effect on the nervous system, particularly the neocortex and reticular formation. They are still widely used as hypnotics. At present they are denounced for causing dependence and serious withdrawal symptoms, disturbing the sleeping EEG, interacting adversely with other drugs, and providing an easy means of suicide. While no one will deny that they have great disadvantages, the barbiturates are unexcelled in acute anxiety, and as hypnotics for some insomniacs.

Phenobarbitone causes and enhances depression, and should not be used for psychiatric syndromes. Barbiturates are particularly likely to cause confusion in elderly patients. They are contra-indicated in patients with porphyria.

Barbiturates are broken down in the liver by microsomal enzymes, and in the process the activity of these enzymes is increased. As a result, other drugs metabolised by them, tricyclic antidepressants and phenothiazines for example, are broken down more rapidly. Barbiturates also interact with coumarin anticoagulants. Their withdrawal from a patient anticoagulated with warfarin is potentially hazardous.

Benzodiazepine derivatives. Introduced in the early 1960s, these drugs have largely replaced barbiturates and meprobamate. They are less likely to cause physical dependence, are less sedating, are safe even after huge overdoses, and do not interact appreciably with other drugs.

Chlordiazepoxide was the first, and there are now a number of derivatives. They are used widely as anxiolytics and hypnotics. Diazepam, lorazepam, clorazepate, oxazepam, medazepam are all closely related pharmacologically and chemically. They are broken down in the liver to common active metabolites, of which desmethyldiazepam is the most important. Their differences rest more in their half-life than in their anxiolytic properties.

There is little point in changing from one to another if the first does not relieve anxiety. Clorazepate is useful at night as a hypnotic, and because of its long action a sedative effect extends into the next day. Oxazepam and lorazepam are better for short-lived and intermittent anxiety.

These drugs act on the limbic lobe and reticular activating system, and do not affect the cortex. They reduce emotional reactions to stress. Their main use is in the treatment of anxiety, both primary and secondary to other conditions. They can be safely combined with any other drug, and used with comparative safety in such conditions as liver failure and heart failure. In larger doses, or as nitrazepam and flurazepam, all the diazepines can be used as hypnotics. None of the diazepines produces REM rebound on withdrawal, which often characterises drugs causing dependency. But physical dependency can occur, and sudden withdrawal after large doses have been ingested for some time can produce fits and confusion and reactivate anxiety and tension symptoms.

Chlordiazepoxide can be given intramuscularly, diazepam and lorazepam both intramuscularly and intravenously. Large doses, up to 800 mg of diazepam, 20 mg of lorazepam a day, are sometimes used to control delirium tremens. Intravenous diazepam, 10 to 30 mg, is useful in alleviating panic attacks, as an adjunct to behaviour therapy, and with ECT to prevent post-ECT confusion and agitation. It is also invaluable in treating status epilepticus. The dosage ranges widely from 2 mg diazepam up to 80 mg or more orally at times of acute anxiety.

Side effects are remarkably few. Drowsiness and tiredness occur with too high a dosage. Ataxia, headache, confusion and agitation are uncommon. Some patients gain a considerable amount of weight. Patients with markedly obsessional personalities sometimes feel depressed and unpleasantly out of control. Rarely, in old people, they cause confusion and hallucination. When given intravenously, diazepam can cause hypotension and apnoea. Amnesia develops for up to 30 minutes afterwards, which is useful in dentistry and gastroscopy. There is still some doubt about the teratogenic effects of diazepam. There have been reports of cleft lip and palate in children born to mothers given diazepam during pregnancy.

Beta-adrenergic blocking agents

Propranolol. *Propranolol* has been compared favourably to chlordiazepoxide in relieving anxiety. In fact, the action of propranolol is probably largely due to peripheral blockade of sympathetically mediated symptoms, like palpitations. The cutting short of such symptoms interrupts a feedback loop which otherwise perpetuates the anxiety. Propranolol is indicated therefore when there are marked somatic symptoms; palpitation, diarrhoea, tremor. The dosage ranges from 30 to 240 mg a day.

The combination of a diazepine derivative with propranolol sometimes has advantages, combatting both the peripheral and central components of anxiety.

Propranolol in very high dosage has been advocated in the treatment of schizophrenia, usually in combination with neuroleptics. Doses of up to 3 g a day have been used. This produces bradycardia, and sometimes severe hypotension and headache, but only rarely improves psychotic symptoms.

Chlormethiazole. A derivative of the thiazole part of thiamin, chlormethiazole is useful both as an anxiolytic and as a hypnotic, especially in elderly patients, in whom it rarely causes hypotension. But its main value is in the treatment of withdrawal states, particularly from alcohol. It is a safe drug, but can cause dependence, and should not generally be given for more than a few weeks.

Up to 16 g of chlormethiazole a day may be needed in the treatment of delirium tremens. It can be given in the form of tablets, syrup, or by infusion. The drug's effects are potentiated by other tranquillisers and neuroleptics. Side effects are few. The most common are sneezing, and nasal and conjunctival irritation.

Antidepressant drugs

Until 1959, amphetamine and related compounds were the only drugs available for treating depression. But they are general euphoriants, without specific antidepressant properties. They have virtually no role today in the treatment of depressive illness; although there is still a place for methylamphetamine abreaction in selected obsessional personality disorders.

The antidepressant drugs all exert their chemical effects by elevating mood, hence the term 'thymoleptic'. But in practice, 'thymoleptic' is restricted to antidepressant drugs that are not monoamine oxidase inhibitors (MAOI).

Tricyclic antidepressants (Dibenzazepines) (see p. 206). All contain a three-ringed nucleus structure (Fig. 27.3). Imipramine was the prototype, introduced 20 years ago. These drugs are thought to act by inhibiting the re-uptake of transmitter amines (see p. 73 and p. 206), thus increasing the availability of the latter at receptor sites within the central nervous system, notably the catecholamines dopamine and noradrenaline, and the indolamine 5 hydroxytryptamine (5HT). There is evidence that some tricyclics preferentially block the re-uptake of 5HT – clomipramine is most potent in this respect – others of noradrenaline. Maprotiline, a tetracyclic, mainly blocks the re-uptake of noradrenaline. Imipramine and amitriptyline have some ability to block both amines. It may be that, in future, treatment of depression will be helped by identifying the biochemical abnormality behind the disorder; at present this is not possible.

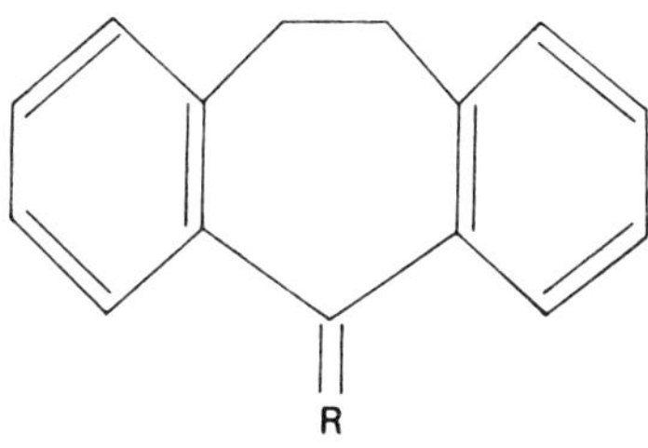

Fig. 27.3 Tricyclic antidepressant structure

The tricyclic antidepressants are broken down in the liver by microsomal enzymes. The breakdown products are numerous, and some of them themselves have antidepressant effects: desimipramine, derived from imipramine, nortriptyline from amitriptyline.

The half-life of all the tricyclic antidepressants is long, 24 hours or more, and this is liable to increase with increasing age of the patient. One dosage a day is sufficient to maintain an adequate steady plasma concentration for 24 hours. The dose is often given at night, which has the additional advantage of helping to lessen sleep disorders. Vivid and sometimes unpleasant dreams upset about 30 per cent of patients. Tricyclic antidepressants are rapidly absorbed and pass into the tissues.

Clinical effects. Depression is protean, and depressive illness probably encompasses a number of different psychological and biochemical conditions. Many depressed and anxious patients respond to tricyclic antidepressants, but particularly those with clinical features of 'endogenous' depression; early morning waking, loss of appetite and weight, marked anergia, lack of libido, feelings of self-blame and guilt, and varying degrees of retardation and agitation.

Apart from their mood lifting effect, some tricyclic antidepressants also sedate, a few markedly so. Where anxiety and agitation are prominent, a sedating antidepressant is obviously preferable. One of the more stimulating tricyclics is indicated when retardation and apathy are prominent.

When depression and agitation are severe, when weight loss is considerable, antidepressant drugs alone are often ineffective, or at least very slow in bringing about improvement. ECT should then be considered. It should never be withheld when there is a risk of suicide.

The antidepressant effects of these drugs become manifest only after several days, usually between 5 and 14, although unwanted side effects occur almost at once. These are often the cause of drug defaulting. Full improvement takes three to four weeks, sometimes up to eight weeks. If there is little or no improvement within approximately three weeks, given an adequate dosage, there is little point in continuing that particular drug.

Antidepressant drugs do not cure, they suppress depressive symptoms. They must be continued until there is spontaneous remission. Most depressions remit sooner or later, within 6 to 18 months, but chronic depressive states occur, mainly in older patients. In such cases, or when depression continues because of adverse, unchangeable circumstances, an effective antidepressant drug may have to be continued for years. Similarly, when there is likelihood of relapse, whether from external or internal causes, continuous medication lessens this risk.

Side effects. Side effects develop rapidly and are mostly dose related. They stem largely from anticholinergic and adrenergic blocking properties which all these drugs possess in variable degrees. Common ones are drowsiness, dry mouth, constipation, difficulty in micturition, impotence, sweating, tremor, blurred vision, tachycardia, and postural hypotension. Weight gain can be excessive and is often difficult to reduce until the drug is stopped. Dysarthria and paralytic ileus are occasional complications.

Central effects include restlessness and agitation, confusion, sleep disturbance, inability to concentrate, overactivity, and psychotic and psychopathic behaviour. Epileptic fits can occur, particularly in known epileptics. Parkinsonism is a rare complication.

Neurodermatitis and, occasionally, urticaria can be troublesome. Agranulocytosis and cholestatic jaundice are rare occurrences, the result of idiosyncrasy, requiring the drug to be stopped.

In usual therapeutic doses, tricyclics may cause ECG changes; flattened T waves, prolonged QT intervals, and depressed ST segments. Because of their anticholinergic actions and the increased levels of circulating catecholamines, all the tricyclics are probably capable of interfering with intracardiac conduction, especially in overdosage or when the heart is already diseased and, occasionally, of causing cardiac arrest and death. Trimipramine and tricyclic based compounds such as doxepin are comparatively safe.

Dosage. The usual effective antidepressant dosage of most of the tricyclics is 150 mg a day. Exceptions are nortriptyline, 100 mg, and protriptyline 40 mg. Their half-life is long enough for them to be given in one dose, except for protriptyline, preferably at bedtime, when any drowsiness caused by the drug is an advantage. However, the more stimulating tricyclics may cause insomnia. There are large individual differences in dose tolerance and efficacy. Some patients respond to a small dose, say 30 mg a day, others require 300 mg or more. Patients treated with the same dosage often show a wide range of blood levels of the drug.

Anything from 10 to 30 times or more the therapeutic dose is liable to be lethal. Overdosage results in delirium, convulsions, hyperpyrexia, hyperreflexia, bowel and bladder paralysis, mydriasis. Tachycardia and arrhythmias can progress to cardiac arrest and death. Coma rarely lasts longer than 24 hours. The most important aspect of treatment is management of cardiac function, and ideally the patient should be admitted as soon as possible to an intensive care unit. Cardiac irregularities can develop several days after the patient has regained consciousness.

Children tolerate tricyclic antidepressants well in small doses. Their main use here, particularly imipramine, is in the treatment of nocturnal enuresis.

Old people are very sensitive to tricyclics and metabolise them slowly. They readily develop toxic confusional states, with vivid visual hallucinations, postural hypotension and urinary retention. The dosage should therefore be very small initially.

Combinations of tricyclics with other drugs and treatments

Electroconvulsive treatment can be safely given with these drugs, which probably reduces the number of treatments required.

Lithium

Only a small proportion of manic depressive attacks are entirely suppressed by lithium. In the majority of patients episodes of depression are reduced in frequency, duration and intensity. If such a modified depression does occur, an antidepressant drug can be usefully combined with lithium and continued until depression lifts. There is some evidence that lithium potentiates the antidepressant drug's effects. Tremor is a common side effect, which is abolished by propranolol. Toxic effects include severe nausea and vomiting and diarrhoea.

Monoamine oxidase inhibitors (MAOI)

The combination of a MAOI with a tricyclic antidepressant can be highly effective in depressed patients unresponsive to other treatments. Those tricyclics that have least effect on the re-uptake of 5HT are safest to use. Trimipramine and tranylcypromine are seemingly the safest and most effective combination. Side effects, particularly postural hypotension, are increased, but there is little risk of a hypertensive crisis provided the patient obeys dietary instructions.

Under no circumstances should tricyclics be given parenterally to a patient on, or within 14 days of stopping, a MAOI. A severe hypertensive crisis, and cerebral overstimulation leading to coma and death, are likely consequences (see p. 361).

Neuroleptics. Antidepressant drugs may be required during treatment of a depressed schizophrenic patient. The antidepressant drug is given in the same dosage as for any other depression. Neuroleptics and tricyclics may also be given together in the treatment of agitated depression, or when depressive paranoid delusions are prominent. Neuroleptic drugs enhance the activity of tricyclic antidepressants.

Anxiolytics, sedatives and hypnotics. Benzodiazepine derivatives are often given with a tricyclic antidepressant to combat anxiety and insomnia. They have no effect on the antidepressant's rate of metabolism and activity. Barbiturates, on the other hand, increase the breakdown of tricyclics and diminish their activity. Similar effects occur with glutethimide.

Contra-indications to tricyclic antidepressants. (a) Confusional states. (b) Recent myocardial damage, particularly if it involves the conduction system. Cardiac failure. Caution is required with glaucoma, liver failure, prostatic enlargement, old age.

Tetracyclic compounds

Maprotiline is structurally like the tricyclics, with a stabilising bond in the middle. It resembles the tricyclics in its metabolism, activity and side effects. Biochemically it specifically blocks the re-uptake of noradrenaline. It has a long half-life, and can be given in one single dose at bedtime. It seems to be an effective antidepressant, particularly in reactive forms of depression, when depression is not too severe and tension is more prominent.

Side effects increase with dosage. Anticholinergic effects are less, dose for dose, than with the tricyclics. Skin rashes occur in about 10 per cent of patients, fits in 1 per cent. Cardiotoxicity is similar to the tricyclics.

Maprotiline overdosage resembles that with tricyclics.

The dosage is 25 to 150 mg a day.

Mianserin, although a tetracyclic compound, has different biochemical activities, and does not affect 5HT and noradrenaline re-uptake. It may act on the presynaptic receptors, which control the release of monoamines at the synapses.

Mianserin has a short half-life and needs to be given at least twice, and possibly three times a day. It has little anticholinergic activity, does not affect the heart or cause fits. *Side effects* are few, mainly drowsiness.

The dosage is 30 to 90 mg a day in three divided doses. A large dose at night improves sleep.

Viloxazine is an oxazine derivative, which does not inhibit monoamine oxidase. It mainly blocks the re-uptake of noradrenaline. Its half-life is short and the drug needs to be taken three times a day. It has an antidepressant and sometimes almost an amphetamine-like effect, which develops within a day or two. Agitation is sometimes increased. Nausea, vomiting and headache are the commonest side effects, and are dose related.

The dose ranges from 150 to 300 mg a day in three divided doses.

Nomifensine is a tetrahydroisoquinoline. It blocks the re-uptake of both dopamine and noradrenaline. Anticholinergic and cardiotoxic effects are small. It has a half-life of four hours. The dosage is 75 to 300 mg a day. It has an alerting, sometimes stimulating effect, so much so that it may increase agitation unless a tranquilliser is added. Limited clinical experience suggests that it is best with reactive depressions.

L-tryptophan. Tryptophan is a precursor of 5HT. It is claimed to have antidepressant properties and to enhance the activity of tricyclic antidepressants. Side effects are few: headache, nausea, anorexia and drowsiness. The dose of L-tryptophan is up to 6 g a day.

Monoamine oxidase inhibitors (MAOI)

Iproniazid, a hydrazine derivative of isonicotinic acid, was first used in the treatment of tuberculosis. It did not succeed in that role, but was found to have remarkable antidepressant effects. It was introduced into psychiatry in 1957.

Iproniazid strongly inhibits monoamine oxidase, which is concerned in the breakdown of monoamines. Iproniazid has toxic effects, particularly on the liver. However, the risk of jaundice is probably small.

A number of analogous compounds have been introduced, all having the ability to inhibit MAO. These are the hydrazine derivatives, phenelzine, isocarboxazid and carbomazepine. The only nonhydrazine MAOI that is an effective antidepressant is tranylcypromine.

The MAOI are readily absorbed and metabolised in the liver. Their half-life is short, and two to three doses a day are usually required. Therapeutic effects take between four and ten days to appear, with the exception of tranylcypromine which sometimes increases alertness and energy, and lifts depression, within 48 hours.

The MAOI have a narrower range of use than the tricyclics. Indeed some people say that they should not be called antidepressants, but are essentially anxiolytics. They are most useful in reactive or neurotic depression, especially when the phobic anxiety is prominent. They are also good in those persistent neurotic depressive states that follow childbirth; when a previously capable woman can no longer cope with her family and complains of constant exhaustion, irritability and loss of zest. Such patients tend to sleep heavily day and night, invariably waking tired and unrefreshed. Many phobic anxiety patients, particularly those with previously capable personalities, respond well to phenelzine in doses of up to 90 mg a day, losing their symptoms as they regain confidence over a period of four to eight weeks. However, the drug has to be maintained, sometimes indefinitely, in order to prevent relapse.

The MAOI are less useful in endogenous depression, particularly severe depression, with the possible exception of iproniazid and tranylcypromine. Tranylcypromine has both MAOI and tricyclic-like properties, and some amphetamine-like effects. Depressed patients who have failed to respond to tricyclic antidepressants may improve with a MAOI, particularly tranylcypromine. Phenelzine and isocarboxazid are not usually effective in endogenous forms of depression.

While therapeutic effects take four to ten days to appear, side effects appear almost at once. They can be troublesome, particularly hypotension, genito-urinary difficulties, constipation, blurred vision, dry mouth, drowsiness, headaches, insomnia.

A hypertensive crisis, due to release of free catecholamines from binding sites, can develop with all MAOIs, but particularly tranylcypromine. Death can result from a hypertensive crisis, usually from rupture of an aneurysm on one of the cerebral vessels. Treatment is with 5 mg phentolamine IV if this is at hand; otherwise it is best to treat the patient conservatively, lying down and sedated. The severe headache usually lifts within an hour, although an unpleasant headache may persist for some days afterwards.

A hypertensive crisis may occur when foods containing tyramine or other pressor amines are eaten. These are normally broken down by MAO in the gut wall and liver, but because MAO is inhibited, they now pass directly into the circulation. Foods to avoid include cheese, yoghurt, yeast and meat extracts, pickled herring, paté, game, chianti wine, broad bean pods and banana skins. Dangerous reactions sometimes develop when drugs with sympathomimetic properties are taken concurrently. These include amphetamines, ephedrine, phenylephrine, phenylpropanolamine, methyldopa, L-dopa, clonidine. Narcotic analgesics like pethidine, morphine, cocaine and procaine may interact dangerously. Most anaesthetists, before cold surgery, require a MAOI to be stopped for a fortnight or so beforehand, in case measures to restore blood pressure are required at operation.

Some tricyclics, particularly those which block re-uptake of 5HT, can cause dangerous central stimulation. And no tricyclic should be given parenterally until at least 14 days have elapsed after stopping a MAOI. However, the combination of one of the sedating tricyclics, usually trimipramine, with a MAOI, usually tranylcypromine, can be highly effective in depression refractory to all other treatments, and is safe provided the patient obeys instructions.

The actions of barbiturates and alcohol are potentiated, and the effects of insulin and hypoglycaemic agents are increased by MAOIs.

The daily dose of phenelzine ranges from 30 to 90 mg, the usual being 45 mg a day. The daily dose of tranylcypromine is usually between 20 and 40 mg.

Contra-indications to MAOIs

1. Severe cirrhosis or liver failure.
2. Concurrently with certain drugs (see above).
3. A past history of subarachnoid haemorrhage.
4. Prostatic enlargement sufficient to cause retention.

Lithium

Lithium is widely used to treat mania and to prevent recurrent affective disorders. The drug's prophylactic value in manic depression, or bipolar affective disorders, is now firmly established. Lithium can sometimes abolish attacks completely. More commonly, the frequency of attacks is lessened, and the severity of symptoms and their duration diminished. Studies have shown that about 30 per cent of manic depressives on lithium relapse over a two-year period, compared to 90 per cent on placebo. A small proportion of patients are not helped. There is no sure way of knowing in advance whether a patient will or will not respond to lithium; only 'rapid cycling' – four or more episodes a year – is definitely associated with a poor response.

Recurrent depression, or unipolar affective disorders, also respond to lithium, although probably not so well as manic depression. There is disagreement about the actual antidepresant activity of lithium. But most clinicians agree that a depressed patient is better treated with antidepressant drugs or even ECT than with lithium alone. However, many clinicians combine lithium with an antidepressant when treating recurrent depression. There is evidence that this combination is more effective than either drug alone.

Long-term lithium should not be prescribed without good reason. Three episodes of manic depression within two years, or an attack of depression every year for three years, unresponsive to maintenance treatment with antidepressants, are good reasons for considering giving lithium. Once begun, lithium may have to be given indefinitely. Mild swings of depression and hypomania often occur during maintenance treatment, and call for a temporary increase of lithium and/or addition of haloperidol or an antidepressant.

The dosage of lithium, in the form of lithium carbonate, ranges from 400 to 1600 mg a day, preferably at bedtime. The aim is to achieve a steady serum concentration of between 0.6 and 1.2 mmol/litre. Careful observation and monitoring of the serum lithium concentration are needed for the first few weeks, but these can be gradually extended to 6 monthly intervals, provided the patient and, just as important, her family, know the warning signs of toxicity, and can be relied upon to stop the drug and report at once.

Lithium is excreted unchanged through the kidneys, although there is considerable individual variation. Serious renal disease is usually an absolute contra-indication to lithium. Lithium can be given at any age. *Side effects* are dose related. Common are a fine tremor (which is sometimes severe and can be controlled by propranolol), sleepiness, tiredness, nausea, indigestion and diarrhoea. Many patients feel thirsty, and a small number of patients develop nephrogenic diabetes insipidus – extreme thirst and polyuria. Oedema is sometimes troublesome, usually of the face or legs. Thiazide diuretics control nephrogenic diabetes insipidus and oedema, although great care is needed with this combination, otherwise toxicity will result. Increase of weight is common, and is sometimes the reason for a patient stopping the drug. Acne and maculopapular cutaneous eruptions can occur, and psoriasis be made worse.

A benign diffuse goitre occurs in a substantial proportion of patients. Hypothyroidism develops in about 5 per cent of patients, particularly females on long-term lithium. It may well be that lithium must be continued, combined if necessary with thyroxine. It has been suggested that thyroid function should be evaluated before starting treatment, and repeated each year.

Changes in the ECG are not uncommon, and bundle branch block can occur. Patients with pre-existent arrhythmias should be watched carefully. Rarely, a confusional state develops in the first two or three weeks of treatment, which rapidly clears up when lithium is withdrawn.

Signs of toxicity develop when the serum lithium concentration exceeds 2 mmol/litre, but some patients occasionally develop toxic signs at lower levels. The onset of severe tremor, twitching, nausea, vomiting, anorexia and diarrhoea, slurred speech, unsteadiness and some degree of disorientation are indications for immediately stopping the drug. Increasing toxicity results in oligorenal failure, confusion, fits, coma and eventually death. Toxicity is liable to develop in a patient previously stabilised on lithium if (a) there is cardiac failure, (b) the sodium balance is upset by a low salt diet or a diuretic, (c) there is a rise of lithium levels, which sometimes occurs when a patient switches rapidly from mania into depression, and (d) suicide is attempted by overdose.

There is doubt about the safety of lithium in pregnancy and in general it is best to stop the drug during this time.

Miscellaneous drugs

Disulfiram and citrated calcium carbimide acts as deterrents to the alcoholic. Disulfiram is longer lasting than citrated calcium carbimide, and only one dose a day is required. Reaction to alcohol is more violent. Symptoms come on rapidly within ten minutes or so, and include vasodilation, palpitations, headache, tachycardia, breathlessness and nausea and vomiting. If much alcohol is drunk the blood pressure drops, cardiac arrhythmias may develop and the patient collapses and may even die. It is therefore essential to warn the patient of the consequences of drinking with these drugs, and indeed they only work through fear (see p. 166). *Side effects* are largely dose related. These include fatigue, nausea, halitosis, constipation, and reduction of libido. Peripheral neuritis, cardiotoxicity and, rarely, psychotic reactions can occur.

Contra-indications to both drugs are cardiac failure, coronary artery disease, psychotic conditions and pregnancy.

The dose of disulfiram ranges from 200 to 600 mg a day, in one dose. The dose of citrated calcium carbimide is 50 to 100 mg twice a day.

Drugs for dementia

Claims have been made for several so-called 'cerebral vasodilators' or 'cerebral activators' in arresting intellectual decline and improving the behaviour of patients who are developing dementia. These drugs include cyclandelate, dihydroergoamine mesylate, meclofenoxate, cosaldon and naftidrofuryl. Trials of these drugs have given variable results. Mood and behaviour often improve, perhaps as a result of increased attention, but memory and intellectual functioning are not greatly changed. It seems doubtful that they can arrest intellectual decline.

Drugs for sexual problems

No drug acts as a specific aphrodisiac, nor will any drug specifically alter sexual object choice. But drugs are now used to reduce or remove male libido. Drugs used for this include stilboestrol, benperidol, and cyproterone acetate. Stilboestrol has the disadvantage of producing gynaecomastia. Benperidol may cause drowsiness and extrapyramidal side effects. Cyproterone acetate can also cause gynaecomastia, and irreversible atrophy of the testicles (see Medico-legal chapter, p. 388).

Electroconvulsive Therapy (ECT)

In 1933 von Meduna revived an old treatment and induced fits in his patients by injecting camphor. Camphor was replaced by cardiazol and pictrotoxin, and in 1937 therapeutic fits were produced by passing an electric current across two electrodes placed on the head. Its effectiveness in relieving depression became immediately apparent, and it has remained standard treatment for psychotic depressive illness; at times it can be lifesaving. It is important that the patient's psychiatrist discusses with him his reasons for prescribing ECT, the therapeutic effects, how long these may take, the possible side effects and risks, and the actual procedure. Nurses and other staff must also understand why the patient is to have ECT, so that they can answer questions and reassure the patient and his relatives.

In the vast majority of cases patients accept the need for ECT and agree to the treatment. The consent form is signed, as before any operation. But sometimes the patient may be unwilling, or too disturbed to come to a reasonable decision. Often other methods of treatment are able to bring about recovery, although they take longer to do so than ECT. But if the psychiatrist considers ECT to be a lifesaving or urgent necessity he cannot delay; he must arrange for his patient to be sectioned, if not already so, and he should seek written agreement from the nearest relative. He must obtain another consultant opinion.

Patients having ECT are anaesthetised and given a muscle relaxant by a trained anaesthetist. The responsibility for seeing whether a patient is physically fit for ECT is the psychiatrist's, and he must weigh the possible risks of ECT against the probable benefits of treatment. Chest X-ray, ECG and other tests may be required, and advice obtained from a physician if doubt exists.

There are several contra-indications to ECT. The more important are cardiac failure, a recent myocardial infarct or cerebrovascular accident, and severe pulmonary disease. Old age itself is no contra-indication.

ECT should be administered, ideally, in one particular room;

and adjoining it should be a comfortable waiting rom, preferably fitted with TV or radio. The ECT room should have two doors, one from the waiting room, and a separate door into a recovery room, so that waiting patients do not see the treated patient. In the ECT room are the anaesthetist and psychiatrist, and the nursing staff. Nursing staff ideally should consist of a staff nurse experienced in ECT and two junior nurses.

The patient is reassured as he enters the ECT room, and the anaesthetist checks that the patient has had nothing to eat or drink for the previous five hours. A very anxious patient can be calmed with a tranquilliser given one to two hours before treatment. Dentures are taken out and (usually) shoes taken off.

The dangers of ECT are few, and mainly cardiac, but emergency equipment should be present in the ECT room, including a sucker, reserves of oxygen, telephone and a defibrillator, where possible.

Anaesthetic induction

Atropine is given first, usually intravenously. This not only dries up secretions but lessens the risk of arrhythmias and of vagal overstimulation.

Thiopentone is often preferred to methohexitone because of its longer action, allowing the patient to sleep longer and therefore be more relaxed on waking. Patients should be allowed to waken naturally, rather than be roused by a nurse, if space permits.

A muscle relaxant such as *succinylcholine* is given immediately after the anaesthetic. The dosage varies, depending on a patient's size and medical condition. It is important that the dosage is not so large that the physical convulsion is totally abolished. All the evidence is that the efficacy of ECT is dependent upon the seizure; a subconvulsion or non-generalised seizure is not only therapeutically less effective, but may be positively harmful. It is vital to *see* that a bilateral convulsion always occurs. Rarely a patient is deficient in plasma pseudocholinesterase, the enzyme concerned with metabolising succinylcholine. The paralying effect of succinylcholine is then prolonged, so that return of natural respiration is delayed, sometimes for several hours.

The patient is now oxygenated; this procedure lessens the chance of memory disturbances after ECT. A mouth gag is inserted.

Type of ECT given. There is convincing evidence that unilateral ECT, given to the *nondominant hemisphere,* produces less memory disturbance than bilateral ECT, or unilateral ECT given to the dominant hemisphere. When depression is not severe, and when laterality is not in doubt, it is preferable to use unilateral ECT. But many psychiatrists feel that for *severe* depression, bilateral ECT is preferable, that it acts more rapidly, and fewer treatments are therefore required.

The therapeutic effect of ECT is dependent upon producing a generalised fit. The amount of current needed is as small as possible; just enough to cause a fit. Memory disturbance following ECT is directly related to the amount of current given.

There are various machines for giving ECT. One with a choice of waveforms, and automatic timing, is preferable since this allows the current to be kept at the minimum needed to produce a convulsion. Should a convulsion not occur the procedure should be repeated, up to three times, until the patient fits. A subconvulsion is liable to leave a patient anxious, and with headache and other side effects.

The standard practice for bilateral ECT is to position electrodes over the fronto-temporal areas. For unilateral ECT the electrodes are placed over the mastoid and frontal regions of the non-dominant hemisphere side. After the fit the patient is oxygenated, with an airway in situ, and remains in the ECT room under the care of the anaesthetist until respiration returns and he recovers consciousness. He needs close nursing observation, for this is the risk time when patients can choke, stop breathing or arrest. He is then moved to the recovery room.

A nurse should be in attendance in the recovery room. Reassurance and explanation as the patient recovers help to minimise anxiety. Although each patient has treatment alone he may recover in the company of others due to lack of space. Once he has woken completely and is orientated, he is helped from the recovery room to a comfortable chair in the ante room or, if an inpatient, back to his bed in the ward. He is given tea and sandwiches, and rests for an hour or so. An analgesic is helpful if he complains of headache.

There is no set number of treatments. Patients are seen by a psychiatrist before each treatment. The usual number of treatments is around six, but in refractory cases it may be necessary to give twelve or more over a period of several weeks. Daily or twice daily fits (although occasionally still used in otherwise uncontrollable mania) do not increase the rate of recovery from depression. Most psychiatrists give ECT twice a week. Spacing ECT closer than 48 hour intervals probably increases memory disturbance, with little or no additional therapeutic gain.

There is no particular problem about giving outpatients ECT, provided the total circumstances of the patient are taken into consideration, including age, physical state, distance from hospital to home, and availability of a responsible person to take the patient home. The psychiatrist administering ECT is responsible for assessing these factors, and when the patient is fit to leave after treatment.

Behavioural psychotherapy

Behavioural psychotherapy utilises modern theories of learning to help people rid themselves of undesirable behaviour, and to replace this with one that is more satisfactory, not only to the individual but often to others. The term 'behaviourist' has unfortunate connotations. Behavioural psychotherapy does not simply concern itself with behaviour. It also embraces cognitions, emotions and, perhaps less successfully, volition. Its concern is not only with people's activities but also with their experiences; with the washing rituals of an obessive/compulsive patient, the terror of the phobic individual, the depressive's gloomy evaluation of his existence and future, and his tendency to shun all satisfying activities.

Behavioural psychotherapy revolves around two apparently simple notions (see p. 11):

1. When two events occur together in time, they become linked in the mind. This is, of course, the basic principle of classical conditioning. The hungry dog salivates when offered food. If a buzzer goes off at the same time, sooner or later the dog salivates when he hears the buzzer alone.
2. Those activities which are pleasurable are more likely to be repeated than those which are not (operant conditioning).

Behavioural psychotherapy conjures up the spectre of a powerful technology capable of almost anything; in totalitarian institutions, of brain-washing. In reality, the successes of behavioural psychotherapy are modest. The initial reports of near 100 per cent success have given way to more realistic estimates of its therapeutic value.

Behavioural and interpretive psychotherapists have been equally contemptuous of each other's efforts in the past. Behaviourists have mocked the search for meaning of those who look for insight in psychotherapy. The belief that non-specific elements in the relationship between patient and therapist are more important than the belief system of interpretive psychotherapists. The latter, in their turn, see behavioural psychotherapists' pre-occupation with conscious experience and observable activity as blinkered. The combativeness of the two therapeutic approaches is passing and a rapproachment is under way. Therapists of both schools are seeking to understand, within their own conceptual frameworks, what the others are doing. They are trying to enhance the effectiveness of treatment by borrowing from each other's methods.

Behavioural analysis

The patient, unable to help himself despite encouragement and aid from friends and relations, comes for therapy, often with a sense of shame. The behaviour therapist's first task is to delineate in detail the size and shape of the problem presented. This has been called the *behavioural analysis*, with feelings and cognitions subsumed under that heading. The sequence of actions, emotions, and thoughts complained of by the patient, is elicited in detail, together with the changes wanted. A search is made for what precedes the sequence and what follows it, what originated it in the past, and what seems to be maintaining it in the present.

> A business man had been drinking heavily in the evenings for over seven years. He was in his early fifties, and further promotion in his organisation was unlikely. Younger and abler men were surpassing him. His son had dropped out of university, and openly criticised him. His wife was irritated and bored by him, and their sexual relationship had ended years ago, partly because of his drinking.
>
> His drinking was confined to the early evening, but was rapid and continued to drunkenness. Reasonable conversation was only possible with his wife and son in the early stages. Verbal violence developed later, usually during the evening meal. This was succeeded by a heavy sleep, often on the floor. The patient awoke in the early hours, remorseful, with no desire for alcohol. He went to bed, but remained wakeful and fretful until dawn, when sleep supervened; just before he had to face another day, an alienated family, and a competitive work situation with which he could now barely cope.

Any behavioural approach that disregarded the complex problems apparent above is not likely to succeed for long.

Therapy objectives

An important feature of behavioural psychotherapy is the defining of a specific aim of treatment agreed on by patient and therapist: the *therapeutic target.* This has the advantage of forcing patient and therapist, and outsiders, to assess progress and ultimately to see whether the target has been achieved or not. A patient with a dog phobia may set herself the objective of stroking a neighbour's terrier for 5 minutes. An obsessional may aim to reduce hand washing from 80 to less than 7 times a day, with no wash to last more than a minute. An exhibitionist may aim to masturbate in his room without his 'hunt–flash–masturbate–escape' sequence.

Baseline levels of the activities, emotions and cognitions that are involved in therapy are recorded, often graphically for visual impact. For example, the number of deviant urges, fantasies and actions may be charted by the fetishist alongside his more normal sexual activity. It is against this baseline – and recording it may have its own impact on behaviour – that the results of treatment are charted.

Motivation for change

The patient and therapist have understandably been evaluating each other during the behavioural analysis and objective-setting. The therapist's competence, trustworthiness, confidence in his methods, interest, perhaps even humanity, are scrutinised by the patient. The therapist, alongside his other tasks, has been trying to estimate the motivation and capacity for change of his patient and, where possible, to heighten it.

If the question, 'Why do you want to change?', is answered by 'To be more normal' the therapist has reason to be uneasy. The wish for more specific advantages to be derived from changes in the direction targeted carry greater hopes of success. Many therapists outline in unsparing detail the steps that therapy can take, and assess the patient's motivation from how he receives this.

Action change

Activity acquisition. When the problem is to help the patient behave in a *new* way, the therapist must be sure that the patient is *capable* of this. A patient may be highly anxious under certain social circumstances. His anxiety may interfere with his social behaviour and conceal the fact that this is reasonably sophisticated. By contrast, another man may be markedly deficient in this field. Deficiency in social skills may exist irrespective of social anxiety; for example, in the mentally handicapped or chronically institutionalised patient. Therapy may be either on an individual basis or in groups, but in both events it encourages the patients to develop those roles they habitually fear and shirk. Some patients find it difficult to assert themselves. They behave passively, and are liable to be bullied by other people; and occasionally they explode inappropriately.

The mentally impaired and schizophrenics, who lack basic social skills, are helped by rehearsing increasingly sophisticated social roles with the therapist, or in groups. Other members of a social skills group may contribute to this process, perhaps modelling for the patient appropriate ways of dealing with whatever situation is presented. Modelling, as well as feedback on the patient's own performance, is an important part of therapy, as is the therapist's approval of desirable activities in the patient. The whole procedure may be enriched by the use of video tape. The patient's behaviour can be reviewed and commented on, not least by the patient himself.

Role rehearsal can be supplemented by *role reversal.* A simple example is provided by the patient who is reluctant, through timidity, to return a pair of defective shoes to the shop and ask for his money back. He first of all rehearses several ways of approaching the shopkeeper; then he himself assumes the role of the shopkeeper. This gives the patient a wider view of the problem and allows him to modify his behaviour and develop self-confidence. Ultimately, play activity must be replaced by the real life task of actually returning a pair of shoes to the shop. Some social skills groups have actually bought goods in order to return them to the shop, to enable patients to acquire the self-confidence that, up until now, has eluded them.

Activity increase. When a patient performs some necessary action only very infrequently – and reluctantly – an increase of this activity may become the objective of therapy. In marital therapy, for example, conducted on behavioural lines, the couple may describe activities that they wish to encourage in each other. The wife wants to talk longer about the events of her husband's day when he arrives home in the evening. The husband expects a greater show of affection when he comes through the door. Each partner draws up a list of changes he and she would like to see in the other. Exchanges are then agreed upon, each item in the husband's list being matched by one in his wife's. Charts are kept of the frequency of such agreed activities. These are not discussed between sessions, but are examined with the therapist who, in his objective role, can constructively point out of the deficiencies of either or both.

Sometimes the increase in desirable behaviour also requires changes in its nature. This may be helped by the use of what is known as *shaping*. The final target is approached by a series of ever-nearer approximations, each stage being rewarded and therefore reinforced when attained. A self-charted record of the patient's progress, combined with his therapist's approval or otherwise, may be sufficient.

Token economy, which is based on shaping, has been extensively used to increase the range and desirability of the activities of many patients; for example, in the rehabilitation of chronic schizophrenics. Treatment objectives are set for individual patients, designed to start 'from where the patient is at'. When unwanted activities are reduced and replaced by more suitable behaviour, tokens are given. They are exchanged in the ward shop for cigarettes, sweets, beverages and items of clothing.

Alongside reward and punishment, *aversion relief* therapy has a useful part to play. When an unpleasant stimulus stops, the patient feels pleasurable relief. The unpleasant stimulus can be terminated by a patient himself, under the right circumstances. For instance, a paedophile is sexually aroused by the picture of a child. He receives continuous, aversive electrical stimulation, via his forearm, during the showing of the photograph. This can be ended at any time by his substituting the slide of a reasonably attractive (for him) adult for that of the child, with immediate relief from discomfort.

Activity decrease. Habit disorders may involve any one or more of a number of undesirable activities: smoking, drinking, overeating, hair pulling and nose picking are examples. Only by understanding the situations and factors that contribute to such behaviour can the patient and therapist construct a realistic therapeutic plan of action.

Consider, for instance, a patient with alcoholism. The amount drunk, and when, is delineated. Given reasonable motivation it is sometimes possible to reduce significantly the amount drunk by altering the patient's drinking ritual; alcohol may be drunk in an unusual room, from a less attractive glass or container, and in a less pleasant form (absinthe say, instead of gin). The approval of his spouse, his workmates and his therapist when he stays clear of alcohol, or strictly controls his drinking, enhances the patient's morale and self-respect.

Biofeedback techniques, utilising blood levels of alcohol (from apparatus like the breathalyser), may be used in the training of chronic alcoholics who are unwilling to become completely teetotal. The knowledge that their blood alcohol has not risen above, say, 60 mg per cent during a sociable evening both encourages and trains them to keep their drinking within clearcut limits. Exceeding the agreed intake may carry a *response-cost* in the shape of some self-imposed deprivation. A donation of money to charity is sometimes used as penalty.

Where total abstinence is the objective, some form of conditioning may be tried. It is comparatively easy to associate an electrical stimulus in time with the smell or taste of a favourite alcoholic drink. It need not be particularly painful and can be self-administered. The objective is to couple an unpleasant sensation with the drink, and to develop an avoidance response. Apomorphine induces nausea and vomiting, and may be similarly paired with alcoholic drink. It requires the assistance of medical personnel for the injection and its timing is less precise than electrical stimulation but it is more effective. The induction of terrifying paralysis by intravenous scoline immediately after the patient has poured himself a drink and taken a sip is another, although rarely used, method.

Self-regulatory techniques include *covert sensitisation*. The patient imagines the shameful consequences of his undesirable actions; the alcoholic sees the dead victim of his drunken driving and the consequences; the paedophile conjures up pictures of prison and his family's shame.

Activity loss. In successfully treated cases a steady decrease in unwanted activities is succeeded by their total disappearance. A paedophile, for example, heterosexual or homosexual, well motivated, may come for treatment. After baseline charting, electrical shock aversion, using paedophilic images and photographs, may start the treatment. Alternatively, sexual arousal, initially induced by slides and pictures of children, may be coupled with showing pictures of sexually attractive adults of the preferred sex. The procedure of *fading* aims gradually to increase the arousing properties of adults and to decrease that of children. Any deficiency of social skills in the paedophile relating to dating or mating behaviour must be rectified. The effect of the patient's behaviour on his family and friends must be understood, and appropriate measures, where indicated, undertaken. When behavioural psychotherapy alone is not successful in such cases, reduction in sexual interest may be achieved by use of drugs; benperidol, or the antiandrogen, cyproterone.

Obsessive/compulsive rituals, which are often concerned with contamination and harm, have been reduced by *response-prevention*. In this form of therapy, the anxiety which is aroused when the patient is unable to complete his senseless ritual is prolonged, so that ultimately it is reduced and extinguished. The drive to perform the compulsive behaviour is thereby lessened.

Cognition change

Increasingly, behavioural psychotherapy looks for help from the patient's imagery, thoughts and beliefs. Observable behaviour is properly seen as only part of human activity and experience.

Take a model represented by ABC. C is the unwanted activity or emotional state the patient wishes to discard. A represents the circumstance or event which produces this feeling state or activity. B is the irrational linking belief which therapy aims to change. For example, if A is a forthcoming examination, and C is the anxiety associated with it, the belief, B, may include a considerable underestimation by the patient of his preparedness for the examination, and of his intellectual abilities. He may have unrealistic ideas of the attitudes of the examiners, and of the standards expected of candidates. The aim of therapy is to counter such distorted beliefs; in effect, to change the language he uses as faces the problem.

Meichenbaum has extensively explored inner language (cognitive therapy), attempting to get patients to think positively, to substitute a coping language in their own words for the non-coping, defeatist language they use to describe various fear-inducing situations. The latter are delineated, as usual, in the behavioural analysis. The patient then learns to express his thoughts, both to himself and others, in more realistic terms. He makes less awesome predictions about the outcome, focuses on his strengths rather than assumed weaknesses, and reminds himself of past successes. He substitutes a 'but language' (I feel panicky *but* I will cope) for an 'and language' (I feel panicky *and* I will pass out).

Emotion Change

The management of emotions by changing inner language has also been applied to the self control of anger and depression. A coping, managing language is fashioned, away from the anger producing circumstances, but for use later within them. Repeated, carping criticism, from a colleague at work, for instance, can be coolly disregarded with the prepared, but obviously credible thought that, 'His fault-finding is necessary to bolster his low self-confidence; he's an inadequate man.'

The repetitive self-denigrations of the depressive need to be supplanted by increasingly confident and positive thinking. This can be encouraged by linking positive thinking to common everyday activities, such as drinking, smoking or eating. The patient must repeat to himself that he is capable, likeable, has good prospects for the future, and so on, whenever he starts and finishes a cigarette, a drink or a meal.

The treatment of phobic anxiety invariably requires some form of exposure to the phobic stimulus. This may be imagined, or occur in real life circumstances. Either exposure may be made in a graded fashion, moving from the least to the most terrifying aspects of the situation or object which is feared, or it may happen rapidly by immediate confrontation with the most terrifying elements in the hierarchy.

Imaginal desensitisation, with or without a relaxation procedure, involves imagining items in a hierarchy, starting with the less terrifying; when an item can be thought of without anxiety, the patient moves to the next one. This 'within-the-head' exposure therapy allows the patient to habituate to the induced anxiety, and thus learn to adapt better. He is able to develop his own, more realistic language.

The *graded exposure in vivo* of the phobic patient starts with real life encounters which he can barely tolerate. He gradually habituates to the anxiety, and proves to himself that his fearful predictions are only shadows. As fear steadily decreases he climbs the hierarchical tree, until eventually he can face the situation which previously most terrified him. The agoraphobic who has managed to walk from his home to the bus stop, with consequently decreasing anxiety, may now find it comparatively easy to catch a bus and stay on it, until he no longer feels in the least anxious. Travel by underground train may now become possible.

Intravenous methohexitone sodium, a rapidly acting, short-lived barbiturate, may help a patient face a dreaded situation. As its effect wears off, and the patient stays in the phobic situation, the opportunity occurs to habituate on exposure. Diazepam, but only if blood levels of the drug are waning, also enhances the effect of exposure. The last dose should be taken no closer than 3 hours before the exposure exercise.

The imaginary confrontation of the most terrifying items in the phobic patient's hierarchy is called *implosion*. Sometimes the therapist provides a fear-inducing narrative, but in general it is better to let the patient provide one for himself, for this is bound to be more realistic and terrifying to him. He describes his story in the present tense, and the therapist prompts and keeps him to the task, and does not allow him to deviate from his fearful path. The narrative is prolonged until the patient becomes habituated to his anxiety. This exposure has then of course to be tested, as does any imaginal method, in real circumstances.

Flooding in vivo is the real life confrontation by a patient of what he most fears. It is only for the most determined of patients.

It is often better to start treatment of a seriously phobic patient with phenelzine and a tranquilliser, provided the patient's personality is a reasonable one and there are no psychopathic features, or other contra-indications. These drugs have the effect of gradually reducing anxiety, improving the patient's morale and self-confidence, and allowing him perhaps to assert himself more at home, even venturing a few steps further afield than usual.

At the same time, a psychotherapeutic approach aims to encourage the patient to examine the deeper nature of his fears, to explore his relationship with his spouse and family, and discuss his desire and potential for development. The spouse, or parent may also be seen, alone or with the patient, and their capacity for change and adaptation assessed and utilised. At this point, some form of exposure therapy may be valuable.

The MAOI and tranquillisers controlling anxiety and accompanying autonomic symptoms need to be continued during the period of desensitisation, and for a variable time subsequently. When an agoraphobic patient has been virtually housebound for many years, he has numerous habits to break before he can be considered to be fully recovered and able to lead a full life. In some cases, when say, neither patient nor spouse are prepared to adapt realistically to changed circumstances, drug therapy may need to be continued for years, perhaps indefinitely. Many others need a tranquilliser from time to time to cope with periodic upsurges of anxiety, which may cause maladaptive patterns to reappear.

Biofeedback techniques

Biofeedback is the conversion of changes in physiological functions into perceptible signals. This information is then used by motivated patients to alter the physiological function in the direction desired.

A great deal of interest and apparatus has surrounded attempts to control heart rate and rhythm, blood pressure, electromyographic and electroencephalographic activity, and skin temperature. Inflated claims have been made for the control of cardiac arrhythmias and epileptic fits, the alleviation of migraine, tension headaches, anxiety and insomnia. The induction of a so-called 'alpha state' comparable to that found in meditation, by training alpha rhythms on the EEG, has been claimed. Controlled trials have been few, though it must be said that sham feedback has, on the whole, been less helpful than true feedback in the conditions mentioned. Blood pressure has been reduced 'to a statistically but not clinically significant' level (by about 10 mmHg) in hypertensives. No doubt the present day intense research activity will eventually show just what place the modality has in therapy. At the time of writing, its contribution seems unlikely to be large.

Criticisms of behavioural psychotherapy

Three main themes can be seen in the criticisms levelled against behavioural psychotherapy. The first is that it is too powerful and inhuman a technology, its future development must be watched with care. The second is that it is too weak to be relevant to human difficulties, because it deals only with symptoms and not with causes; symptom-elimination will simply be followed by symptom-substitution. The third is that the results of behavioural psychotherapy are further proof of the gullibility and suggestibility of some human beings at the hands of others.

The power of behavioural psychotherapy has been over-estimated, not least by therapists themselves. Initial 'cure' rates above the 90 per cent mark have, in recent years, been replaced by more moderate claims of success in individuals who are 'sufficiently motivated' for change. The counter-controls a person can exert over his would-be therapist are great in any free situation. Even in the total-control situation of prison and prisoner-of-war camps, few adult brains were, and are, lastingly brainwashed.

Behavioural psychotherapists do not find it necessary to conceptualise the actions and experiences they try to change as 'symptoms' of some underlying conflict or illness. Change is rarely followed by new unwanted substitute behaviour. No new decontaminating or other ritual replaces hand-washing in the obsessional. Relapse, on the other hand, is not uncommon, and booster sessions to maintain earlier treatment gains are often needed.

Although symptom substitution is not a serious problem, it needs to be said that the cure of a patient may create difficulties in those closely involved with him or her. For instance, hostility and jealousy may develop or increase in the husbands of agoraphobic wives, as the latter improve. They become insecure and alarmed as their wives become more independent. The therapist who is aware of this possibility will take steps to deal with this at an early stage of treatment.

The third criticism suggests that the non-specific aspects of the transactions between patient and therapist are more important than the therapeutic. The hope of the patient, the self-confidence of the therapist, his interest in his patient, the nature of the relationship they build, are, on this view, the essential elements of therapy. Most so-called controlled studies in behavioural psychotherapy fail to allow for the therapist's and patient's belief in the efficacy of the treatment. If, together, they achieve results they both appreciate, that would seem to be justification enough.

Non-physical treatments

Psychotherapy

This includes every form of therapeutic communication between doctor and patient. In this sense all doctors and nurses practise psychotherapy with their patients.

There are different forms or 'levels' of psychotherapy.

1. *Authoritative.* The therapist helps the patient to reorganise his life and to deal with his major problems. It is essential that the therapist thoroughly understands his patient's personality and circumstances.

2. *Abreactive.* This is akin to the confessional box, the psychiatrist taking the place of the priest. The patient pours out his troubles, releasing a good deal of emotion in the process.

These two forms of psychotherapy are usually combined in some degree, and are sometimes referred to as *supportive psychotherapy*. Supportive psychotherapy is simpler and less time consuming than interpretative psychotherapy. By encouragement, reassurance and support the patient is helped to face and overcome his problems. The therapist, be he doctor or nurse, must be careful to view the patient's problems objectively, and not to see the patient as himself. The effectiveness of such treatment is directly related to the patient's trust and belief in the omniscience of his therapist.

3. *Interpretative*. The patient's symptoms and behaviour are interpreted to him in terms of his personality, background and current needs, with the object of giving him insight into and bringing about a radical change in his attitude and behaviour.

4. *Psychoanalysis* also aims to give a patient understanding of his behaviour and feelings, but treatment is more intense and prolonged. The patient 'free associates', that is, he says whatever comes into his mind. He is seen by the therapist up to five times a week. *Transference* describes the projection by a patient of his feelings, needs and wishes on to the analyst. A strong transference, which alternates between 'positive' and 'negative', develops in the patient for the analyst. The material brought up and the transference situation are used by the analyst in his interpretations. It must be noted that the therapist may develop likes and dislikes, in turn, for his patient: counter-transference. Unless aware of these, his treatment may be affected, to the detriment of his patient.

Group psychotherapy. Individual psychotherapy is time consuming, and to overcome this problem groups of eight to ten patients are treated together. Techniques vary. The therapist may assume an authoritarian attitude to the group, lead the discussions and explain symptom formation and other problems. Or he may adopt a more passive role and encourage the members of the group to conduct their own discussions, only intervening to interpret at the appropriate moment.

A marital therapy group consists of four or five married couples, each with marital difficulties. The group may be a closed one, the same members meeting together for anything up to two or three years at regular, usually weekly, intervals. Some groups are 'open-ended', its members changing continually.

Family therapy

Family therapy has arisen out of the increasing importance attributed to the family in the formation of psychiatric disorders and maladaptive behaviour among its members, particularly the children. The whole family may be seen together regularly, husband and wife only, or with one or more children. Therapists vary enormously in their approach; some concentrate on the psychodynamics of the various individuals; others are interested mainly in the ways in which members of the family communicate with each other, manipulate one another, and psychologically protect themselves. More than one therapist may take part in the group meetings.

Transaction analysis was devised by Eric Berne, the author of *Games People Play*. The method focuses on interpersonal communications, and what is *really* being said and done. It is a method that is particularly useful in marital therapy.

Encounter groups developed out of methods for training psychiatrists, paramedical and other mental health workers in group therapy. Release of emotion is encouraged, physical contacts permitted, and disinhibited discussions of feelings generated by members of the group for one another may continue for hours, or even days. Its value remains uncertain.

Modified prefrontal leucotomy

Prefrontal leucotomy was introduced in 1935 by Moniz. The object of the operation is to interrupt connections between the frontal cortex and the limbic system (see Fig. 7.2, p. 74), and so reduce emotional tension. The operation was at first too extensive and resulted in severe personality changes and epilepsy. Present-day operations have been greatly modified. Stereotactic methods have improved the accuracy of the operation. In well-selected cases personality changes are minimal. Intelligence is generally unaltered, as judged by intelligence tests. Under Section 57 of the 1983 Mental Health Act the treatment can only be given if the patient consents and a second opinion agrees (see p. 388).

Indications

1. Chronic, intractable tension and anxiety states.
2. Severe, long-standing obsessional states.
3. Depressive states which are severe, chronic, associated with tension and refractory to treatment.

Symptoms should have lasted for *at least* five years, be disabling, and have failed to respond to any other treatment. Success or failure of the operation depends on being able to exclude all patients with inadequate or psychopathic personality traits. Aggressive and antisocial traits are liable to increase after operation.

Results

Successful operation relieves tension and depression. Obsessional thoughts are less compelling and may gradually fade from lack of reinforcement. There is usually some slight blunting of sensitivity, but whether it is noticeable depends upon the patient's background and way of life.

Patients usually stay in hospital for about a month after operation, so that post-operative inertia can be dealt with and old maladaptive patterns of behaviour broken. Improvement continues for six to twelve months after operation in good results.

28
Medico-Legal

Until the *Mental Treatment Act of 1930*, allowing for voluntary admission, patients requiring admission to mental hospitals had to be certified insane. By the 1950s, although most admissions were voluntary, the ancient laws were proving increasingly inadequate. Accordingly, in 1954 the Government set up a Royal Commission on 'the Law relating to Mental Illness and Mental Deficiency', which resulted in the 1959 *Mental Health Act*.

The Mental Health Act of 1959 broke the artificial legal barrier that separated psychiatry from the rest of medicine. A patient suffering from a mental illness now became entitled to receive the same facilities for treatment as any other type of patient, i.e. those with physical illness, and to enter any hospital without legal formality. It also introduced the concept of Community Care for the mentally ill.

The 1959 Act remained virtually unaltered until the *Mental Health (Amendment) Act*, 1982. The two were then incorporated into the *Mental Health Act*, 1983. The main changes are as follows:

Section 1. Definition of Mental Disorder. A patient cannot be admitted compulsorily to hospital, or guardianship contemplated, unless he or she is suffering from *mental disorder*. The Act defines this term as 'mental illness, arrested or incomplete development of mind, psychopathic disorder and any other disorder or disability of mind'. The latter can obviously cover a wide range of behaviour, but the Act specifically excludes promiscuity or other immoral behaviour, sexual deviancy, or dependence on alcohol or drugs.

Mental impairment has replaced the term *subnormality*. *Severe mental impairment* means a *state of arrested or incomplete development of mind* which includes severe impairment of intelligence and social functioning and *is associated with abnormally aggressive or seriously irresponsible conduct* on the part of the person concerned. *Mental impairment* means a *state of arrested or incomplete development of mind* which includes significant impairment of intelligence and social functioning and *is associated with abnormally aggressive or seriously irresponsible conduct* on the part of the person concerned. The term *mental handicap* remains a useful one, and includes most people suffering simply from arrested or incomplete development of mind, and are in no way dangerous or seriously irresponsible.

Psychopathic disorder means a persistent disorder or disability of mind (whether or not including significant impairment of intelligence) which results in abnormally aggressive or seriously irresponsible conduct on the part of the person concerned. This definition is similar to the one in the 1959 Act, but whereas it was only possible to detain such a person compulsorily if he or she was under 21, the age limit is abolished by the new Act. *But, as in the case of mental impairment, it must seem that treatment is likely to alleviate or prevent a deterioration of his condition.*

Admission to Hospital. The vast majority of hospital admissions today are informal. Any person over the age of 16 wishing to admit himself to hospital, and who is offered a bed, can do so. If he or she is a minor, under the age of 16, he needs the authority of his parents or guardian. The legal rights of an informal psychiatric patient are similar to those of non-psychiatric patients, including the common law right to refuse treatment. They are free to leave hospital any time they wish, unless holding powers or common law powers (see below) are employed.

Compulsory admission to hospital and guardianship.

Section 2 of the 1983 Act replaces Section 25 of the 1959 Act which covered admission for observation. This is changed to *Admission for Assessment*, or *Assessment followed by medical treatment*. The patient can be detained for 28 days. *Assessment, followed by medical treatment*, is a new clause, and clears away the ambiguity of the old Section 25, admitted for observation, when it was unclear whether active treatment was authorised.

The application for admission has to be made by the nearest relative or an approved social worker, and must be supported by two medical recommendations, one of whom must be approved by the Secretary of State for Social Services 'as having special experience in the diagnosis or treatment of mental disorder'. They must agree that (a) the patient is suffering from mental disorder of a nature or degree which warrants his detention in a hospital for assessment (or for assessment followed by medical treatment) for at least a limited period; and (b) he ought to be so detained in the interests of his own health or safety or with a view to the protection of others.

Such a patient has the right to apply to a *Mental Health Review Tribunal* within 14 days of admission. His nearest relative can discharge the patient at any time, subject to the responsible Medical Officer objecting.

Section 3 deals with *Admission for Treatment*, replacing Section 26. This order lasts for a maximum of 6 months, renewable for a further 6 months, and then for a year at a time. The application is made by the nearest relative or an approved social worker (who can only do so if the nearest relative does not object. If he does object, the only course open to the approved worker is to ask the County Court to displace the nearest relative), supported by two doctors, one of them 'approved', who must give the grounds for their opinion and why no other methods of dealing with the patient are appropriate.They must certify that (a) the patient is suffering from mental illness, severe mental impairment, psychopathic disorder or mental impairment and his mental disorder is of a nature or degree which makes it appropriate for him to receive medical treatment in a hospital; and (b) in the case of psychopathic disorder or mental impairment, such treatment is likely to alleviate or prevent deterioration of his condition; and (c) it is necessary for the health or safety of the patient or for the protection of other persons, that he should receive such treatment and it cannot be provided unless he is detained under the Section.

The patient can apply to a Mental Health Review Tribunal within the first 6 months, or one during each subsequent renewal period.

Section 4 replaced Section 29, *Admission for Assessment in Cases of Emergency*. The application is made by the nearest relative or approved social worker, supported by *one* doctor, preferably one who is already acquainted with the patient, such as his general practitioner. The patient must have been seen by the relative or approved social worker and the doctor within 24 hours of the recommendation being made. And the patient must be admitted within 24 hours of being medically examined or the application made, whichever is the earlier. The application must state that it is of *urgent necessity* to admit the patient, and that admission under Section 2 would entail undesirable delay. The order lasts 72 hours unless the hospital managers receive the second medical recommendation required under Section 2.

Emergencies on a Hospital Ward.
Detention of an informal patient in hospital.
Section 5 (2). The doctor in charge of the case – or his nominated deputy, in practice usually the duty doctor of the day – can detain any informal *inpatient* for 72 hours, including one receiving treatment for a physical illness in a general hospital, if he is

considered to be a danger to self or others. After 72 hours he is free to leave hospital unless Sections 2 or 3 have been utilised.

Section 5 (4). Nurse's holding powers.
A registered mental nurse, including registered nurses for mental handicap, can detain for 6 hours (2 hours in Scotland) a patient already receiving treatment for mental disorder in hospital until a doctor is found. The nurse must certify that (a) the patient is suffering from mental disorder of such a degree that it is necessary for his health or safety or for the protection of others, for him to be immediately restrained from leaving hospital and (b) that it is not practicable to secure the immediate attendance of a practitioner for the purpose of formulating a report under Section 5 (2). Once the doctor arrives the nurse's holding power lapses. If the doctor signs an application under Section 5 (2) the 6 hour period, or however long it was if shorter, counts as part of the 72 hours.

Common law powers of detention. It is possible to imagine an emergency occurring when neither a doctor nor a registered mental nurse is immediately available. Under common law, anyone of the ward staff is entitled to apprehend and restrain an individual who is mentally disordered and an immediate danger to himself or others, or would be if he left the hospital. Bodily force, mechanical restraints, or seclusion may be necessary. But obviously this must be the minimum necessary to end the emergency. Nurses should not give sedation to an unwilling patient unless it is *specifically* prescribed by a doctor. A nurse giving a *PRN* medication may later have difficulty in justifying his action, if challenged in a court of law.

Other Methods of Compulsory Admission.

Section 135. A police constable or other authorised persons may, on a Magistrate's Warrant applied for by an approved social worker, enter premises and remove a person believed to be suffering from mental disorder who has been (a) ill-treated or neglected or not kept under proper control or is (b) unable to care for himself and is living alone. The order lasts 72 hours.
Section 136. A police constable can remove a person from a public place to a place of safety if he appears to be suffering from mental disorder, and is in immediate need of care and control, and the constable considers he should be detained in his own interests or for the protection of others. He can be detained for 72 hours. He must

be examined by a doctor and interviewed by an approved social worker as soon as possible.

Mentally Abnormal Offenders.

Section 35 allows a Crown Court or Magistrates' Court to remand an accused person to a specified hospital for a report. The order lasts 28 days, renewable at 28 day intervals for up to 12 weeks.

Section 36 empowers the Crown Court to remand a person awaiting trial for an imprisonable offence, other than murder, to a hospital for treatment. The order lasts for 28 days, renewable up to 12 weeks.

Section 47. The Home Secretary may agree to a sentenced prisoner's transfer to a hospital for treatment.

Section 48 authorises transfer of other prisoners, including those on remand, in urgent need of treatment. It is limited to mental illness and *severe* mental impairment.

Restriction order (Section 41). A Crown Court can impose a Restriction Order on an offender transferred to hospital, after hearing *oral* evidence from one of the two doctors concerned with his sectioning. This is to protect the public from 'serious harm'. The order can be without time limit or for a specified period. The effect is to prevent the patient having leave of absence, being transferred or discharged without the consent of the Home Secretary.

Guardianship (Section 7. Application for Guardianship).

A patient aged 16 or more may be placed under the supervision of a guardian. The guardian has the power to:

1. require the patient to reside at a specified place.
2. require him to attend at specified places and times for medical treatment, occupation, education or training.
3. require access to the patient to be given, at the patient's residence, to any doctor, approved social worker, or other specified person.

The application is made by the nearest relative or approved social worker to the local social services authority, and is supported by two doctors, one being 'approved', who confirm that the patient has one of the forms of mental disorder. The order lasts 6 months, renewable for a further 6 months, and then at yearly intervals.

Mental Health Review Tribunals.

Tribunals were originally established by the 1959 Act. If a patient or his relative did not accept that he should be detained, he was able to apply to a Tribunal to examine his case. Under the 1983 Act, patients have increased opportunities to apply to a Tribunal, and are also entitled now to be legally represented. There are usually three members of the Tribunal, a lawyer who is president, a doctor, and a layman.

The function of the Tribunals is to hear the applications and references by patients detained in hospital or subject to guardianship, and if apposite, to discharge the patient from detention, or order delayed discharge. The Tribunal can also recommend leave of absence and transfer to another hospital. Usually the patient or his nearest relative makes the application. But if a patient admitted for treatment has not applied within 6 months of admission to hospital, he must be automatically referred to a Tribunal by the hospital managers.

In the case of a patient transferred from prison to hospital, with a restriction order, the Tribunal will decide whether he would be entitled to an absolute or conditional discharge. The Tribunal then recommends to the Home Secretary whether he stays in hospital or returns to prison.

The Mental Health Act Commission.

A special health authority, known as the Mental Health Act Commission, has been set up by the 1983 Act, with a general responsibility to protect the rights of detained patients. There are around 80 part-time members, made up of nurses, lawyers, doctors, psychologists, social workers and lay people. All hospitals are visited regularly by a team, and detained patients are interviewed and complaints investigated. The Commission has few actual powers, and cannot discharge a patient. It reports directly to the Secretary of State, who can take appropriate action if need be.

Consent to Treatment by Detained Patients.

Under the 1959 Act, the legal right of detained patients to refuse treatment was unclear. (Informal patients of course had the same right to refuse treatment as any other patient under common law.) It was sometimes assumed that if he needed to be compulsorily admitted for treatment, the patient was unlikely to be competent to decide whether or not he should have treatment. The 1983 Act assumes that a detained patient may well be competent to give 'informed' consent to treatment. In cases where a patient *detained for treatment* (Section 2, as well as 3 is included here) either refuses treatment, or is incompetent to give his permission, the Act sets out certain conditions and procedures. The new legislation does not apply to patients on short-term orders of 72 hours of less, or to those remanded for report, or under guardianship.

Treatment is divided into three categories:

1. (Section 57) where both the patient's consent *and* a second opinion is required. This applies to an irreversible treatment such as psychosurgery, and a hazardous treatment or one insufficiently established such as a surgical implantation of hormones to reduce male sex drive. These treatments are only possible if the patient gives his written consent, an independent doctor and two laymen – appointed by the Mental Health Commission – has confirmed that the patient has consented, knowing the nature, purpose and likely effect of the treatment, and thirdly, the independent doctor confirms that the treatment is appropriate. He must consult with two other people who have been concerned professionally with the patient's treatment, one of whom must be a nurse, the other neither a nurse nor a doctor.

This procedure applies both to detained and informal patients.

2. (Section 58). The treatment requires the patient's consent *or* if he refuses it, a second opinion. Treatment includes ECT, and medication if given for more than 3 months. The patient's consent must be recorded by the responsible Medical Officer, or the independent doctor appointed by the Mental Health Act Commission. And the independent doctor must certify that the patient is either not capable of understanding the nature, purpose and likely effects of the treatment, or has not given consent but that, having regard to the likelihood of its alleviating or preventing deterioration of his condition, the treatment should be given. As with Section 57, the doctor giving the second opinion must consult with two professionals involved in the patient's care, one of whom must be neither a nurse nor a doctor.

If at any time the patient withdraws the consent originally given, the treatments included under Section 57 must stop, and those included under Section 58 require the above procedure to be set in motion at once.

3. Other treatments, which require no consent.

Urgent treatment without the patient's consent, or the need for a second opinion, may be given under Section 62 (a) for the purpose of immediately saving the patient's life, (b) (not being an irreversible treatment) is immediately necessary to prevent a serious deterioration of the patient's condition, (c) (not being irreversible or hazardous) is immediately necessary and represents the minimum interference necessary to prevent the patient from behaving violently or being a danger to himself or others.

Approved Social Workers (ASW).
Approved social workers have taken over the duties of mental welfare officers. They are approved by local authorities as 'having appropriate competence in dealing with persons who are suffering from mental disorder'. Their duties include deciding on whether compulsory admission to hospital is the most appropriate way of dealing with a case. And when a patient is admitted at the request of the nearest relative, it is incumbent on the hospital managers to ask for a report from ASW as soon as possible.

Detained inpatients' rights.
Leave of absence. A patient compulsorily detained can be granted leave from the hospital by the responsible Medical Officer, either indefinitely or for a specified time. The responsible Medical Officer can recall him at any time by informing the patient, or the person temporarily in charge of him, in writing. If such a patient absents himself without leave from hospital he can be taken into custody by the police and returned to the hospital.

Correspondence.

Post sent to or by an informal patient cannot be read or withheld.

Post sent *to* a detained patient cannot be read or withheld. Post sent *by* a detained patient can only be withheld if the addressee has specifically requested this.

There are special provisions relating to post sent to and by patients in special hospitals.

Voting rights.

Some long stay detained patients in mental hospitals may now vote. They must make a 'patient's declaration', which allows them to have their names entered on the electoral register for an address given, which must be outside the hospital.

Special hospitals.

Four special hospitals – Broadmoor, Rampton, Moss Side and Park Lane – exist for detained patients whose 'dangerous, violent or criminal propensities' required them to be treated in a setting of special security. Unlike other hospitals they are managed directly by the Secretary of State for Social Services.

Regional Secure Units.

Only a few of these exist. They are meant for patients who are too difficult to treat in mental or mental handicap hospitals, yet their behaviour does not merit admission to a Special Hospital.

Glossary

Abreaction Reliving past events with a release of emotion.
Amnesia Loss of memory.
Animism Thinking of external objects as 'alive' and having feelings similar to your own.
Anxiety state A continual and irrational feeling of anxiety in the absence of any justifiable cause.
Behaviour therapy Behaviour therapy is based on the theory that neurotic symptoms or patterns of behaviour are learned, unadaptive responses to a conditioned stimulus, and can be 'unlearned' by certain methods.
Belle indifference The unconcern shown by a hysterical patient about his symptoms.
Character A person's qualities, attitudes and expected behaviour.
Clouding of consciousness A mental state in which awareness is diminished or lost.
Complex Ideas which are emotionally unacceptable and have therefore been repressed, but continue to influence behaviour and thought.
Compulsive neurosis An impulse or movement which an individual feels compelled to carry out, usually repetitively, in spite of a strong urge to resist.
Confabulation A word describing the fabrication which a patient with loss of memory may employ to fill in the gaps in his memory.
Conditioned reflex A simple reflex which has been modified so that it is now evoked by a stimulus different from the 'natural' one.
Continuous narcosis A form of treatment in which the patient is kept asleep for up to twenty hours a day.
Conversion Changing a repressed wish into a bodily symptom, as occurs in hysteria.
Culture The values, beliefs, accepted patterns of behaviour and customs accumulated by a society.
Cyclothymic personality An individual whose mood constantly fluctuates, often for little or no apparent cause, between elation and depression.
Deconditioning Abolishing a conditioned reflex by applying another stimulus between the conditioned stimulus and the expected response.
Déjà vu The sense of familiarity, associated with a feeling of

'having been there before', or reliving experiences from some earlier state of existence.

Delirium A state of reversible confusion.

Delusion A false belief.

Dementia A state of permanent, and sometimes progressive, intellectual impairment.

Depersonalization A feeling that you have changed, and the world is seen as though in a dream.

Dipsomania A form of alcoholism.

Displacement A mental mechanism whereby anxiety is switched from what is really feared to some apparently unconnected object or situation.

Dissociation A mental mechanism which results in 'splitting of consciousness' so that inconsistencies in thought or behaviour are overlooked.

Ego A psychoanalytical term for the conscious part of the mind.

Egocentric thought Thought which is controlled more by inner needs and wishes than by reality. It is typical of young children.

Eidetic imagery A vivid form of visual imagery, in which past scenes are reproduced with almost photographic accuracy and clearness.

Emotion A subjective feeling combined with certain bodily changes.

Extravert A sociable, outgoing person.

Fugue Loss of memory in a patient who has 'wandered' off from home.

Group psychotherapy A form of treatment in which groups of patients discuss one another's problems, as well as their own.

Hallucination Percepts that occur in the absence of any external stimuli. They cannot therefore be perceived by other people.

Heterosexuality Sexual attraction for someone of the opposite sex.

Homeostasis Maintaining the 'internal environment' of the body.

Homosexuality Sexual attraction for someone of the same sex.

Hypnogogic hallucination Hallucinations experienced at the moment of dropping off to sleep.

Hypnopompic hallucination Short-lived persistence of dream image on wakening.

Hypochondriasis Preoccupation with one's own bodily functions and sensations.

Hysteria A disorder in which physical symptoms or certain

mental disturbances occur in the absence of organic disease.
Hysterical personality An emotionally shallow, selfish, demanding person.
Ideas of reference Delusional beliefs that certain external events are especially related to the individual.
Identification Imitating an admired person.
Illusion An error of perception whereby stimuli are wrongly interpreted.
Imagery The process of seeing with the 'mind's eye' something that is not actually real or present at the time.
Instinct Unlearned, inherited patterns of behaviour.
Intelligence The ability to reason and to think rationally and purposefully.
Intelligence quotient (IQ) The ratio of mental age over chronological age × 100.
Introvert A reserved, rather unsociable type of person.
Mania A condition characterized by elation and overactivity.
Memory A mental process consisting of registering, retaining, recalling and recognizing 'information'.
Mental age The age at which the 'average' child would have passed the intelligence tests the individual concerned has passed.
Mental defect This term has now been replaced by mental impairment.
Neurasthenia A state of inexplicable fatigue.
Neurosis A condition in which the patient recognizes that he is mentally ill.
Nursing process A problem solving approach which is applied to individual patient's nursing care.
Obsessional neurosis An obsession is a thought, impulse or movement which an individual feels compelled to carry out, usually repetitively, in spite of a strong urge to resist.
Obsessional personality Someone who tends to be over-conscientious and self-exacting.
Occupational therapy Therapeutic work.
Omnipotence Feeling of tremendous power.
Paraphrenia A form of schizophrenia starting relatively late in life, where the personality is well preserved.
Perception The process of selection and organization of stimuli by the brain whereby we become aware of what is happening around and in our bodies.
Personality This is the *whole* person, his attitudes, moods, characteristic behaviour, the way he parts his hair, the type of girl friend he has, the books he likes.

Phantasy Undirected, uncontrolled thought.
Phobia A specific fear of something.
Prejudice Fixed beliefs which are unfavourable to the objects concerned.
Presenile dementia Dementia occurring usually between the ages of forty and sixty.
Primary nursing The term used when one nurse is primarily responsible for an individual patient's care.
Projection Displacing unacceptable attitudes and feelings on to someone else.
Psychiatry The study and treatment of disordered mental processes.
Psychoanalysis A form of treatment in which unconscious memories are brought to light by 'free association', by allowing thoughts to wander without conscious direction.
Psychology The study and understanding of normal mental functions and behaviour.
Psychopath An individual who has little or no sense of right and wrong, and who appears unable to learn from experience.
Psychopathology The past events in a patient's life which may have contributed to his present illness.
Psychosis An illness in which the patient does not recognize that he is ill, and his whole personality is involved in and changed by the illness.
Psychosomatic Physical conditions or symptoms for which emotional factors are responsible, or in which they play a major role.
Psychotherapy Treatment depending on therapeutic discussions between doctor and patient.
Reaction formation A mental mechanism by which unconscious wishes result in the opposite attitudes and behaviour being adopted consciously.
Reasoning Thought controlled and directed purposefully.
Reflex (simple) An inborn, involuntary, automatic response to a stimulus.
Regression Returning to earlier, more childish, forms of behaviour.
Repression The involuntary process by which ideas unacceptable to the conscience, or super-ego, are pushed out of consciousness.
Schizoid personality A solitary individual lacking emotional warmth.
Stereotype Groups of fixed, oversimplified and generalized

conceptions. When these conceptions are unfavourable they are linked with prejudice.

Sublimation Directing undesirable tendencies into socially acceptable channels.

Super ego Psychoanalytical term for conscience.

Temperament The characteristic mood of an individual.

Thought Conscious mental activity.

Thought blocking Interference with the 'normal' train of thought; it occurs in schizophrenia.

Transference A term used to describe the dependent and often childlike relationship which sometimes forms between patients and medical staff.

Unreality A feeling that the world, rather than you, has 'changed', and become colourless and meaningless.

References

ALTSCHUL, A. T. 1977. Use of the nursing process in psychiatric care. *Nursing Times* **73** (36): 1412–13.

BATES, B. 1979. *A Guide to Physical Examination*, 2nd ed. Philadelphia: F. A. Davis.

GREEN, B. 1983. Primary nursing in psychiatry. *Nursing Times* **79** (3): 24–7.

HENDERSON, V. 1977. *Basic Principles of Nursing Care*. Basel: Karger.

MARKS-MARAN, D. 1978. Patient allocation vs. task allocation in relation to the nursing process. *Nursing Times* **74** (10): 413–16.

MARRAN, G. D. *et al.* 1974. *Primary Nursing – a model for individualised care*. St. Louis: C. V. Mosby & Co.

MCFARLANE, J. & CASTLEDINE, G. 1982. *A Guide to the Practice of Nursing Using the Nursing Process*. St. Louis: C. V. Mosby.

MENZIES, I. 1970. *The Functioning of Social Systems as a Defence against Anxiety*. Tavistock Pamphlet No. 5.

MILLER, E. 1981. Learning to communicate. *Nursing* 27: 1197–9.

OREM, D. 1971. *Nursing: Concepts of Practice*. New York: McGraw-Hill Book Co.

ROBB, B. 1967. *Sans everything*. London: Nelson.

ROGERS, C. 1967. *On Becoming a Person – a Therapist's View of Psychotherapy*. London: Constable.

ROPER, N. 1976. A model for nursing and nursology. *Journal of Advanced Nursing* **1**: 219–27.

ROPER, N., LOGAN, W. W. & TIERNEY, A. J. 1980. *The Elements of Nursing*. Edinburgh: Churchill Livingstone.

ROY, C. 1982. *In* Riehl, J. P. & Roy, C. (Ed.) *Conceptual Models for Nursing Practice*, 2nd ed. East Norwalk, Conn: Appleton-Century Croft.

STOCKWELL, F. 1984. *The Unpopular Patient*. Edinburgh: Churchill Livingstone.

WALK, A. 1961. The history of mental nursing. *The Journal of Mental Science* **107**.

Further Reading

A *Psychiatric Nursing*

ALTSCHUL, A. & SIMPSON, R. 1977. *Psychiatric Nursing*, 5th ed. Eastbourne: Baillière Tindall.

POTHIER, P. 1980. *Psychiatric Nursing – A Basic Text*. Boston: Little, Brown & Co.

STUART, G. & SUNDEEN, S. J. 1983. *Principles and Practice of Psychiatric Nursing*, 2nd ed. St. Louis: C. V. Mosby.

B *Community Psychiatric Nursing*

CARR, P. J., BUTTERWORTH, C. A. & HODGE, B. E. 1980. *Community Psychiatric Nursing*. Edinburgh: Churchill Livingstone.

C *Sociology*

COX, C. 1983. *Sociology*. London: Butterworth.

D *Psychiatry*

ANDERSON, E. W. & TRETHOWAN, W. H. 1978. *Psychiatry*, 3rd ed. London: Baillière Tindall.

DARCY, P. T. 1984. *Theory and Practice of Psychiatric Care*. Sevenoaks: Hodder and Stoughton.

WILLIS, J. 1979. *Lecture Notes on Psychiatry*, 5th ed. Oxford: Blackwell Scientific Publications.

E *Psychology*

HILGARD, E., ATKINSON, R. C. & ATKINSON, R. L. 1980. *Introduction to Psychology*, 7th ed. New York: Harcourt Brace Jovanovich Inc.

WATTLEY, L. & MULLER, D. 1984. *Investigating Psychology: A practical approach for nursing*. London: Harper & Row.

Index